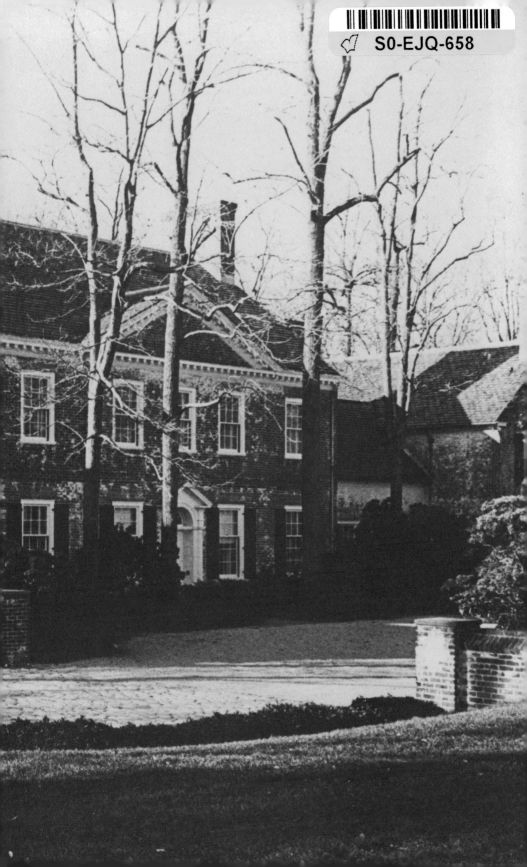

Nongenotoxic Mechanisms in Carcinogenesis

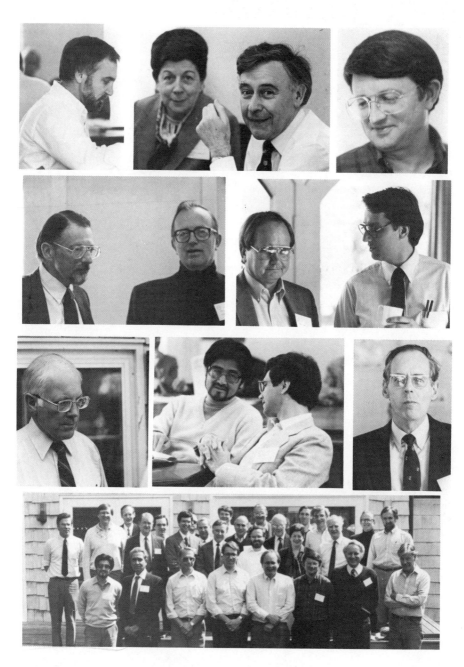

Row 1: W.F. Greenlee; L. Diamond, M.M. Coombs; B.E. Butterworth
Row 2: R.H. Reitz, H.C. Pitot; T.J. Slaga, A. Sivak
Row 3: P.N. Magee; H. Yamasaki, C.J. Boreiko; E.D. Wachsmuth

Nongenotoxic Mechanisms in Carcinogenesis

Edited by

BYRON E. BUTTERWORTH
Department of Genetic Toxicology
Chemical Industry Institute of Toxicology

THOMAS J. SLAGA
Department of Carcinogenesis
The University of Texas System Cancer Center
Science Park–Research Division

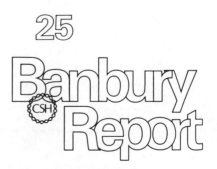

COLD SPRING HARBOR LABORATORY
1987

Banbury Report 25: Nongenotoxic Mechanisms in Carcinogenesis

Library of Congress Cataloging-in-Publishing Data

Nongenotoxic mechanisms in carcinogenesis.

(Banbury report, ISSN 0198-0068 ; 25)
Based on a conference held at and sponsored by the
Banbury Center of the Cold Spring Harbor Laboratory in
the spring of 1986.
Includes bibliographies and indexes.
1. Carcinogenesis—Congresses. 2. Carcinogenicity
testing—Congresses. I. Butterworth, Byron E. II. Slaga
Thomas J. III. Banbury Center. IV. Series. [DNLM:
1. Carcinogens—toxicity—congresses. 2. Mutagenicity
Tests—congresses. 3. Neoplasms, Experimental—
chemically induced—congresses. W3 BA19 v.25 /
QZ 202 N812 1986]
RC268.6.N66   1987   616.99'4071   87-899
ISBN 0-87969-225-1

All Cold Spring Harbor Laboratory publications may be ordered directly from Cold Spring Harbor
Laboratory, Box 100, Cold Spring Harbor, New York 11724. (Phone: 1-800-843-4388) in New York State
(516) 367-8425.

BANBURY REPORT SERIES

Banbury Report 1: Assessing Chemical Mutagens
Banbury Report 2: Mammalian Cell Mutagenesis
Banbury Report 3: A Safe Cigarette?
Banbury Report 4: Cancer Incidence in Defined Populations
Banbury Report 5: Ethylene Dichloride: A Potential Health Risk?
Banbury Report 6: Product Labeling and Health Risks
Banbury Report 7: Gastrointestinal Cancer: Endogenous Factors
Banbury Report 8: Hormones and Breast Cancer
Banbury Report 9: Quantification of Occupational Cancer
Banbury Report 10: Patenting of Life Forms
Banbury Report 11: Environmental Factors in Human Growth and
Development
Banbury Report 12: Nitrosamines and Human Cancer
Banbury Report 13: Indicators of Genotoxic Exposure
Banbury Report 14: Recombinant DNA Applications to Human
Disease
Banbury Report 15: Biological Aspects of Alzheimer's Disease
Banbury Report 16: Genetic Variability in Responses to Chemical
Exposure
Banbury Report 17: Coffee and Health
Banbury Report 18: Biological Mechanisms of Dioxin Action
Banbury Report 19: Risk Quantitation and Regulatory Policy
Banbury Report 20: Genetic Manipulation of the Early Mammalian
Embryo
Banbury Report 21: Viral Etiology of Cervical Cancer
Banbury Report 22: Genetically Altered Viruses and the Environment
Banbury Report 23: Mechanisms in Tobacco Carcinogenesis
Banbury Report 24: Antibiotic Resistance Genes: Ecology, Transfer,
and Expression
Banbury Report 25: Nongenotoxic Mechanisms in Carcinogenesis

Participants

Robert L. Anderson, The Procter & Gamble Company, Miami Valley Laboratories

J. Carl Barrett, Laboratory of Pulmonary Pathobiology, National Institute of Environmental Health Sciences

Craig J. Boreiko, Department of Genetic Toxicology, Chemical Industry Institute of Toxicology

K. Gerhard Brand, Department of Microbiology, University of Minnesota Medical School

Byron E. Butterworth, Department of Genetic Toxicology, Chemical Industry Institute of Toxicology

Peter A. Cerutti, Department of Carcinogenesis, Swiss Institute for Experimental Cancer Research, Lausanne, Switzerland

Samuel M. Cohen, Eppley Institute for Research on Cancer and Allied Diseases, University of Nebraska Medical Center

Maurice M. Coombs, Imperial Cancer Research Fund Laboratories, London, England

Leila Diamond, Wistar Institute of Anatomy and Biology

John DiGiovanni, Science Park-Research Division, The University of Texas System Cancer Center

Amiya Ghoshal, Departments of Pathology and Biochemistry, University of Toronto, Ontario, Canada

William F. Greenlee, Department of Cell Biology, Chemical Industry Institute of Toxicology

Henry d'A. Heck, Department of Biochemical Toxicology and Pathobiology, Chemical Industry Institute of Toxicology

David J. Loury, Chemical Industry Institute of Toxicology

Peter N. Magee, Fels Research Institute, Temple University School of Medicine

Paul M. Newberne, Department of Pathology, Boston University School of Medicine

Wolfram Parzefall, Institut für Tumorbiologie-Krebsforschung, Vienna, Austria

Henry C. Pitot, McArdle Laboratory for Cancer Research, University of Wisconsin

Richard Henry Reitz, Mammalian and Environmental Toxicology Laboratory, Dow Chemical Company

Francis J.C. Roe, London, England

Herbert S. Rosenkranz, Department of Environmental Health Sciences, Case Western Reserve University School of Medicine

Dittakavi S.R. Sarma, Department of Pathology, University of Toronto, Ontario, Canada

Harvey E. Scribner, Department of Toxicology, Rohm and Haas Company

Andrew Sivak, Arthur D. Little, Inc.

Thomas J. Slaga, Science Park-Research Division, The University of Texas System Cancer Center

Donald E. Stevenson, Westhollow Research Center, Shell Development Company

James A. Swenberg, Department of Biochemical Toxicology and Pathobiology, Chemical Industry Institute of Toxicology

Raymond W. Tennant, Cellular and Genetic Toxicology Branch, National Institute of Environmental Health Sciences

Benjamin F. Trump, Department of Pathology, University of Maryland School of Medicine

Ernst Dieter Wachsmuth, Pharmaceuticals Division, Ciba-Geigy Limited, Basel, Switzerland

I. Bernard Weinstein, Institute of Cancer Research, Columbia University College of Physicians and Surgeons

Gary M. Williams, American Health Foundation

Hiroshi Yamasaki, International Agency for Research on Cancer, Lyon, France

This volume is dedicated to the memory of
Steve Prentis
who was Director of Banbury Center
at the time of this conference.
He will be remembered as a
knowledgeable colleague
and warm personal friend.

Preface

Every year, a large number of long-term animal assays are conducted to identify environmental carcinogens. It is clear that many carcinogens are mutagens and that at least one step in the complex process of carcinogenesis may involve alteration of the information encoded in the DNA. Over the past few years, the recognition that oncogenes may be activated by mutational events has resulted in models for carcinogenesis that are dominated by genotoxic events. In addition, the success of short-term tests in predicting carcinogenic activity has led to the development of risk assessment models, many of which are a measure of genotoxicity. However, a large and growing list of experimental carcinogens share some of the following characteristics: (1) The agent is nongenotoxic as defined by the lack of reactivity of the parent compound or its metabolites with DNA; (2) the database for short-term tests, such as mutagenesis and clastogenesis, is substantially negative; (3) tumors are often seen only in one organ of one sex of one species (e.g., induction of mouse liver tumors only); and (4) massive doses beyond 500 mg/kg/day for a lifetime are required to produce only a small increase in tumor induction.

As the field of chemical carcinogenesis progresses, it is important to ask whether we can do a better job in defining the mechanism and predicting the risk of such agents. This, in fact, was a goal of the conference from which this volume was generated. In putting together the program, we were fortunate to have such a good response from so many experts in so many fields. Our only disappointment was not being able to include as many of the important areas and investigators as we would have liked.

This volume describes the wide variety of valuable studies that are being directed toward nongenotoxic mechanisms of carcinogenesis. The information presented is exciting and in many cases can be applied to practical areas of predicting carcinogenic potential and risk assessment. Still, we are left with the sobering recognition of how much we do not know and how much research remains to be done in this important area.

The organizers gratefully acknowledge the financial and organizational support of the American Industrial Health Council, Inc. We also appreciate the effort, skill, and enthusiasm of everyone involved in making this meeting run smoothly, especially Bea Toliver, Banbury Center administrative assistant, Katya Davey, hostess of Robertson House, and Judith Blum and Chris Nolan, editors of this volume. Finally, we are grateful to the late Steve Prentis, who as Director of Banbury Center decided to sponsor this conference on nongenotoxic mechanisms in carcinogenesis.

B. E. Butterworth
T. J. Slaga

Contents

Participants, vii

Preface, xi

Nongenotoxic Carcinogens: Prologue / Andrew Sivak,
Muriel M. Goyer, and Paolo F. Ricci   1

SESSION 1: PROMOTION

**Tumor Promotion and Progression in the Mouse Skin
Model** / John F. O'Connell, Joel B. Rotstein, and
Thomas J. Slaga   11

**Studies on the Skin Tumor Promoting Actions of
Chrysarobin** / John DiGiovanni, Francis A. Kruszewski,
and Kristine J. Chenicek   25

Multistage Carcinogenesis of the Rat Hepatocyte /
Henry C. Pitot, David G. Beer, and Suzanne Hendrich   41

Bladder Tumor Promotion / Samuel M. Cohen,
Leon B. Ellwein, and Sonny L. Johansson   55

Cell Injury, Ion Regulation, and Tumor Promotion /
Benjamin F. Trump and Irene K. Berezesky   69

SESSION 2: FORCED CELL PROLIFERATION

**Orotic Acid, a Novel Liver Tumor Promoter: Studies on Its
Mechanism of Action** / Ezio Laconi, Shanthi Vasudevan,
Prema M. Rao, Srinivasan Rajalakshmi, and
Dittakavi S. R. Sarma   85

**Role of Stimulation of Liver Growth by Chemicals in
Hepatocarcinogenesis** / Rolf Schulte-Hermann,
Wolfram Parzefall, and Wilfried Bursch   91

Role of Cytotoxicity in the Carcinogenic Process /
Richard H. Reitz   107

The Value of Measuring Cell Replication as a Predictive Index
of Tissue-specific Tumorigenic Potential /
David J. Loury, Thomas L. Goldsworthy, and
Byron E. Butterworth   119

Chemically Induced Cell Turnover in the Kidney and Its
Possible Role in Carcinogenesis / Ernst D. Wachsmuth   137

Influence of Cytotoxicity on the Induction of Tumors /
James A. Swenberg and Brian G. Short   151

SESSION 3: RODENT BIOASSAYS

Nongenotoxic Mouse Liver Carcinogens / Paul M. Newberne,
Vora Suphakarn, Phaibul Punyarit, and
Joao de Camargo   165

Induction of Cancer by Dietary Deficiency without Added
Carcinogens / Amiya Ghoshal, Thomas Rushmore, and
Emmanuel Farber   179

The Problem of Pseudocarcinogenicity in Rodent Bioassays /
Francis J. C. Roe   189

SESSION 4: SOLID STATE CARCINOGENESIS

Solid State Carcinogenesis / K. Gerhard Brand   205

Biogenic Silica Fibers and Skin Tumor Promotion /
Tarlochan Bhatt, Maurice Coombs, and Charles O'Neill   215

Bladder Stones and Bladder Cancer: A Review of the
Toxicology of Terephthalic Acid / Henry d'A. Heck   233

SESSION 5: EXAMPLES OF NONGENOTOXIC CARCINOGENS

TCDD: Mechanisms of Altered Growth Regulation in Human
Epidermal Keratinocytes / William F. Greenlee,
Rosemarie Osborne, Karen M. Dold, Lisa Ross,
and Jon C. Cook   247

Genetic Toxicology of Di(2-ethylhexyl)phthalate /
    Bryon E. Butterworth   257

The Mechanism of Urinary Tract Tumorigenesis of
    Nitrilotriacetate / Robert L. Anderson   277

SESSION 6: CELL CULTURE MODELS

Modulation of Transformed Focus Formation in Cultures of
    C3H/10T1/2 Cells / Craig J. Boreiko   287

The Role of Cell-to-Cell Communication in Tumor Promotion/
    Hiroshi Yamasaki   297

Genetic and Epigenetic Mechanisms of Presumed
    Nongenotoxic Carcinogens / J. Carl Barrett,
    Mitsuo Oshimura, Noriho Tanaka, and Takeki Tsutsui   311

Genotoxic Oxidant Tumor Promoters / Peter A. Cerutti   325

SESSION 7: REGULATORY CONSIDERATIONS

Some Implications and Limitations of In Vitro Genetic
    Toxicity Data in Regulatory Decisions /
    Raymond W. Tennant   339

Practical Approaches to Evaluating Nongenotoxic Car-
    cinogens / Harvey E. Scribner, Kay L. McCarthy, and
    David J. Doolittle   355

Definition of a Human Cancer Hazard / Gary M. Williams   367

Concluding Discussion   381

Author Index   387

Subject Index   389

Nongenotoxic Carcinogens: Prologue

ANDREW SIVAK, MURIEL M. GOYER, AND PAOLO F. RICCI
Arthur D. Little, Inc.
Cambridge, Massachusetts 02140

INTRODUCTION

The concept that cancers could be induced by nongenotoxic influences would very likely have met with disbelief and possible scorn in the early days of the Ames assay, a decade or so ago. However, a considerable amount of data has been developed to force us to deal with the reality that there are, in fact, animal carcinogens without apparent genotoxic activity. These results have raised significant scientific questions with respect to our understanding of the process of carcinogenesis, and they pose significant regulatory dilemmas relating to the assessment of risk to humans from exposure to apparently nongenotoxic chemicals (Ricci and Melton 1985). Much of this volume will address these issues, and, hopefully, it should enable us to make some progress toward their resolution.

In earlier times when we had more confidence in the generality of models for carcinogenesis, the study of biological mechanisms and application of regulatory decisions were often the province of different constituencies. Now we realize that these two areas, and their uncertainties, demand a close collaboration between scientists engaged in studies of mechanism of cancer induction and the regulators upon whose shoulders rest the difficult choices (Ricci and Cirillo 1985). This collaboration is needed to provide the most appropriate basis for human risk analysis and for the regulatory stances that utilize the scientific results and models for cancer induction. Although these are easy words to say, we have no illusions about the difficulties of carrying out the alliances that are needed. Several factors complicate the forging of this alliance. Some of these are (1) the litigious environment that pervades the regulatory scene and seems to subvert the process of developing scientific risk analysis; (2) the disinclination to surrender long-held and comfortable mechanistic views related to the genetic origin of cancer, which have been so much a part of cancer research for decades; and (3) the general reluctance to give up a set of algorithms for risk assessment, even though they work poorly for nongenotoxic carcinogens, and thus enter an even more uncharted sea.

GENOTOXIC VERSUS NONGENOTOXIC CARCINOGENS

To focus more acutely on the nature of these problems, it is useful to examine the nongenotoxic carcinogens to determine what the thought processes were that went into the analyses of their carcinogenic effects and, with the benefit of hindsight, to ascertain whether our present state of knowledge could have resulted in a different

Banbury Report 25: Nongenotoxic Mechanisms in Carcinogenesis
© Cold Spring Harbor Laboratory. 0-87969-225-1/87. $1.00 + .00

outcome. Indeed, following the deliberations of the meeting on which this volume is based, our conclusions might well be different than the ones we currently accept.

Some examples of the potential problems in comparing carcinogenic and genotoxic activities have been summarized by Tennant et al. (1986) using data from the National Toxicology Program. There is a distinct dichotomy among a set of carcinogens that have trans-species and trans-sex activities (Table 1). The expected strong genotoxic activity of a potent carcinogen is evident for those carcinogens in the upper portion of Table 1; the lower portion depicts the absence of genotoxic activity for other active carcinogens.

There is considerable concern that a number of the compounds that may be nongenotoxic carcinogens are prevalent in the environment and have significant human exposure. Some of these compounds are shown in Table 2. The concern is not so much that human cancer incidence will be markedly increased by exposure to these materials (with the possible exception of the dioxins), but rather that models and concepts to determine effectively the risks to humans have not been developed adequately for this special class of carcinogens. This is so in spite of the fact that considerable amounts of toxicologic and pharmacokinetic data, as well as results from pathological analyses, are available for several of these compounds.

Beyond not inducing genetic damage or forming adducts with DNA, what are some of the characteristics of nongenotoxic carcinogens? Unlike many genotoxic carcinogens, where a tumor response can be observed after a single exposure or, at most, a short course of exposures, long-term continuous exposure to nongenotoxic agents, often at toxicologically and pathologically significant doses, is required to induce tumors. If one looks at the toxicology and pathology resulting from these chronic exposures to nongenotoxic agents, a range of responses is found, from the minimal general effects of long-term saccharin exposure to the severe pathological manifestation of 2,3,7,8-tetrachlorodibenzo-p-dioxin (TCDD), with other responses being intermediate between these two. Similarly, the pharmacokinetic and metabolic findings cover the gamut from saccharin, which is rapidly cleared and

Table 1
Genetic Toxicity versus Trans-Sex/Species Carcinogens

Chemical	Positive	Equivocal	Negative
1,2-Dibromo-3-chloropropane	6	—	5
Diglycidylresorcinol ether	10	—	5
4,4'-Oxydianiline	16	—	5
Ethylene dibromide	9	—	5
Diethylhexylphthalate[a]	1	—	17
TCDD[a]	—	—	13
Polybrominated biphenyls[a]	—	—	15

Data from Tennant et al. (1986).
[a] Hepatic malignant tumors only.

Table 2
Nongenotoxic Carcinogens with
Human Exposure

TCDD
Diethylhexylphthalate
Butylated hydroxyanisole
Saccharin
Dichloromethane
Nitrilotriacetic acid

essentially not metabolized, through diethylhexlyphthalate and dichloromethane, which undergo extensive metabolic conversion and fairly rapid clearance, to TCDD, which exhibits limited metabolism, but marked retention and storage, especially in fatty tissues. Thus, except for the need for long-term exposure, there do not seem to be any general characteristics common to this set of nongenotoxic carcinogens. A key area that needs attention is the development of risk models and algorithms based on the actual, biologically plausible mechanisms of cancer induction for these materials, rather than forcing all carcinogens into a single genotoxic model that has its root in the quintessential genotoxic carcinogen, ionizing radiation. For the present, the model for cancer risk generally used is the multistage model, initially developed by Armitage and Doll (1961), and subsequently modified by Crump and others (Crump 1979).

A look at the data available for TCDD may be instructive in attempting to relate the animal experiments to the human situation since human exposure estimates and tissue levels have been reported. Comparing the relationship between exposure and fat burden in a chronic oral rat study, the ratio is reasonably constant across the two orders of magnitude of the dose range (Table 3). Although the uncertainties are considerable in making similar calculations for humans, there are no serious order-of-magnitude differences between the rat and human data, especially if one considers the estimates based on the consumption of Great Lakes fish being at the upper end of the scale.

If the relationship between experimental animal dose and tumor incidence is examined and compared to likely human doses using the scaling factors employed by the Environmental Protection Agency, the individual excess lifetime cancer risk levels above background associated with the FDA-estimated intake levels of TCDD are between 10^{-5} and 10^{-6}. These values are obtained with the linearized multistage model that has, as its biological basis, the assumption of a genetically based induction of tumors. The calculations lead to a conclusion that exposure to TCDD from the most likely source (food) may result in increased cancer risks of 10^{-5} to 10^{-6}, which are not readily detectable by epidemiological means and which lie in the range of regulatory acceptability. There is considerable uncertainty over whether the genotoxic model faithfully represents the actual biological mechanisms

Table 3
TCDD Exposure and Tissue Burdens

TCDD Exposure	TCDD burden (ppt)		Exposure/fat burden
(μg/kg/day)	liver	fat	ratio
Rat[a]			
0.1	24,000	8,100	1.2×10^{-5}
0.01	5,100	1,700	0.6×10^{-5}
0.001	540	540	0.2×10^{-5}
Human			
0.00078[b]	—	6.4[c]	12.2×10^{-5}
0.00003[d]	—	6.4	0.5×10^{-5}

[a] Data from Kociba et al. (1978).
[b] EPA estimate based on consumption of Great Lakes fish.
[c] Data from Center for Biology of Natural Systems.
[d] FDA estimates based on consumption of beef and dairy products.

by which this nongenotoxic carcinogen produces tumors. The resolution of this dilemma is not at all clear on the basis of current information, and even the assembly of a research agenda to test hypotheses is no simple task. Indeed, one key goal of this volume is to identify some concepts for experimental verification and the definition of some actual experimental models to test the hypothesis that non-genotoxic cancer induction differs mechanistically from genotoxic induction of tumors.

One possible concept that requires serious examination is the proposal that nongenotoxic carcinogens are tumor promoters. Although this idea avoids the question of how the initiation events occur, the common properties of long-term exposure and a toxic and/or proliferative response in the target organ are certainly consistent with this view. Indeed, saccharin (Cohen et al. 1979), TCDD (Pitot et al. 1980; Poland et al. 1983), and butylated hydroxyanisole (Imaida et al. 1983) are well-demonstrated tumor promoters in several organ systems. With applicable animal experimental models available to address this initial question, the issue would appear to be more a matter of generating interest in doing the studies and obtaining resources to carry them out rather than devising new models. With a demonstration of the generality of the proposal that nongenotoxic carcinogens act as tumor promoters, the more difficult studies of specific mechanism could be undertaken.

One other concept that seems worthy of examination is that nongenotoxic carcinogens are, in fact, genotoxic, but our tools to measure genetic alteration have been inappropriate. There is some reason to explore this issue based on observations that aneuploidy and possibly nondisjunction may be important events in tumor induction (Oshimura et al. 1984). So far, the data are restricted to cell culture systems; however, demonstration of the phenomenon in vivo is within experimental grasp.

Finally, the idea must be entertained that multiple events, including those listed

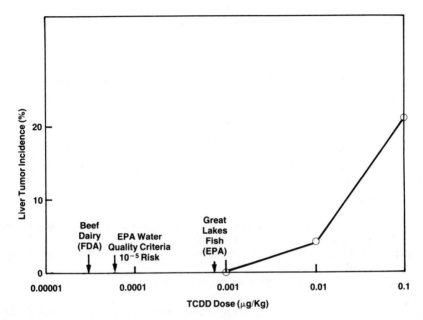

Figure 1
Dose-response of rat liver tumor incidence vs. administered dose. Data from Kociba et al. (1978).

above and others yet unrecognized, act together to generate a neoplastic response by the special class of carcinogens that are the subject of this volume. We have all stood under the banner of the multifactorial and multistep nature of the carcinogenic process, and there is no reason to believe that nongenotoxic carcinogens behave differently.

If a charge should be offered at the beginning of this volume, one could ask that we leave our preconceptions and biases behind and view the papers and their subsequent discussions with a healthy skepticism, following the data to wherever they lead. Our most important mission should be to frame the next set of questions, questions that can lead us to a more rational and biologically plausible way to evaluate the potential carcinogenic effects on the human population from apparently nongenotoxic carcinogens.

REFERENCES

Armitage, P. and R. Doll. 1961. Stochastic models for carcinogenesis. In *Proceedings of the 4th Berkeley Symposium on Mathematical Statistics and Probability* (ed. LeCam and Neyman), p. 19. University of California Press, Berkeley.

Cohen, S.M., A. Masayuki, J.B. Jacobs, and G.H. Friedell. 1979. Promoting effect of saccharin and DL-tryptophan in urinary bladder carcinogenesis. *Cancer Res.* **39:** 1207.

Crump, K.S. 1979. Dose-response problems in carcinogenesis. *Biometrics* **35:** 157.

Imaida, K., S. Fukushima, T. Shirai, M. Ohtani, K. Nakanishi, and N. Ito. 1983. Promoting activities of butylated hydroxyanisole and butylated hydroxytoluene on 2-stage urinary bladder carcinogenesis and inhibition of γ-glutamyl transpeptidase-positive foci development in the liver of rats. *Carcinogenesis* **4:** 895.

Kociba, R.J., D.G. Keyes, J.E. Beyer, R.M. Carreone, C.E. Wade, D.A. Dittenber, R.P. Kalnins, L.E. Frauson, C.N. Park, S.D. Barnard, R.A. Hammel, and C.G. Humiston. 1978. Results of a two-year chronic toxicity and oncogenicity study of 2,3,7,8-tetrachlorodibenzo-p-dioxin in rats. *Toxicol. Appl. Pharmacol.* **46:** 279.

Oshimura, M., T.W. Hesterberg, T. Tsutsui, and J.C. Barrett. 1984. Correlation of asbestos-induced cytogenetic effects with cell transformation of Syrian hamster embryo cells in culture. *Cancer Res.* **44:** 5017.

Pitot, H.C., T. Goldsworthy, H.A. Campbell, and A. Poland. 1980. Quantitative evaluation of the promotion by 2,3,7,8-tetrachlorodibenzo-p-dioxin of hepatocarcinogenesis from diethylnitrosamine. *Cancer Res.* **40:** 3616.

Poland, A., D. Palen, and E. Glover. 1983. Tumour promotion by TCDD in skin of HRS/J hairless mice. *Nature* **300:** 271.

Ricci, P.F. and M.C. Cirillo. 1985. Uncertainty in health risk analysis. *J. Hazard. Mater.* **10:** 433.

Ricci, P.F. and L.S. Melton. 1985. Regulating cancer risks. *Environ. Sci. Technol.* **19:** 473.

Tennant, R.W., S. Stasiewicz, and J.W. Spalding. 1986. Comparison of multiple parameters of rodent carcinogenicity and in vitro genetic toxicity. *Environ. Mutagen.* **8:** 205.

COMMENTS

STEVENSON: In your genotoxic definition, do you include compounds that do not bind to DNA but set up a chain of events at the end of which DNA is affected?

SIVAK: I think there is ample evidence for this. Asbestos is one, with Barrett's work as an example. We have repeated it in our laboratory. One gets altered chromosomes. They are puffy and the aneuploidy that results may be at least as significant as traditional clastogenic effects. It would be useful to reread the paper that Peter Newell wrote on chromosomal changes and instability in relation to cancer. This sort of general genetic instability may in fact be much more important than the typical genetic changes. The gene mutations and the DNA adducts may not result in the change of specific gene loci, but for cancers they may induce the genetic instability that ultimately evolves into whatever this lesion becomes.

SARMA: I would like to echo your sentiments on the need for a term for nongenotoxic carcinogens, but I am not quite comfortable with the term nongenotoxic for two reasons. First, gene is the term given for a functional attribute of the DNA, and when you say genotoxic, you only mean that the chemical interacts with the DNA, either physically or chemically. Second, the term toxicity is not well-defined either. Maybe we should come up with a different term for chemical carcinogens which apparently do not interact with DNA.

SIVAK: Nongenotoxic implies nondirect or indirect. I think that one of our problems may be that we try to put things in boxes, and we do not go back and look at our basic biology. We have to find some ways to describe what we see. I have no great discomfort with genotoxic and nongenotoxic, except with the understanding that there is some gray area in between, and things are not always as genotoxic or nongenotoxic as we would like. We need words to describe what we see. In the absence of any better words, I am comfortable with those.

ROE: I am uncomfortable with the free use of the term tumor-promoting. In the case of a highly malignant cancer, it is easy to accept that there is something wrong with the DNA of the cells involved. Furthermore, some of the agents that cause such tumors clearly damage DNA from the start. In the case of tumors which eventually develop after a prolonged period of reversible hyperplasia, it seems that any genetic damage involved is occurring in the wake of nongenotoxic damage, i.e., as a late event and not as the first event. Therefore, to use the term promoter for describing the nongenotoxic part of this process seems wrong. The same is true for tumors that appear as a late consequence of long-standing tissue damage and repair. It is for these reasons that the term nongenotoxic carcinogens appeals to me.

SIVAK: I don't know that I share that view completely. I think you are right in the first two examples, that in something like TCDD one gets early liver lesions. But I think that one has to understand that as a long-term experiment goes on, you get these changes before, during, and after. I think the key is that you may have induced some proliferative change in the liver, and some genetic change may be made, but then the TCDD is fed for the rest of the lifetime. There is no reason that materials cannot do many things. There is a nice little experiment that we did at NYU about 20 years ago, where we initiated mouse skin with a single dose of dimethylbenzanthracine. We then gave a dose of benzo[a]pyrene that was noncarcinogenic in its own right and administered it to the initiated skin repeatedly; there was a very strong tumor promoter response. A single material might be doing several different things, including promotion as broadly defined.

ROE: Your preference for the damage afterwards is unjustified. There are inadequate grounds for thinking that damage that occurs after the genotoxic event is more important than the damage that occurs before it. In hormonal carcinogenesis, proliferation occurs before and as long as exposure continues. Proliferation may or may not go on to benign or malignant tumor development. The development of such a tumor may depend on exposure to a genotoxin either before or after the onset of hormonal imbalance.

SIVAK: That is precisely why the late exposure is important. If you treat with TCDD for 6 months and stop, you do not get tumors. If you treat with saccharine for 6 months and stop, you do not get tumors. This indicates to me that the late events, whatever they are, are very important for the final culmination of the tumor response.

ROSENKRANZ: You seem to imply that we are having problems in defining nongenotoxic. To me there is no problem in defining nongenotoxic as an operational term that simply means that a chemical is not genotoxic. The problem is that we do not agree on how to define genotoxic.

Session 1:
Promotion

Tumor Promotion and Progression in the Mouse Skin Model

JOHN F. O'CONNELL, JOEL B. ROTSTEIN, AND THOMAS J. SLAGA
The University of Texas System Cancer Center
Science Park—Research Division
Smithville, Texas 78957

OVERVIEW

The three stages of mouse skin carcinogenesis are initiation, promotion, and progression. Initiation likely involves the induction of irreversible damage to cellular DNA. Promotion is the specific expansion of initiated cells within the epidermis and appears to involve both direct and indirect mechanisms. Malignant progression is the process by which a benign lesion develops into squamous cell carcinomas. Recent data indicate that both carcinogenic and noncarcinogenic agents can enhance progression. The progression stage of mouse skin carcinogenesis warrants further study especially since the mechanisms involved in malignancy are not clearly understood.

INTRODUCTION

Mouse skin carcinogenesis can be operationally and mechanistically divided into initiation, promotion, and progression. Skin tumors are induced by a single subthreshold dose of a carcinogen (initiation) which, when followed by repetitive applications of a noncarcinogenic, nonmutagenic agent (promotion), produces first papillomas and then squamous cell carcinomas (two-stage tumorigenesis). Tumors that arise from repetitive applications of a carcinogen (complete carcinogenesis) are theoretically the result of both the initiating and promoting abilities of most carcinogens. A good dose-response exists for the activity of common initiators and promoters. Recently we have been able operationally to modulate the progression stage of carcinogenesis, the conversion of benign tumors to malignancy, through the limited or, in some cases, the repetitive applications of agents such as the carcinogen ethylnitrosourea (ENU) or the promoter benzoyl peroxide to papilloma-bearing mice. Since the stages of tumorigenicity are easily delineated and occur sequentially, the mouse skin model offers an excellent opportunity to study mechanisms underlying the individual steps in the carcinogenic process and to investigate the inhibition of tumorigenesis by chemical and dietary agents. The focus of this paper will be to provide an overview of current knowledge related to the stages of carcinogenesis with particular attention to more recent data regarding progression.

Banbury Report 25: Nongenotoxic Mechanisms in Carcinogenesis
© Cold Spring Harbor Laboratory. 0-87969-225-1/87. $1.00 + .00

RESULTS

Initiation

Evidence indicates that initiation involves the induction of permanent genetic damage and is essentially irreversible (Boutwell 1964). A good correlation exists between the carcinogenicity of many carcinogens and their mutagenic activities (McCann and Ames 1976). The critical target for the initiator is likely cellular DNA, and a strong correlation exists between the initiating potency of several polycyclic aromatic hydrocarbons and their covalent binding to DNA (Slaga et al. 1972). Within the epidermis, the regenerative cells or basal cells would seem to represent a likely population within which the initiating event could occur and remain irreversible and stable for about a year.

Promotion

The tumor promotion stage in mouse skin is distinct from the initiation stage by the facts that (1) promoters are nonmutagenic, noncarcinogenic agents and (2) promotion of noninitiated skin fails to yield tumors. Promotion is initially reversible but later becomes irreversible. Promotion can be further subdivided into a first stage, which correlates with the induction of dark, basal keratinocytes, and a second stage, which correlates well with the induction of hyperplasia and ornithine decarboxylase (ODC) activity (Slaga et al. 1980a,b). It is during the second stage of promotion that most of the biochemical events shown to be important in promotion occur.

Table 1 lists the relative potency of agents that can serve as tumor promoters in the mouse skin system. Some skin promoters appear to have a common mode of cellular action—via binding to the natural cellular substrate for diacylglycerol—a phospholipid, calcium-dependent kinase called protein kinase C. Promoters that interact with protein kinase C include 12-O-tetradecanoylphorbol-13-acetate (TPA) (Nishizuka 1984) and related phorbol agents, teleocidin and its analogs, and aplysiatoxins (Fujiki et al. 1984). Other promoters, such as benzoyl peroxide, lauroyl peroxide, hydrogen peroxide, anthralin and its derivative, and palytoxin, do not interact with the protein kinase C and apparently act as promoters via some other mechanism, possibly their ability to generate free radicals. Even with the ability to classify promoters by their interaction with protein kinase C, the mechanisms involved in promotion are not clearly understood. As reported in Table 2, promoters induce a wide variety of cellular and tissue effects when applied to skin. Of the responses mentioned in Table 2, the induction of inflammation and hyperplasia, the increase in dark basal keratinocytes, and the increase in ODC activity demonstrate the best correlation with the potency of a tumor promoter.

Ultimately, the major effect of all promoters, regardless of type, is the expansion of the initiated cell to form visible tumors. Table 3 lists possible mechanisms for the

Table 1
Relative Potency of Skin Tumor Promoters[a]

Promoters	Potency
Croton oil	Strong
Certain phorbol esters in croton oil	Strong
Some synthetic phorbol esters	Strong
Certain euphorbia latices	Strong
7-Bromomethylbenz(a)anthracene	Strong
Teleocidin B[b]	Strong
Aplysiatoxin[b]	Strong
Lyngbyatoxin A[b]	Strong
Palytoxin[c]	Strong
Anthralin	Moderate
Extracts of unburned tobacco	Moderate
Tobacco smoke condensate	Moderate
1-Fluoro-2,4-dinitrobenzene	Moderate
Benzo(e)pyrene	Moderate
Benzoyl peroxide	Moderate
Lauroyl peroxide	Moderate
Hydrogen peroxide	Weak
Certain fatty acids and fatty acid methyl esters	Weak
Certain long-chain alkanes	Weak
A number of phenolic compounds	Weak
Surface active agents (sodium lauryl sulfate, Tween 60)	Weak
Citrus oils	Weak
Iodoacetic acid	Weak

[a] See Slaga (1984) for individual references.
[b] Fujiki and Sugimura (1983).
[c] Fujiki et al. (1986).

Table 2
Summary of Morphological and Biochemical Responses of Mouse Skin to Phorbol Ester and Other Tumor Promoters[a]

Responses

1. Induction of inflammation and hyperplasia
2. Increase in DNA, RNA, and protein synthesis
3. Increase in basal, dark keratinocytes
4. An initial increase in keratinization followed by a decrease
5. Increase in phospholipid synthesis
6. Increase in prostaglandin synthesis
7. Increase in histone synthesis and phosphorylation
8. Increase in ornithine decarboxylase activity followed by an increase in polyamines
9. Increase in histidine and DOPA decarboxylase activity
10. Decrease in the isoproterenol stimulation of cAMP
11. Decrease in the number of dexamethasone receptors
12. Increase in cell division of slowly cycling basal cells[b]

[a] See Slaga (1984) for individual references.
[b] Morris et al. (1986).

Table 3
Mechanisms of Selection of Initiated Epidermal Stem Cell by Skin Tumor Promoters

1. Some tumor promoters may have direct effect on initiated stem cells (dark cells?) causing them to divide and expand in number.
2. Tumor promoters convert some basal keratinocytes to an embryonic phenotype similar to the dark cells and thereby supplying a positive environment for the initiated dark cells to expand in number.
3. Tumor promoters stimulate terminal differentiation of some epidermal cells and thus decrease a negative feedback mechanism on cell proliferation.
4. Some tumor promoters have a selective cytotoxic effect which may cause initiated cells to expand in number.

selection of initiated epidermal cells by tumor promoter. Of the four mechanisms mentioned, evidence supporting each can be found experimentally. Recent studies by Morris (Morris et al. 1986) have demonstrated that slowly cycling basal cells (cells that retain thymidine label) are induced to divide by a single dose of TPA. Many skin tumor promoters increase the presence of dark basal keratinocytes in the epidermis, which correlates well with the activity of first-stage tumor promoters such as TPA, hydrogen peroxide, and calcium ionophore A23187 (Klein-Szanto 1984). The significance of dark basal keratinocytes is not clear, but they appear normally in large numbers in embryonic skin, and their presence in promoted skin may reflect environmental changes within the epidermis, which allows the expansion of cells (including initiated cells) similar to that observed in embryonic tissue (Klein-Szanto 1984). Tumor promoters are potent inducers of terminal differentiation (Reiners and Slaga 1983) and mechanistically may cause the expansion of initiated cells via a decrease in negative feedback signals on cell proliferation. Tumor promoters, especially the free-radical-generating promoters such as benzoyl peroxide and hydrogen peroxide, are highly cytotoxic and may promote by causing a regenerative hyperplasia in the skin similar to the response observed after wounding.

A number of agents, including antioxidants, anti-inflammatory steroids, protease inhibitors, prostaglandin synthesis inhibitors, and the polyamine synthesis inhibitor, difluromethylornithine, have been shown to inhibit promotion (Slaga et al. 1982).

Progression

Many studies have been directed toward understanding the mechanisms involved in tumor initiation and promotion, whereas only a few studies have been performed on the progression stage. The initiation-promotion protocol in mouse skin produces a large number of benign papillomas but only a limited number of squamous cell carcinomas. In this protocol more than 90% of the squamous cell carcinomas appear to develop from papillomas, but the conversion rate is low, approximately 5%.

Several investigators have treated papilloma-bearing mice with the carcinogens, urethane (Roe et al. 1972; Hennings et al. 1983), N-methyl-N-nitro-N'nitrosoguanidine (MNNG), or 4-nitroquinoline-N-oxide (Hennings et al. 1983), and have noted enhanced malignant progression compared to the promoter TPA.

Studies in our laboratory have shown that a limited number of applications of an agent such as ENU to papilloma-bearing mice dramatically enhances malignant progression (O'Connell et al. 1986a). In these experiments, mice were initiated with a low dose of 7,12-dimethylbenzanthracene (DMBA) and promoted with TPA for 16–20 weeks until the papilloma response plateaued. Papilloma-bearing mice were then treated four times with ENU (10 μmoles), four times with MNNG (1 μmole), or with TPA (1.7 nmoles). After the ENU or MNNG treatment, both groups received biweekly TPA treatments for the duration of the experiment (week 40). Mice treated four times with ENU had a higher incidence of carcinomas (74% vs. 38%) and developed 217% more cumulative carcinomas than TPA-treated controls. The incidence of carcinomas in MNNG-treated mice appeared accelerated compared to TPA controls. The ratio of the cumulative number of carcinomas divided by the cumulative number of papillomas at the start of the progression stage (week 20) indicates that ENU was 1.7 times more potent than MNNG and 2.6 times more potent than TPA in causing the progression of papillomas to carcinoma. In a subsequent experiment where the ENU applications (10 μmoles, three times) were not followed by TPA treatment, the percentage of mice with carcinomas was 100% (J.F. O'Connell, unpubl.). In all these studies, once the papillomas' yield had stabilized, there was no increase in cumulative papillomas per group during the progression stage. Thus, the increase in carcinomas was due to an effect of ENU on preexisting papillomas and not the result of the development of new papillomas with a high tendency to become carcinomas.

Other studies have investigated the effect of free-radical-generating agents on progression. Benzoyl peroxide is a free-radical-generating agent used as an industrial polymerizing agent, as a curing agent in cheese, and as an additive in cosmetics and pharmaceuticals, including those used in the treatment of acne (Karaz et al. 1974; Department of Health, Education and Welfare 1977). It is moderately active as a tumor promoter but is inactive as a complete carcinogen or tumor initiator (Van Duuren et al. 1963; Slaga et al. 1981). As shown in Table 4, benzoyl peroxide, like TPA, induces an increase in dark basal keratinocytes, epidermal hyperplasia, and terminal differentiation and inhibits intercellular communication in mouse cells (Slaga et al. 1981; Klein-Szanto and Slaga 1982). However, benzoyl peroxide has only a marginal effect on ODC levels (C.E. Weeks and T.J. Slaga, unpubl.). As is true for other agents, these promotional effects may be related to benzoyl peroxide's ability to generate free radicals. In previous work (Reiners et al. 1984), tumor promotion with benzoyl peroxide (20 mg twice weekly) was found to cause an unexpectedly high rate of carcinomas relative to papillomas.

Recently we have found that the progression of papillomas induced by a

Table 4
Comparison of TPA and Benzoyl Peroxide Promotion in Mouse Skin[a]

	Response	TPA	Benzoyl peroxide
1.	Interacts with receptor (protein kinase C)	yes	no
2.	Hyperplasia	+ + + +	+ + +
3.	Dark cells	+ + + +	+ + +
4.	ODC	+ + + +	+/−
5.	Promotion in SENCAR and CD-1	yes (effective)	yes (effective)
6.	Tumors in SENCAR and CD-1	high number of papillomas low number of carcinomas	moderate number of papillomas moderate number of carcinomas

[a] Slaga et al. (1981); Klein-Szanto and Slaga (1982); T.J. Slaga and C.E. Weeks, unpubl.

standard two-stage protocol (DMBA initiation and TPA promotion) could be enhanced by topical benzoyl peroxide treatment of tumor-bearing mice (O'Connell et al. 1986b). Mice treated with benzoyl peroxide (20 weeks, twice weekly) during the progression stage had a higher incidence of carcinomas (70% vs. 38%) and developed 325% more cumulative carcinomas than did TPA controls. The ratio of the number of cumulative carcinomas per group to the number of papillomas at the start of the progression stage (week 20) indicates that benzoyl peroxide was approximately three times more potent in causing the progression of papillomas to carcinomas than was TPA (0.16 carcinomas/papilloma vs. 0.06 carcinoma/papilloma).

These studies have been further expanded through the use of limited applications of benzoyl peroxide during the progression stage (J.B. Rotstein et al., in prep.). Mice initiated with DMBA and promoted with TPA for 20 weeks were then treated with benzoyl peroxide for various time periods. At the termination of the experiments, the percentage of mice that developed carcinomas was 61%, 74%, and 81% for mice treated with benzoyl peroxide for 4 weeks, 12 weeks, and 20 weeks, respectively, compared to 41% for acetone-treated controls. These studies clearly demonstrate that enhanced progression can occur after a limited number of doses of benzoyl peroxide as was observed with the carcinogen ENU. In the same experiment, papilloma-bearing mice treated repetitively with 15% hydrogen peroxide during the progression stage resulted in a significantly higher percentage of mice with carcinomas than acetone-treated controls (68% vs. 41%).

Studies to determine the potency of both first- and second-stage promoters during the progression stage are summarized in Table 5. Of the promoters tested, the free-radical-generating promoters, benzoyl peroxide and hydrogen peroxide, have the highest activity during the progression stage.

Table 5
Activity of Promoters during Stages of Tumorigenesis[a]

Promoter	Complete carcinogenesis[b]	Initiation[b]	Promotion[b]	Progression[c]
Acetone	—	—	—	weak
TPA	—	—	strong	weak
Mezerein	—	—	moderate (second stage)	weak
Benzoyl peroxide	—	—	moderate	strong
Hydrogen peroxide	—	—	weak	strong
Calcium ionophore 23187	—	—	moderate (first stage)	weak

[a] (—) No activity when tested in specified stage.
[b] See Slaga et al. (1980a, 1982) and Klein-Szanto and Slaga (1982) for individual references.
[c] O'Connell et al. 1986a,b and unpubl.

DISCUSSION

Until recently, most studies using the mouse skin tumorigenesis model have concentrated on the initiating and promoting stage, with few studies specifically addressing progression. We had demonstrated that malignant progression can be enhanced by a limited treatment with noncarcinogenic doses of MNNG or ENU. When applied during weeks 21–22, these agents apparently induced some critical events related to malignancy that led to the appearance of carcinomas predominantly during weeks 30–40. Because of the limited period of treatment with the progressor agent and due to the latency until carcinomas appear, protocols of this type are particularly adaptable to inhibitor studies of the progression stage. Such studies using chemical and dietary inhibitors are presently under way.

Protocols which lead to enhanced progression may also be useful for assessing the carcinogenic risk of environmental chemicals. The need to evaluate chemicals for activity during the progression stage is underscored by the high potency of benzoyl peroxide and hydrogen peroxide in enhancing progression. It is also interesting that although a number of short-term tests exist for initiators, such as the Ames assay (McCann and Ames 1976), and for promoters, such as the cell-cell communication assay (Trosko and Chang 1984) or the induction of hyperplasia on mouse skin (Slaga et al. 1972), there are no short-term tests for the activity of agents during the progression stage of carcinogenesis. When tested on mouse skin, benzoyl peroxide and hydrogen peroxide were not active as tumor initiators or complete carcinogens and are moderately (benzoyl peroxide) or weakly (hydrogen peroxide) active as tumor promoters. As shown in Table 5, the potency of a promoter during the first stage or the second stage of promotion does not correlate well with its potency during progression.

The mechanisms involved in progression in the mouse skin system are unclear. The carcinogens, ENU and MNNG, and the peroxides are all genotoxic compounds (Saladino et al. 1985). Chromosomal studies have shown that squamous cell carcinomas are highly aneuploid lesions, often exhibiting hyperdiploid stem cell lines (Conti et al. 1986). Although early papillomas (10 weeks of promotion) are diploid, they progressively show chromosomal changes and eventually become all aneuploid after 30–40 weeks of promotion. Additional evidence does indicate that a specific chromosome alteration, a trisomy of chromosome number 2, may be a marker of malignancy present in a high percentage of squamous cell carcinomas (C.M. Aldaz et al., unpubl.). Whether the genotoxic effects of the agents used in progression experiments are able to induce such a specific alteration is not known.

In addition to chromosomal alterations, squamous cell carcinomas exhibit a number of changes in protein expression, including the lack of high-molecular-weight keratins (Klein-Szanto et al. 1983) and filaggrin (Mamrack et al. 1984), and the presence of positive staining for the enzyme γ-glutamyltransferase (GGT) (Klein-Szanto et al. 1983; Chiba et al. 1986). Possibly, these phenotypic changes are the result of the gene alterations and rearrangements and can be induced by genotoxic agents. Histological and cytochemical studies of keratoacanthomas, induced by both ENU and benzoyl peroxide when these agents were used as progressors, showed a high percentage of GGT—positive tumors possibly reflecting a novel expression of this enzyme in benign lesions (O'Connell et al. 1986a,b).

A different mechanism of genetic alteration that could be relevant to progression is changes in the methylation state of DNA. Preliminary evidence from this laboratory has indicated that a gradient in DNA methylation exists from normal mouse epidermis to papillomas to carcinomas, with carcinomas being highly undermethylated (J.N. LaPeyre et al., unpubl.). With regard to the agents used as progressors in these studies, both ENU and MNNG have been shown to inhibit methylation by blocking DNA methyltransferase activity (Wilson and Jones 1983).

An alternate hypothesis for the action of progressor agents is related to their high degree of cytotoxicity. In this model for progression, highly cytotoxic agents may (1) selectively or nonselectively kill cells within a tumor, allowing the growth of more malignant cells, and/or (2) kill normal cells, reducing the constraints against expansion along the border between normal and tumor tissue. Both alternatives assume that cells capable of invasion preexist within the benign tumor or that expansion of tumor clones increases the chance of the natural progression of cells toward malignancy. We are currently testing a number of cytotoxic agents for activity during the progression stage.

SUMMARY

Many mouse skin carcinogenesis studies have concentrated on events during initiation and promotion, with few critical reports on the progression stage of carcinogenesis. Although recent data do not clearly indicate the mechanisms involved in progression, they do suggest that progression proceeds by a selection for rapidly proliferating malignant cells. During progression, chemical agents may be acting through genetic or epigenetic means to provide a selective growth advantage to tumor cells with specific phenotypic alterations. Alternatively, progression may reflect a selection for tumor cells that survive chemically induced cytotoxic events within the tumor and surrounding epidermis. Present studies are addressing the question of the mechanisms involved in the malignant progression stage of mouse skin carcinogenesis.

ACKNOWLEDGMENT

We gratefully acknowledge and thank Christie Hoy, Karen Engel, and Catherine Veninga for their help in preparing this paper.

REFERENCES

Boutwell, R.K. 1964. Some biological aspects of skin carcinogenesis. *Prog. Exp. Tumor Res.* **4**: 207.

Chiba, M., M.A. Maley, and A.J.P. Klein-Szanto. 1986. Sequential study of γ-glutamyltransferase during complete and two-stage mouse skin carcinogenesis. *Cancer Res.* **46**: 259.

Conti, C.J., C.M. Aldaz, J.F. O'Connell, A.J.P. Klein-Szanto, and T.J. Slaga. 1986. Aneuploidy, and early event in mouse skin tumor development. *Carcinogenesis* **7**: 1845.

Department of Health, Education and Welfare (DHEW). 1977. Criteria for a recommended standard occupational exposure to benzoyl peroxide. DHEW/PUB/NIOSH-77/166. U.S. Government Printing Office, Washington, D.C.

Fujiki, H. and T. Sugimura. 1983. New potent tumor promoters: Teleocidin, lyngbyatoxin and aphsiatoxin. *Cancer Surv.* **2**: 539.

Fujiki, H., Y. Tamaka, R. Miyake, U. Kawa, and T. Sugimura. 1984. Activation of calcium-activated, phospholipid-dependent protein kinase (protein kinase C) by new classes of tumor promoters, teleocidin and debromoaplysiatoxin. *Biochem. Biophys. Res. Commun.* **120**: 339.

Fujiki, H., M. Suganuma, M. Nakayasu, H. Hakii, T. Horiuchi, S. Takayama, and T. Sugimura. 1986. Palytoxin is a non-12-0-tetradecanoyl-phorbol-13-acetate type tumor promoter in two-stage mouse skin carcinogenesis. *Carcinogenesis* **7**: 707.

Hennings, H.J., R. Shores, M.L. Wenk, E.F. Spangler, R. Tarone, and S.H. Yuspa. 1983. Malignant conversion of mouse skin tumors is increased by tumour initiators and unaffected by tumour promoters. *Nature* **304**: 67.

Karasz, A.B., F. DeCocco, and J.J. Maxstadt. 1974. Gas chromatographic measurements of benzoyl peroxide (as benzoic acid) in cheese. *J. Assoc. Off. Anal. Chem.* **57**: 706.

Klein-Szanto, A.J.P. 1984. Morphological evaluation of tumor promoter effects on mammalian skin. In *Mechanisms of tumor promotion: Tumor promotion and skin carcinogenesis* (ed. T.J. Slaga), vol. II, p. 41. CRC Press, Boca Raton, Florida.

Klein-Szanto, A.J.P. and T.J. Slaga. 1982. Effects of peroxides on rodent skin: Epidermal hyperplasia and tumor promotion. *J. Invest. Dermatol.* **79**: 30.

Klein-Szanto, A.J.P., K.G. Nelson, Y. Shah, and T.J. Slaga, 1983. Simultaneous appearance of keratin modifications and γ-glutamyltransferase activity as indicators of tumor progression in mouse skin papillomas. *J. Natl. Cancer Inst.* **70**: 161.

Mamrack, M.D., A.J.P. Klein-Szanto, and J.J. Reiners, Jr. 1984. Alteration in the distribution of the epidermal protein filaggrin during two-stage chemical carcinogenesis in the SENCAR mouse skin. *Cancer Res.* **44**: 2634.

McCann, J. and B.N. Ames. 1976. Detection of carcinogens as mutagens in the *Salmonella/ microsome* test: Assay of 300 chemicals: Discussion. *Proc. Natl. Acad. Sci. U.S.A.* **73**: 950.

Morris, R.J., S.M. Fischer, and T.J. Slaga. 1986. Evidence that a slowly cycling subpopulation of adult murine epidermal cells retains carcinogen. *Cancer Res.* **46**: 3061.

Nishizuka, Y. 1984. The role of protein kinase C in cell surface signal transduction and tumor promotion. *Nature* **308**: 693.

O'Connell, J.F., A.J.P. Klein-Szanto, D.M. DiGiovanni, J.W. Fries, and T.J. Slaga. 1986a. Malignant progression of mouse skin papillomas treated with ethylnitrosourea, N-methy-N′-nitro-N-nitrosoguanidine or 12-0-tetradecanoylphorbol-13-acetate. *Cancer Lett.* **30**: 269.

———. 1986b. Enhanced malignant progression of mouse skin tumors by the free-radical generator benzoyl peroxide. *Cancer Res.* **46**: 2863.

Reiners, J.J. and T.J. Slaga. 1983. Effects of tumor promoters on the rate and commitment to terminal differentiation of subpopulations of murine keratinocytes. *Cell* **32**: 247.

Reiners, J.J., S. Nesnow, and T.J. Slaga. 1984. Murine susceptibility to two-stage skin carcinogenesis is influenced by the agent used for promotion. *Carcinogenesis* **5**: 301.

Roe, F.J., R.L. Carter, B.C. Mitchley, R. Peto, and E. Hecker. 1972. On the persistence of tumor initiation and the acceleration of tumor progression in mouse skin tumorigenesis. *Int. J. Cancer* **9**: 264.

Saladino, A.F., F.C. Willey, J.F. Lechner, R.C. Grafström, M. LaVeck, and C.C. Harris. 1985. Effects of formaldehyde, acetaldehyde, benzoyl peroxide, and hydrogen peroxide on cultured human bronchial epithelial cells. *Cancer Res.* **45**: 2522.

Slaga, T.J. 1984. Mechanisms involved in two-stage carcinogenesis in mouse skin. In *Mechanisms of tumor promotion: Tumor promotion and skin carcinogenesis* (ed. T.J. Slaga), vol. 1, p. 1. CRC Press, Boca Raton, Florida.

Slaga, T.J., S.M. Fischer, L.L. Triplett, and S. Nesnow. 1972. Comparison of complete carcinogenesis and tumor initiation and promotion in mouse skin: The induction of papillomas by tumor initiation-promotion a reliable short term assay. *J. Environ. Pathol. Toxicol.* **4**: 1025.

Slaga, T.J., S.M. Fischer, K.G. Nelson, and G.L. Gleason. 1980a. Studies on the mechanism of skin tumor promotion: Evidence for several stages in promotion. *Proc. Natl. Acad. Sci. U.S.A.* **77**: 3659.

Slaga, T.J., S.M. Fischer, K.G. Nelson, and S. Major. 1980b. Studies on mechanism of anti-tumor promotion agents: Their specificity in two-stage promotion. *Proc. Natl. Acad. Sci. U.S.A.* **77**: 2251.

Slaga, T.J., A.J.P. Klein-Szanto, L.L. Triplett, L.P. Yotti, and J.E. Trosko. 1981. Skin tumor-promoting activity of benzoyl peroxide, a widely used free radical-generating compound. *Science* **213**: 1023.

Slaga, T.J., S.M. Fischer, C.E. Weeks, A.J.P. Klein-Szanto, and J.J. Reiners. 1982. Studies on the mechanisms involved in multistage carcinogenesis in mouse skin. *J. Cell Biol.* **18**: 99.

Trosko, J.E. and C. Chang. 1984. Role of intracellular communication in tumor promotion In *Mechanisms of tumor promotion: Cellular responses to tumor promoters* (ed. T.J. Slaga), vol. IV, p. 119. CRC Press, Boca Raton, Florida.

Van Duuren, B.L., N. Nelson, L. Orris, E.D. Palmes, and F.L. Schmitt. 1963. Carcinogenicity of epoxides, lactones, and peroxy compounds. *J. Natl. Cancer Inst.* **31**: 41.

Wilson, V.L. and P.A. Jones. 1983. Inhibition of DNA methylation by chemical carcinogens in vitro. *Cell* **32**: 239.

COMMENTS

ROE: In your comparison of benzoyl peroxide and TPA for converting papillomas to carcinomas, did you start at the same place, i.e., with animals that had been identically exposed up to the time point when your comparison started?

SLAGA: Yes. We randomized the mice with papillomas generated by DMBA-TPA and tried to get an equal number of tumors. As a matter of fact, we even tried to map the tumors to make sure that when you give benzoyl peroxide or the third treatment, you are not generating new papillomas. We have done enough studies that we are sure that we are not generating new papillomas.

PITOT: When you did your chromosomal studies, what do the keratoacanthomas look like?

SLAGA: You mean histologically?

PITOT: Are they aneuploid or euploid?

SLAGA: Preliminary data suggest that they are aneuploid.

CERUTTI: Norbert Fusenig has now reported that after 48 hours of TPA treatment of mouse skin, explants are full of chromosomal aberrations. Later on (e.g., in the papillomas), these cells may not be viable. Nevertheless, I wonder whether you have actually looked at banding patterns in the papillomas.

SLAGA: We are presently doing six-banding on papillomas and should have some data very shortly.

CERUTTI: Fusenig finds aberrations soon after TPA application. Because cytogenetics, even with banding, is a very crude measure, there may very well be DNA rearrangements and genetic changes which cannot be seen. The result remains that very early after TPA treatment, cells are full of aberrations. It is conceivable that in the papillomas there may be sequence changes which are not detectable by cytogenetic means.

SLAGA: I agree. It is a very superficial way to look, but it is a starting point. It is only recently that we have been able to do cytogenetic studies in solid tumors. Hopefully, we can do more detailed studies to look for different types of rearrangements.

MAGEE: You said that all tumor promoters induce hyperplasia, but there are agents that induce hyperplasia that are not tumor promoters. Is there anything in the character of hyperplasia that distinguishes between the two?

SLAGA: Yes. You always have to have a sustained hyperplasia. There are agents, like acetic acid, that will cause hyperplasia by their cytotoxic effect but are not promoters. If you keep giving acetic acid, the skin adapts to it, in which case you do not get as much damage with acetic acid nor do you get a sustained hyperplasia from it. So, in general, as has been stated by a number of investigators, sustained hyperplasia is really one of the keys.

MAGEE: I was asking that question in relation to the very earliest experiments by Paton Rous on wound healing. What was the characteristic of that?

SLAGA: Wound healing does give you some tumors after initiation, but it is very difficult to relate it to a chemical promoter because you are given a wound which only involves regeneration in a very narrow area; so it is hard to relate the number of tumors per area and it always seems to be inefficient. It may actually be very efficient, but superficially it appears to be inefficient because you only get one tumor once in a while. When you are treating with TPA, the whole back of the skin can get tumors. If one could come up with some kind of mathematical conversion there, it may be as efficient or more so.

ROE: But there was one feature about wound healing: in order for it to be effective, the wound had to be through the dermis as well as the epidermis.

SLAGA: That was correct the way the initial experiments were done, but Arygus has removed the epidermis down to the basement membrane by the abrasion technique and has produced a reasonable tumor response. As a matter of fact, that is one of the best stimulants for hyperplasia that I have ever seen.

SIVAK: What about the convertibility of keratoacanthomas to CAs versus papillomas?

SLAGA: We have not done that yet.

SIVAK: Because with benzoyl peroxide it is clear that keratoacanthomas predominate.

SLAGA: In complete carcinogenesis studies and in the conversion studies using benzoyl peroxide, we do get some keratoacanthomas. But under normal DMBA-TPA, they are not that common.

SIVAK: So, when benzoyl peroxide is treated as a classical promoter and as a progressor, you get phenotypically different kinds of lesions that predominate?

SLAGA: Yes. The tumor response is more like complete carcinogenesis.

SIVAK: I wanted to discuss the C57 black mice that give weak promoting response for phorbol ester. Do you have any more background on that with respect to its genetics or to the physiology?

DIGIOVANNI: We have some data with the anthrone class of compounds that we are working on.

SIVAK: With an inbred strain like that, you might be able to get another inbred strain that is very strong and do the appropriate genetic studies.

DIGIOVANNI: I will present some data on that. For now, I will say that there are marked differences in the responses of various inbred mouse strains to phorbol ester tumor promotion. However, in several instances, such as benzoyl peroxide and chrysarobin, animals that are nonresponsive to TPA respond to these other classes of promoters. These data imply that different mechanisms may be operating for different classes of tumor promoters.

SARMA: Orotic acid is an excellent tumor promoter in the liver as well as in the intestine. It does not induce cell proliferation.

SLAGA: I didn't intend to mention other tissues because when you get to the liver, things change.

TENNANT: Tom [Slaga], in the plateauing of the benzoyl peroxide doses, have you done experiments where you hold the animals longer in the absence of treatment? Do you see a progression or regression of lesions?

SLAGA: We have compared within 2 weeks after the last TPA treatment versus 2 months and there was basically no difference. That is not a big time difference, but it is a reasonable one.

TENNANT: How do you interpret that data in terms of the concept that a fundamental distinguishing property of a promoter is the regression of lesions in the absence of the chemical?

SLAGA: The degree of regression of papillomas is a function of when you stop your treatment and of which mouse you are using.

Studies on the Skin Tumor Promoting Actions of Chrysarobin

JOHN DIGIOVANNI, FRANCIS H. KRUSZEWSKI, AND KRISTINE J. CHENICEK
The University of Texas System Cancer Center
Science Park–Research Division
Smithville, Texas 78957

OVERVIEW

Anthrone derivatives are effective skin tumor promoters in sensitive mice; however, little is known about their mechanism(s) of skin-tumor-promoting action. The present work has demonstrated that anthrone tumor promoters are very efficient tumor promoters. At optimum promoting doses, the anthrone tumor promoter chrysarobin (1,8-dihydroxy-3-methyl-9-anthrone) produces a lower papilloma response compared with the response in 12-O-tetradecanoylphorbol-13-acetate (TPA)-treated mice. However, the final carcinoma incidence and the number of carcinomas per mouse are very similar. Hence, anthrone promoters appear to be more selective for a critical population of papillomas with a high probability of becoming carcinomas. Several morphological and biochemical responses known to be elicited by TPA have been analyzed following treatment with chrysarobin. In each case significant differences between the two types of promoters have been found. The results suggest one of two possibilities: (1) that the promoting action(s) of anthrone derivatives occurs through an initial mechanism clearly distinct from that of the phorbol esters or (2) that some of the known effects of the phorbol esters may be less important for their promoting actions on mouse skin. In either case, the study of non-phorbol ester tumor promoters has provided important insight into mechanisms of skin tumor promotion.

INTRODUCTION

Skin tumor promotion and the phenomenon of tumor promotion in general have been extensively studied using the phorbol esters such as TPA (Slaga 1984; Diamond 1985). The promotion response to phorbol esters appears to be mediated in part by their interaction with protein kinase C (PKC) (Blumberg et al. 1984; Diamond 1985). A number of compounds that differ in chemical structure but induce many of the same cellular and biochemical responses as the phorbol esters include the teleocidins and the aplysiatoxins (Fujiki and Sugimura 1983). Despite differences in chemical structure, these compounds appear to interact with the phorbol ester receptor and thus to exhibit a similar mechanism of action (Fujiki and Sugimura 1983). Many other compounds possess skin-tumor-promoting activity (Slaga 1984; Diamond 1985), for example, free-radical-generating peroxides (e.g., benzoyl peroxide) (Slaga et al. 1983), certain polycyclic hydrocarbons with weak

Banbury Report 25: Nongenotoxic Mechanisms in Carcinogenesis
© Cold Spring Harbor Laboratory. 0-87969-225-1/87. $1.00 + .00

tumor-initiating activity (e.g., benzo[e]pyrene and 7-bromomethylbenz[a]anthracene) (Slaga et al. 1979; Scribner and Scribner 1980), and several anthrone derivatives such as anthralin and chrysarobin (Segal et al. 1971; DiGiovanni et al. 1985). These latter derivatives are considered the next most potent skin tumor promoters after the phorbol esters (and other compounds capable of interacting with PKC) (Fujiki and Sugimura 1983; Slaga 1984; Diamond 1985).

Work in our laboratory has focused on the anthrone class of skin tumor promoters. Several lines of evidence suggested that these compounds might be useful tools for studying the mechanism(s) of skin tumor promotion. First, anthralin does not interact directly with the phorbol ester receptor (Blumberg et al. 1984). Second, at optimum promoting doses, the time course and magnitude of epidermal ornithine decarboxylase (ODC, EC 4.1.1.17) induction by chrysarobin are markedly different from those of the phorbol esters (DiGiovanni et al. 1985; Kruszewski et al. 1986). In addition, when chrysarobin was applied twice weekly for 2 weeks followed by mezerein, in a two-stage promotion protocol, no stage I promoting activity was detected (DiGiovanni et al. 1985). Thus, the available data suggest that anthrone-type tumor promoters work in part by a mechanism distinct from that of the phorbol esters.

The general procedures and approaches used in our studies of the skin-tumor-promoting actions of these anthrone derivatives have been as follows: (1) to examine in detail the dose-response relationships for the formation of skin papillomas and carcinomas in SENCAR mice using the classical two-stage protocol; (2) to perform structure-activity studies; (3) to examine the ability of anthrone-type tumor promoters to produce several morphological and biochemical changes in mouse epidermis known to be produced by phorbol esters; and (4) to examine the effects of various modifying factors (both chemical and genetic) on tumor promotion by anthrone derivatives.

RESULTS

Dose-response Relationships for Papilloma and Carcinoma Formation in SENCAR Mice

A complete knowledge of the dose-response relationships for the biologic effects of anthrone-type tumor promoters is necessary to understand fully their promoting actions. A good dose-response relationship was observed for promotion of both papilloma and carcinoma formation between 25 nmole and 100 nmole per mouse (Table 1). Doses above 100 nmole were essentially maximal promoting doses. We next compared the efficiency of promotion with chrysarobin and TPA. The term efficiency is used here to refer to the maximal number of papillomas formed and the number that progress to carcinomas under the influence of a particular promoter and is expressed as the ratio of carcinomas to papillomas. As shown in

Table 2, chrysarobin and 1,8-dihydroxy-3-methyl-6-methoxy-9-anthrone (physcion anthrone, a derivative of chrysarobin with similar promoting activity) gave higher ratios of carcinomas to papillomas than did TPA (by at least a factor of 2). Therefore, since the final carcinoma response between TPA- and chrysarobin-promoted mice was very similar, tumor promotion with chrysarobin appears to be more selective for a critical population of papillomas with a high probability of becoming carcinomas.

Structure-Activity Relationships

A limited number of structure-activity studies have been performed in our laboratory. Our initial studies have examined two derivatives of chrysarobin with substituents at carbon-6 of the anthrone nucleus. A hydroxy group in place of hydrogen at carbon-6 completely abolished promoting activity (DiGiovanni et al. 1985), whereas a methoxy group (physcion anthrone) at this position gave activity similar to that of chrysarobin (Table 2). The fact that slight structural changes can bring about significant changes in biological activity suggests the possibility that a specific receptor mechanism may exist for these compounds. Further work is in progress with other structural analogs to test this hypothesis.

Receptor-binding Studies

We have examined in detail the ability of a series of anthrone analogs to interact with the phorbol ester receptor in mouse epidermal particulate fractions. These

Table 1
Dose Response for Skin-tumor-promoting Ability of Chrysarobin in SENCAR Mice[a]

Dose (nmole/mouse)	Papillomas per mouse[b]	Mice with papillomas (%)	Carcinomas per mouse[c]	Mice with carcinomas (%)[c]
25	0.73	36	0.12	12
50	2.04	58	0.42	38
75	4.07	63	1.04	67
100	4.70	92	0.78	59
220	5.42	92	0.96	67
440	4.85	96	0.73	58

[a] Each experimental group contained 30 preshaved mice. Animals were initiated with 25 nmole 7,12-dimethylbenz(a)anthracene (DMBA) followed 2 weeks later by twice-weekly applications of chrysarobin. Animals receiving DMBA at initiation followed by twice-weekly applications of acetone (0.2 ml), or acetone (0.2 ml) at initiation followed by twice-weekly applications of 220 nmole chrysarobin, had 0.0 papillomas/mouse and 0.04 papillomas/mouse, respectively, after 60 weeks of treatment.

[b] Average number of papillomas/mouse at plateau. For doses above 50 nmole/mouse, the papilloma response plateaued after 25 weeks of promotion. For the 50-nmole dose, the papilloma response plateaued after 36 weeks of promotion and the 25-nmole dose group did not reach a plateau; so the data are given at 60 weeks.

[c] Average number of carcinomas per surviving mouse and percentage of surviving mice with carcinomas based on the number of surviving mice at the time of appearance of the first carcinoma. Data are given at 60 weeks of promotion.

Table 2
Comparison of the Efficiency of Skin Tumor Promotion with Chrysarobin and TPA[a]

Dose of DMBA at initiation	Promoter	Dose of promoter (application frequency per week)	Mice with carcinomas (%)	Carcinomas per mouse	Ca/Pa[b]
10 nmole	TPA	3.4 nmole (2×)	20	0.20	0.01
10 nmole	chrysarobin	220 nmole (2×)	22	0.30	0.07
25 nmole	TPA	3.4 nmole (2×)	48	0.90	0.05
25 nmole	chrysarobin	220 nmole (2×)	67	0.96	0.18
25 nmole	chrysarobin	220 nmole (1×)[c]	69	1.23	0.13
25 nmole	physcion anthrone	220 nmole (2×)	52	0.59	0.12

[a] Each experimental group contained 30 female SENCAR mice. Data for the 10 nmole DMBA groups are given after 45 weeks of promotion. Data for the 25 nmole DMBA groups are given after 60 weeks of promotion.

[b] $Ca/Pa = \dfrac{\text{average number of carcinomas per mouse at 45 weeks or 60 weeks}}{\text{average number of papillomas per mouse at plateau}}$

[c] Animals in this group received chrysarobin treatments only once weekly.

results are shown in Figure 1. To date, none of the structural analogs tested competed with ^{3}H-labeled phorbol-12,13-dibutyrate (PDBu) for binding sites in epidermal particulate fractions. The compounds tested included chrysarobin, physcion anthrone, and 10-myristoyl-anthralin. Teleocidin, on the other hand, effectively competed with ^{3}H-labeled PDBu for binding sites. Mezerein also inhibited the binding of ^{3}H-labeled PDBu but was less potent than teleocidin. The results with teleocidin and mezerein are similar to previous published data (Blumberg et al. 1984). Since anthralin and chrysarobin undergo autooxidation in solution (Segal et al. 1971; Van Duuren et al. 1978; Krebs et al. 1981), the anthraquinone oxidation product (1,8-dihydroxy-3-methyl-9,10-anthraquinone or chrysophanic acid) was tested. As shown in the figure, chrysophanic acid did not compete with ^{3}H-labeled PDBu for binding sites. In addition to the anthraquinone, a variety of other oxidation products are known to be formed (Segal et al. 1971; Van Duuren et al. 1978; Krebs et al. 1981). We therefore allowed solutions of chrysarobin to stand at room temperature for up to 2 hours prior to addition to the binding assay. Under these conditions, solutions of 1×10^{-5} M chrysarobin that had been standing for 1 hour or more inhibited binding of ^{3}H-labeled PDBu by ~50%. This finding raises the possibility that further breakdown products of chrysarobin may influence the binding of ^{3}H-labeled PDBu in epidermal particulate fractions. Interestingly, the ability of anthralin to inhibit glucose-6-phosphate dehydrogenase activity in solution is time-dependent and correlates with the appearance of further breakdown products (Cavey et al. 1981). Thus, the autooxida-

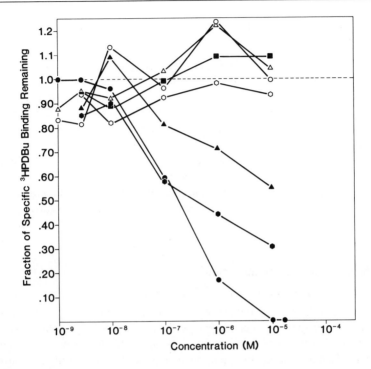

Figure 1

Inability of anthrone derivatives to compete directly for ^{3}H-labeled PDBu receptors in a mouse epidermal particulate fraction obtained from SENCAR mice. ^{3}H-labeled PDBu was added at a final concentration of 60 nM and specific binding was calculated as the difference between ^{3}H-labeled PDBu bound in the absence and presence of 30 μM unlabeled PDBu. (●) PDBu; (▲) mezerein; (◆) teleocidin; (○) chrysarobin; (○) chrysophanic acid; (■) physcion anthrone; and (△) 10-myristoylanthralin.

tion of anthralin or chrysarobin in vivo could potentially generate molecules (or intermediates) capable of altering the functional activity of a variety of cellular constituents.

Weinstein et al. (1981) have suggested that binding of certain compounds (e.g., polycyclic hydrocarbons) to the Ah receptor induces a pleiotropic response which includes biochemical and molecular effects similar to those induced by the phorbol esters. Due to the similarity in structure of anthrone tumor promoters and polycyclic hydrocarbons, we thought it possible that they might interact with the cytosolic Ah receptor. However, over a broad concentration range (1 × 10^{-8} to 1 × 10^{-4} M), chrysarobin was unable to displace [^{3}H]2,3,7,8-tetrachlorodibenzo-p-dioxin (TCDD) from its cytosolic receptor in preparations of rat hepatic cytosol (data not shown).

Genetic Differences in Response to Phorbol Ester or Chrysarobin Skin Tumor Promotion

We have recently shown that TPA is an effective skin tumor promoter in the inbred mouse strain DBA/2 (DiGiovanni et al. 1984). The inbred mouse strain C57BL/6, on the other hand, is highly resistant to phorbol ester skin tumor promotion (DiGiovanni et al. 1984; Reiners et al. 1984). A comparison of the promotion sensitivity of DBA/2, C57BL/6, and SENCAR mice to chrysarobin was examined and is summarized in Table 3. Interestingly, chrysarobin was a much more effective tumor promoter in C57BL/6 mice than TPA, giving a dose-dependent increase in papillomas in this inbred strain. Recently, C57BL/6 mice have been reported to be sensitive to benzoyl peroxide promotion (Reiners et al. 1984). Therefore, C57BL/6 mice may be sensitive to classes of tumor promoters whose mechanism is different from that of the phorbol esters. Further work along these lines would seem warranted.

Ornithine Decarboxylase Induction

Following a single topical application with either 220 nmole chrysarobin or 3.4 nmole TPA, both the time course and magnitude of induction of epidermal ODC differed between the two compounds (Fig. 2A). Whereas chrysarobin gave a single peak of ODC activity of 0.19 nmole CO_2/mg protein/60 min at 56 hours after treatment, TPA application produced a single peak of ODC activity measuring 2.53 nmole CO_2/mg protein/60 min at 6 hours after treatment.

Figure 2B presents representative time courses for the induction of ODC activity in mouse epidermis following five topical applications of 220 nmole chrysarobin when given at different application frequencies. The induction of ODC activity by chrysarobin following a twice-weekly application frequency protocol yielded a multiphasic response over the 72-hour time course examined. Interestingly, the maximum response with the twice-weekly protocol was shifted to earlier time points and there was little or no potentiation in the induction response. This latter observation differs from the observation with TPA (O'Brien 1976), where multiple applications elicit a potentiated induction response. O'Brien (1976) also demonstrated that both single and multiple applications of TPA induce ODC activity with the same time course. Although the data are not shown in Figure 2, five applications of 3.4 nmole TPA in a twice-weekly application protocol gave a single peak of ODC activity measuring 9.12 nmole CO_2/mg protein/60 min at 6 hours after the last application.

The lack of potentiated induction of ODC following twice-weekly applications of chrysarobin and the markedly delayed response after a single application suggested that a less frequent application protocol might yield a greater induction response. Figure 2B shows that a once-weekly application protocol also yielded a multiphasic induction response over the 72-hour time course. Significantly, an overall higher level of ODC activity was sustained throughout the 72-hour time course, with peak activities at least twofold higher than with the twice-weekly application protocol. We have recently found that a once-weekly application frequency of chrysarobin

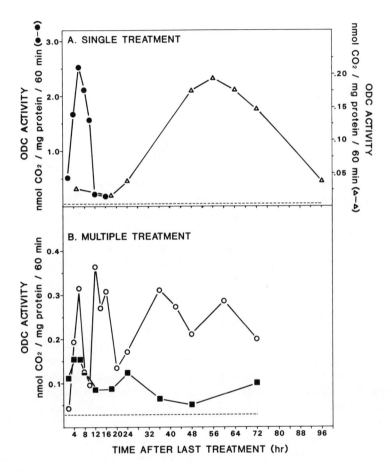

Figure 2

Time-response curves for the induction of epidermal ODC activity by chrysarobin. Groups of five mice were treated topically with either 0.2 ml acetone or the test compound dissolved in acetone (0.2 ml) and were killed at the time indicated after a single treatment or after the last of five multiple treatments. Each point represents the mean of triplicate determinations of enzyme activity (variation < 10%). Graphs are representative responses from experiments that were repeated several times with similar results. (A) ODC activity following a single treatment with 220 nmole chrysarobin (△); 3.4 nmole TPA (●); or 0.2 ml acetone control (----) (right-hand scale). (B) ODC activity following the last of five multiple treatments with 220 nmole chrysarobin given at an application frequency of once weekly over a 5-week period (○) or twice weekly over a 2½ week period (■). (----) Mean of the acetone control groups from the two different application frequencies.

gives an approximately twofold higher papilloma response in SENCAR mice initiated with DMBA (Kruszewski et al. 1986, 1987).

DISCUSSION

The goal of our studies has been to critically examine the mechanism(s) of skin tumor promotion by anthrone-type promoters. Although these compounds show some similarities with the phorbol-ester-type tumor promoters, there are also some very significant differences. We have shown that the anthrone-type promoters are very efficient in that they produce a relatively low papilloma response while giving a similar carcinoma response when compared with the phorbol esters. These data suggest that there may be differences in the mechanism by which anthrone tumor promoters select for initiated cells in the epidermis. This hypothesis is supported by a number of studies. For example, although anthralin and chrysarobin are capable of producing hyperplasia, the kinetics and magnitude of the induced hyperplasia are different from those with TPA (DiGiovanni et al. 1985 and unpubl.). Argyris (1981) has suggested that TPA-induced hyperplasia is essentially a regenerative type. However, Klein-Szanto et al. (1984) have shown that TPA produces only moderate, sublethal damage to epidermal keratinocytes. We have found that chrysarobin (A.J.P. Klein-Szanto and J. DiGiovanni, unpubl.) produces significant epidermal toxicity after a single application. Again, however, the time course of epidermal toxicity with chrysarobin was delayed compared to that with TPA (Klein-Szanto et al. 1984) and followed the delayed hyperplasiogenic response to chrysarobin. These data suggest that the hyperplasia induced by anthrone-type tumor promoters may be more like a regenerative hyperplasia. In addition, these data suggest that some metabolic processes must take place prior to the actions of chrysarobin. Our studies comparing once-weekly and twice-weekly applications of chrysarobin for both ODC induction and tumor promotion also suggest that epidermal toxicity may play an important role in the promotion response to anthrone-type promoters. The role of epidermal toxicity in tumor promotion by anthrone derivatives deserves further investigation.

Further evidence that anthrone derivatives may work by a mechanism distinct from that of the phorbol esters comes from the observation that anthralin does not compete for phorbol ester binding sites in epidermal particulate fractions or on newborn epidermal cells in culture (Blumberg et al. 1984). Our data, obtained using highly purified chrysarobin (DiGiovanni et al. 1985) and several structural analogs, clearly show that none of these compounds compete for phorbol ester receptors in epidermal particulate fractions (Fig. 1). Parkinson and Emmerson (1982) have shown that anthralin and benzoyl peroxide are incapable of producing the same effects on human keratinocyte proliferation (inhibition), morphology, and differentiation as produced by TPA. Driedger and Blumberg (1978) demonstrated that a variety of non-phorbol ester skin tumor promoters, including anthralin, did not

Table 3
Tumor-promoting Activity of Chrysarobin and TPA in Different Stocks/Strains of Mice[a]

Promoter (dose)	Mouse strain[b]		
	SENCAR	C57BL/6	DBA/2
TPA (6.8 nmole)	10.60 (97)*	0.07 (7)*	7.53 (100)*
Chrysarobin (220 nmole)	3.41 (76)[+]	1.35 (72)[+]	0.26 (19)[+]
Chrysarobin (440 nmole)	3.72 (90)[+]	1.84 (89)[+]	1.04 (44)[+]
Chrysarobin (880 nmole)	3.00 (85)[+]	3.19 (100)[+]	2.00 (75)[+]

[a] Each experimental group contained 30 mice. All animals were initiated with DMBA as follows: SENCAR, 10 nmole; C57BL/6, 400 nmole; and DBA/2, 400 nmole. One week later, mice began receiving twice-weekly applications of promoter as indicated.
[b] Values represent the average number of papillomas per mouse after 21* or 31[+] weeks of promotion. Numbers in parentheses represent the percentage of mice with papillomas.

mimic the actions of TPA on chicken embryo fibroblasts. Additionally, in our studies, chrysarobin was found (Table 3) to be a skin tumor promoter in C57BL/6 mice, a mouse strain highly resistant to phorbol ester skin tumor promotion (DiGiovanni et al. 1984; Reiners et al. 1984). These latter data are similar to results of Slaga and co-workers (Reiners et al. 1984), showing that C57BL/6 mice are sensitive to benzoyl peroxide but not to TPA promotion. Finally, anthralin has been shown to be only a weak inducer of dark basal keratinocytes when examined over a 96-hour time course (Klein-Szanto and Slaga 1981). A summary of phorbol ester actions that are not mediated, or are mediated in a significantly different manner, by anthrone derivatives on mouse skin is listed in Table 4. The information currently available has led us to speculate that skin tumor promotion by anthrone derivatives may be more like the promotion stage that occurs during complete carcinogenesis (DiGiovanni et al. 1985).

One must now ask the question, What is the mechanism of skin tumor promotion by anthrone derivatives? A number of possibilities exist that need to be explored. The mechanism must take into account the delayed actions of chrysarobin (or anthralin) when applied to mouse skin. An interesting hypothesis that we are currently exploring in detail is based on the knowledge that anthrone derivatives such as anthralin and chrysarobin undergo autooxidation in solution and biological fluids (Segal et al. 1971; Martinmaa et al. 1978; Sae ē Melo et al. 1983). During autooxidation of anthralin, a semiquinone intermediate is believed to be formed which, upon further oxidation, yields 1,8-dihydroxy-9,10-anthraquinone (Martinmaa et al. 1978; Sae ē Melo et al. 1983). During this process, O_2 can be reduced to O_2^- (Martinmaa et al. 1978; Sae ē Melo et al. 1983). Therefore, these breakdown products (semiquinone and quinone) could participate in redox cycles leading to a prooxidant state. Cerutti (1985) has recently reviewed the literature suggesting a role for prooxidant states in tumor promotion. Furthermore, Slaga et al. (1983) have shown that anthralin inhibits both superoxide dismutase (EC 1.15.1.1) and catalase

Table 4
Phorbol Ester Actions Not Mediated, or Mediated in a Significantly Different Manner, by Anthrone-type Promoters on Mouse Skin

Action	Comparison with TPA	Reference
Complete promotion	higher ratio of carcinomas/papillomas	DiGiovanni et al. (1985)[a]
Hyperplasia/edema	markedly delayed time course and lower magnitude with peak between 4 and 7 days after single application; more effective at producing edema than TPA	DiGiovanni et al. (1985)[b]
ODC induction	very weak inducer, peak induction at 56–64 hr after a single application; little or no potentiation after multiple treatments	DiGiovanni et al. (1985); Kruszewski et al. (1986)
Phorbol-ester-receptor binding	do not compete	Blumberg et al. (1984)[c]
Mouse strain sensitivity	C57BL/6 mice are sensitive to chrysarobin but not to TPA	Table 3
Dark-cell induction	weak inducers	Klein-Szanto and Slaga (1981)
Stage I promotion	inactive, TPCK does not inhibit promotion by chrysarobin	DiGiovanni et al. (1985)[b]

[a] J. DiGiovanni et al. (unpubl.) and Tables 1 and 2.
[b] J. DiGiovanni et al. (unpubl.).
[c] Figure 1.

(EC 1.11.1.6) activities in mouse epidermis, consistent with the hypothesis that anthrone-promoter-induced prooxidant state(s) may be an important component of their mechanism of action. The fact that the 1,8-dihydroxy-9,10-anthraquinone was devoid of promoting activity when tested at a single dose (Segal et al. 1971) casts some doubt on this hypothesis. However, this may be related to pharmacokinetic differences between the two compounds, or it may indicate that the process of autooxidation itself (generating free radicals) is the critical process for tumor promotion. Work in our laboratory is focusing on the role of anthrone autooxidation in skin tumor promotion by this class of promoters.

SUMMARY

Anthrone-type skin tumor promoters, such as chrysarobin, are highly efficient promoters producing in initiated mice a population of papillomas that have a high probability of progressing to carcinomas. Anthrone promoters do not compete with ^{3}H-labeled PDBu for receptors in epidermal particulate fractions, nor do they compete for the [^{3}H]TCDD receptor in rat hepatic cytosol preparations. Furthermore, the induction of epidermal ODC by anthrone tumor promoters is markedly different, in both magnitude and time course, from that by the phorbol esters. C57BL/6 mice, which are highly resistant to phorbol ester skin tumor promotion, are sensitive to chrysarobin promotion. Taken together, these data support the hypothesis that anthrone-type skin tumor promoters work through an initial mechanism distinct from that of the phorbol esters.

ACKNOWLEDGMENTS

Original research was supported by National Institutes of Health grant CA-37111. The authors wish to thank Joyce Mayhugh for her help in preparing the manuscript.

REFERENCES

Argyris, T.S. 1981. The regulation of epidermal hyperplastic growth. *CRC Crit. Rev. Toxicol.* **9:** 151.

Blumberg, P.M., J.A. Dunn, S. Jaken, A.Y. Jeng, K.L. Keach, N.A. Sharkey, and E. Yeh. 1984. Specific receptors for phorbol ester tumor promoters and their involvement in biological responses. In *Mechanisms of tumor promotion. Tumor promotion and carcinogenesis in vitro* (ed. T.J. Slaga), vol. 3, p. 185. CRC Press, Boca Raton, Florida.

Cavey, D., J.C. Caron, and B. Shroot. 1981. Anthralin: Chemical instability and glucose-6-phosphate dehydrogenase inhibition. *Br. J. Dermatol.* (Suppl. 20) **105:** 15.

Cerutti, P.A. 1985. Prooxidant states and tumor promotion. *Science* **227:** 375.

Diamond, L. 1985. Tumor promoters and cell transformation. *Pharmacol. Ther.* **26:** 145.

DiGiovanni, J., W.P. Prichett, P.C. Decina, and L. Diamond. 1984. DBA/2 mice are as sensitive as SENCAR mice to skin tumor promotion by 12-0-tetradecanoylphorbol-13-acetate. *Carcinogenesis* **5:** 1493.

DiGiovanni, J., P.C. Decina, W.P. Prichett, J. Cantor, K.K. Aalfs, and M.M. Coombs. 1985. Mechanism of skin tumor promotion by chrysarobin. *Cancer Res.* **45:** 2584.

Driedger, P.E. and P.M. Blumberg. 1978. Non phorbol mouse skin tumor promoters do not mimic phorbol myristate acetate in its effects on chick embryo fibroblasts. *Int. J. Cancer* **22:** 63.

Fujiki, H. and T. Sugimura. 1983. New potent tumor promoters: Teleocidin, lyngbyatoxin A and aplysiatoxin. *Cancer Surv.* **2:** 539.

Klein-Szanto, A.J.P. and T.J. Slaga. 1981. Numerical variations of dark cells in normal and chemically induced hyperplastic epidermis with age of animal and efficiency of tumor promoter. *Cancer Res.* **41:** 4437.

Klein-Szanto, A.J.P., M. Chiba, S.U. Lee, C.J. Conti, and D. Thetford. 1984. Keratinocyte damage produced by 12-0-tetradecanoylphorbol-13-acetate in rodent epidermis. *Carcinogenesis* **5:** 1459.

Krebs, A., H. Schaltegger, and A. Schaltegger. 1981. Structure specificity of the antipsoriatic anthrones. *Br. J. Dermatol.* (Suppl. 20) **105:** 6.

Kruszewski, F.H., K.J. Chenicek, and J. DiGiovanni. 1986. Effect of application frequency on epidermal ornithine decarboxylase induction by chrysarobin in SENCAR mice. *Cancer Lett.* **32:** 263.

Kruszewski, F.H., C.J. Conti, and J. DiGiovanni. 1987. Characterization of skin tumor promotion and progression by chrysarobin. *Cancer Res.* **47:** (in press).

Martinmaa, J., L. Vanhala, and K.K. Mustakallio. 1978. Free radical intermediates produced by autooxidation of 1,8-dihydroxy-9-anthrone (dithranol) in pyridine. *Experientia* **34:** 872.

O'Brien, T.G. 1976. The induction of ornithine decarboxylase as an early, possibly obligatory, event in mouse skin carcinogenesis. *Cancer Res.* **36:** 2644.

Parkinson, E.K. and A. Emmerson. 1982. The effects of tumor promoters on the multiplication and morphology of cultured human epidermal keratinocytes. *Carcinogenesis* **3:** 525.

Reiners, J.J., S. Nesnow, and T.J. Slaga. 1984. Murine susceptibility to two-stage carcinogenesis is influenced by the agent used for promotion. *Carcinogenesis* **5:** 301.

Sae ē Melo, T., L. Dubertret, P. Prognon, A. Gond, G. Mahuzier, and R. Santus. 1983. Physicochemical properties and stability of anthralin in model systems and human skin. *J. Invest. Dermatol.* **80:** 1.

Scribner, N.K. and J.D. Scribner. 1980. Separation of initiating and promoting effects of the skin carcinogen 7-bromomethylbenz(a)anthracene. *Carcinogenesis* **1:** 97.

Segal, A., C. Katz, and B.L. Van Duuren. 1971. Structure and tumor promoting activity of anthralin (1,8-dihydroxy-9-anthrone) and related compounds. *J. Med. Chem.* **14:** 1152.

Slaga, T.J. 1984. Mechanisms involved in two-stage carcinogenesis in mouse skin. In *Mechanisms of tumor promotion. Tumor promotion and skin carcinogenesis* (ed. T.J. Slaga), vol. 2, p. 1. CRC Press, Boca Raton, Florida.

Slaga, T.J., V. Solanki, and M. Logani. 1983. Studies on the mechanism of action of antitumor promoting agents: Suggestive evidence for the involvement of free radicals in promotion. In *Radioprotectors and anticarcinogens* (ed. O.F. Nygaard and M.G. Simic), p. 471. Academic Press, New York.

Slaga, T.J., L. Jecker, W.M. Bracken, and C. Weeks. 1979. The effects of weak or non-carcinogenic polycyclic hydrocarbons on 7,12-dimethylbenz(a)-anthracene and benzo(a)pyrene skin tumor initiation. *Cancer Lett.* **7:** 51.

Van Duuren, B.L., A. Segal, S.S. Tseng, G.M. Rusch, G. Loewengart, U. Mate, D. Roth, A. Smith, S. Melchionne, and I. Seidman. 1978. Structure and tumor promoting activity of analogues of anthralin (1,8-dihydroxy-9-anthrone). *J. Med. Chem.* **21:** 26.

Weinstein, I.B., A.D. Horowitz, R.A. Mufson, P.B. Fisher, V. Invanovic, J. Laskin, and E. Greenebaum. 1981. Biochemical effects of the phorbol ester tumor promoters and their implications for polycyclic aromatic hydrocarbon carcinogenesis. In *Polycyclic hydrocarbons and cancer* (ed. H.V. Gelboin and P.O.P. Ts'O), vol. 3, p. 293. Academic Press, New York.

COMMENTS

REITZ: Has chrysarobin been tested to see if it has any direct action on DNA, for example in the Ames test?

DIGIOVANNI: Yes. We performed several experiments in collaboration with John Reiners, also at Science Park, to determine whether or not these compounds are mutagenic in the Ames assay. We could never demonstrate any mutagenicity with chrysarobin in either the presence or absence of S9.

One of the problems with these compounds is that they are very cytotoxic to the bacteria and it caused problems in trying to quantitate mutagenic activity. When we did the experiments under conditions of reduced toxicity, we still could not measure any mutagenic activity. We have done experiments where groups of mice were treated with different doses of chrysarobin for 60 weeks to test its complete carcinogenic activity. Under these conditions, we see fewer tumors with chrysarobin than we see with just TPA alone. Therefore, we have little evidence to suggest any complete carcinogenic activity.

SLAGA: You always make your compound up fresh. Have you compared leaving it on the bench for a while for a defined period of time versus difference in activity?

DIGIOVANNI: No, we have not tried that. It would be an interesting experiment. Several of the oxidation products, i.e., the antraquinone and dimer formed from anthralin, were tested by Van Duuren and shown to be inactive. There are, however, many other oxidation products that may possess some biological activity.

ROSENKRANZ: With respect to the question about the genotoxicity of anthralin, there is a very interesting report that a derivative, 1,2,3-trihydroxyanthraquinone, is mutagenic in *Salmonella*, but not in strains deficient in nitroreductase, a bacterial enzyme that may be the analog of xanthine oxidase. It may therefore be that the free-radical mechanism that you have suggested is operative.

DIGIOVANNI: These compounds are known to intercalate into DNA with a mechanism similar to that of ethidium bromide. In fact, in yeast, for example, they do have effects on mitochondrial DNA and can produce petite mutations similar to those produced by ethidium bromide. At one time it was thought that they could produce other types of DNA damage, but there have been several studies that looked at this idea carefully and there is no evidence that they cause any direct DNA damage.

SIVAK: Do you have any protein kinase data?

DIGIOVANNI: We just have some preliminary data that we have done with Curt Ashendel at Purdue University. He has looked at all of the derivatives that we looked at for competition with ^{3}H-labeled PDBu in particulate fractions. We could not find any evidence of activation of PKC in vitro with any of these derivatives.

COOMBS: You found your 10-acetyl compound less active. Van Duuren found them more active with respect to the original compound. Do you think that is due to less oxidation in your sample?

DIGIOVANNI: I think the problem with the Van Duuren paper is that they only used one dose. It is very difficult to make any comparisons based on a single dose because of biologic variation. In our studies currently in progress, we are comparing three doses where we have doses higher and lower than the parent compound. Under these conditions, even though the experiment is only at the twelfth week of promotion, we can already categorize to what extent these compounds are producing their effects. The 10-acetyl derivative is more potent than the myristoyl derivative, but less potent than anthralin.

COOMBS: Did you say that the acetyl compound is a very toxic compound?

DIGIOVANNI: The 10-acetyl derivative does appear quite toxic. However, these compounds as a class are generally quite toxic.

STEVENSON: Do you rule out the free-radical mechanism interacting with DNA?

DIGIOVANNI: At the present time, we do not have any data to rule out that possibility. The only available data suggest that these compounds have a very high affinity for the cell surface membrane, and the chance of any of the autooxidation products (or active oxygen species) getting into the nucleus may be fairly small. We do not think that there is a direct DNA damage mechanism involved here, but further work is necessary to substantiate this.

SLAGA: Do antioxidants have an effect on chrysarobin?

DIGIOVANNI: We are currently examining the ability of a variety of antioxidants to modify skin tumor promotion by chrysarobin. The only compound that we presently have data for is BHA. Interestingly, when we did the experiments, BHA caused significant enhancement in the tumor-promoting activity of chrysarobin. Presently, we do not have an explanation for these results; however, further work is in progress. One possibility is that BHA may reduce some of the toxicity of chrysarobin.

REITZ: Or prevent the autooxidation.

DIGIOVANNI: Yes, that's a distinct possibility. That would go against the idea that autooxidation is involved in the mechanism of promotion by these derivatives. So, obviously, much more work is necessary to understand the role of autooxidation in skin tumor promotion by anthrone derivatives.

SCRIBNER: What strain did you use for the BHA experiments?

DIGIOVANNI: SENCAR mice.

STEVENSON: You know, with BHA there is the possibility of external growth factors simply because when you hepatectomize an animal, you get an increased response. Do you rule out any of those effects or are you thinking in terms of direct effect on the cell?

DIGIOVANNI: That's a difficult question.

CERUTTI: All these antioxidants—at least the simple ones like BHA and BHT—are indeed antioxidants; but at the same time they are being oxidized and become oxidants. Only a wonderful compound such as vitamin E represents an exception because an inactive product is formed. I could envision that with enough autooxidation of your anthralin compounds, it might not be effective to just add a compound such as BHA. That could explain this paradox.

DIGIOVANNI: We certainly could rule that out by looking at a series of other compounds that would not undergo that type of reaction. That is a very good point.

Multistage Carcinogenesis of the Rat Hepatocyte

HENRY C. PITOT, DAVID G. BEER, AND SUZANNE HENDRICH
McArdle Laboratory for Cancer Research
The Medical School
Departments of Oncology and Pathology
University of Wisconsin
Madison, Wisconsin 53706

OVERVIEW

Carcinogenesis, defined as the natural history of neoplastic disease, occurs in two or more sequential stages and has now been shown to occur in a number of histogenetic systems both in vivo (Scribner and Süss 1978; Pitot and Sirica 1980) and in vitro (Mondal et al. 1976; Barrett 1980; Yuspa et al. 1981). Implicit in multistage carcinogenesis are (1) characteristics distinguishing each stage, (2) ordering of the stages relative to each other in time and sequence, and (3) selective action of carcinogenic agents at one or more of the distinguishable stages. This paper will consider each of these areas, primarily in relation to several models of multistage hepatocarcinogenesis in rodents, but also with relation to the natural history of the development of other histogenetic neoplasms where appropriate.

CHARACTERISTICS OF THE STAGES OF HEPATOCARCINOGENESIS

In most of the models of multistage hepatocarcinogenesis in the rat, at least three different stages can be distinguished on the basis of their biological characteristics. These stages and their characteristics are noted in Table 1. The first stage, initiation, is irreversible as judged from an extended separation between the point of initiation and that of the beginning of the second stage, promotion (Peraino et al. 1977; Pitot 1978). Recent studies (Glauert et al. 1986) have shown that enzyme-altered foci (EAF) initiated by a single dose of diethylnitrosamine (DEN) and promoted by phenobarbital (PB) are lost in large measure on cessation of the administration of the promoting agent. Other studies (Goldsworthy and Pitot 1985a) have demonstrated that extended feeding (6 months) of a crude grain-based diet in the absence of PB, following initiation and promotion for 4–6 months, results in a reappearance of essentially the entire population of foci. More recent studies (Table 2) have demonstrated that, under more controlled conditions, removal of the promoting agent results in a rapid loss of EAF, which can then be recovered even after a number of days in the absence of the promoting agent by refeeding of the promoter. From these studies, as well as earlier investigations (Hanigan and Pitot 1985) on the transplantation of cells of EAF into livers of rats treated with PB, altered hepato-

Banbury Report 25: Nongenotoxic Mechanisms in Carcinogenesis
© Cold Spring Harbor Laboratory. 0-87969-225-1/87. $1.00 + .00

Table 1

Biological Characteristics of the Stages of Initiation, Promotion, and Progression in Hepatocarcinogenesis in the Rat

Initiation	Promotion	Progression
Irreversible with constant "stem cell" potential	Reversible	Irreversible. Measurable and/or morphologically discernible alteration in cell genome's structure
Efficacy sensitive to xenobiotic and other chemical factors	Promoted cell population existence dependent on continued administration of the promoting agent	Growth of altered cells sensitive to environmental factors during early phase
Spontaneous (fortuitous) occurrence of initiated cells can be quantitated	Efficacy sensitive to dietary and hormonal factors	Benign and/or malignant neoplasms characteristically seen
Requires cell division for "fixation"	Dose response exhibits measurable threshold and maximal effect dependent on dose of initiating agent	"Progressor" agents act to advance promoted cells into this stage but may not be initiating agents
Dose response does not exhibit a readily measurable threshold	Relative effectiveness of promoters depends on time and dose rate to reach maximal effect and dose rate	
Relative effect of initiators depends on quantitation of focal lesions following defined period of promotion		

cytes populating such foci appear to be dependent for their existence on the continued presence of the promoting agent.

The sensitivity of the stage of initiation during hepatocarcinogenesis to modulation by exogenous factors is now well known. Williams (1984) has reviewed a number of examples of the inhibition of hepatocarcinogenesis during the stage of initiation by the administration of a variety of chemicals, many exhibiting promoting activity in multistage hepatocarcinogenesis. 5-Azacytidine (Denda et al. 1986) and inhibitors of poly(ADP) ribosylation (Takahashi et al. 1984) enhance the process of initiation during hepatocarcinogenesis in the rat. The process of initiation

Table 2

Effects of Withdrawal and Reintroduction of Phenobarbital on Enzyme-altered Foci

	Percentage of liver occupied by EAF[a] ± SE	Number of EAF per liver ± SE
PB for 4 months[b]	0.47 ± 0.09	10,794 ± 1813
PB for 4 months. NIH diet for 30 days	0.97 ± 0.09	5,354 ± 658
PB for 4 months. NIH diet for 30 days. PB for 4 months	2.96 ± 0.79	14,497 ± 3682

[a] The focal volumes and numbers per liver were obtained by quantitative stereology of three serial sections of liver tissue, stained consecutively for canalicular ATPase, γ-glutamyltranspeptidase, and glucose-6-phosphatase according to the method of Campbell et al. (1986). These data represent total foci comprising all possible combinations of phenotypes.

[b] 0.05% phenobarbital in laboratory chow.

during hepatocarcinogenesis is a linear, dose-related phenomenon that does not exhibit a readily measurable threshold (Scherer and Emmelot 1975; Laib et al. 1985). Furthermore, as discussed below, the relative effect of initiating agents can be established from the stereologic quantitation of EAF following a defined period of promotion (Table 3). Important in all of these considerations of initiation is the presence of EAF (the progeny of initiated cells) in livers of animals not treated with exogenous initiating agents (Schulte-Hermann et al. 1983; Popp et al. 1985). Such foci have similar, if not identical, biochemical characteristics to those induced by specific exogenous initiating agents.

The stage of tumor promotion is characterized by its reversibility during hepato-carcinogenesis. In essentially all model systems of multistage hepatocarcinogenesis, this phenomenon has been characteristic of the stage of promotion (Takahashi et al. 1982; Moore et al. 1983; Tatematsu et al. 1983; Glauert et al. 1986). As one might expect from this characteristic, the dose-response relationship exhibits a measurable threshold or no-effect level for the action of the promoting agent on the initiated cell population (Goldsworthy and Pitot 1985a). Furthermore, the action of PB demon-strates a maximal effect in promoting a finite number of cells initiated by a finite dose of initiating agent (Goldsworthy and Pitot 1985a). The relative effectiveness of promoting agents depends on the time required for a specific dose of promoting agent to reach this maximal effect (Table 3).

The stage of progression during hepatocarcinogenesis is one which as yet has not been clearly defined. However, based on the action of promoting agents and analogous to the studies of multistage carcinogenesis in other tissues, this stage during multistage hepatocarcinogenesis is irreversible and is the stage at which irreversible benign and/or malignant neoplasms are characteristically seen (Schulte-Hermann 1985). Progression has been defined (Pitot 1986) as that stage of

Table 3
Initiating and Promoting Potencies of Several Agents as Hepatocarcinogens in the Rat

	Initiating index[a]	Promoting index[b]
Diethylnitrosamine	6.6	0.7[c]
Dimethylbenzanthracene	6.6	—
L-Ethionine	2.5	—
Phenobarbital	0.0	324
Tetrachlorodibenzo-p-dioxin (TCDD)	0.0	8.7×10^6
WY-14,643[d]	—	29
1-Hydroxysafrole[e]	2.5	680

[a] Log (foci/liver/mmole).
[b] $V_f V_c$/mmole/wk. See text for further explanation.
[c] Calculated from Kunz et al. (1983).
[d] In female Fischer 344 rats. All others in Sprague-Dawley female rats.
[e] Calculated from data of Boberg (1986).

carcinogenesis exhibiting measurable (by recombinant DNA techniques) and/or morphologically discernible (karyotypic) changes in the activity or structure of the cell genome. Environmental alterations during the stage of progression may produce effects on the growth rate of the cells during this stage, but only during the early or "responsive" phase. Agents that act only during the early stage of hepatocarcinogenesis or those that advance a cell from the promotion stage to the progression stage have not yet been definitively characterized. Theoretically, it should be those agents which are capable of inducing the genetic changes required for the entrance of a cell into the progression stage. Examples of such agents are clastogenic agents and complete carcinogens, i.e., agents capable of inducing the entire process of hepatocarcinogenesis to and including malignant neoplasia.

Although multistage carcinogenesis in other tissues, especially skin (Pitot 1980), closely resembles that in liver, the stages of hepatocarcinogenesis form a reasonable working format in which logical quantitative experiments can be carried out to characterize further the individual stages. Furthermore, the mechanism of action of agents that act at one or more of these stages during multistage hepatocarcinogenesis may more readily be approached.

SEQUENTIAL ORDER OF STAGES IN HEPATOCARCINOGENESIS

As yet there have been relatively few studies that examine the importance of the sequence of initiation, promotion, and progression during hepatocarcinogenesis. Most studies that have been reported are concerned with the simultaneous administration of the initiating agent and promoting agent. For example, Schwarz et al. (1983) demonstrated that the simultaneous administration of PB and DEN resulted in a marked lowering of the tumor incidence as compared with sequential administration of DEN followed by PB. Since most known promoting agents during hepatocarcinogenesis also act to increase specific xenobiotic metabolic reactions, one obvious mechanism for this effect is the increased metabolism of the initiating agent to noninitiating metabolites. Specific examples of reversal of the initation-promotion sequence have shown the same depression of tumor induction (Williams and Furuya 1984).

On the other hand, hepatocarcinogenesis is also observed even with the omission of the stage of initiation specifically induced by exogenous agents, but with only the chronic administration of promoting agents. The hepatic promoting agents PB (Ross et al. 1977), dioxin (TCDD) (Kociba et al. 1978), and peroxisomal proliferating compounds (Reddy et al. 1983) have all been shown to induce hepatocellular carcinomas on long-term, chronic feeding but do not exhibit appreciable initiating action as judged from in vivo studies (Pitot et al. 1978, 1980; Glauert et al. 1986) or in vitro studies (McCann et al. 1975; Wassom et al. 1977/1978; Reddy et al. 1983).

Incomplete carcinogenesis, i.e., initiation only, does not result in malignant neoplasms following subcarcinogenic doses of DEN (Pitot et al. 1978) or DMBA (Pitot 1978) or in the absence of subsequent exogenous promotion. Thus, evidence to date in model systems of rat hepatocarcinogenesis has shown that the sequence, initiation followed by promotion, is critical to the eventual development of cancer, and omission of either stage results in no yield or a significantly lower yield of hepatocellular tumors than when the normal sequence occurs.

Absence of the stage of progression results in no yield or a low yield of hepatocellular carcinomas during promotion by PB (Glauert et al. 1986) and clofibrate (Greaves et al. 1986). However, by the characteristics of the stage of progression (Table 1), the presence of any carcinomas indicates that some initiated cells have advanced through all three stages. As yet there are few data on agents (progressors) that act specifically to advance the promoted cell into the stage of progression. Most foci and nodules occurring during the stage of promotion disappear, "remodel" (Enomoto and Farber 1982), or die (Bursch et al. 1984) following removal of the exogenous promoting agent. However, in vivo, endogenous promoting agents (hormones) are continuously present as are those found in the diet. The necessity for promotion to immediately precede progression in hepatocarcinogenesis, the molecular effects of progressor agents, and the critical molecular "boundary" between promotion and progression are not yet clearly characterized.

SELECTIVE ACTION OF CARCINOGENIC AGENTS AT SPECIFIC STAGES DURING HEPATOCARCINOGENESIS

Knowledge of multistage carcinogenesis in mouse skin led to the possible classification of chemical carcinogens as initiators (incomplete carcinogens), promoters, and complete carcinogens. Implicit in such distinctions of carcinogenic agents is their action, predominantly or entirely, at one or both of the stages of initiation and promotion. Incomplete carcinogens, which under no condition induce neoplasms, may exist only rarely if at all. However, subcarcinogenic doses of complete carcinogens, i.e., those which initiate but do not promote, have been demonstrated in several instances (see above) and are likely to occur with all complete hepatocarcinogens. The unequivocal distinction of promoting agents from complete carcinogens has probably not been achieved. However, the reversibility of the promotion stage, a threshold for its induction, and a maximum effect following a specific dose of an initiator should allow such a distinction in many instances.

Complete carcinogens, by definition, possess initiating, promoting, and progressing capabilities. In several model systems of hepatocarcinogenesis in the rat it has been possible to estimate the initiation and/or promotion potency of a chemical. Ito et al. (1980) have classified a number of chemicals on the basis of their activity in promoting EAF and nodules following initiation with DEN using the number/cm^2 and area/cm^2 of focal lesions as the endpoint. We have performed a similar study in a system in which initiation can be completely isolated from promotion for each compound examined using a stereologic method for the quantitation of focal lesions identified by at least three different histochemical stains of serial frozen sections (Campbell et al. 1986). With such a system, it has been possible to determine the relative potency of a chemical as an initiator and/or promoting agent. To express such relative potencies, we have established the following parameters:

Initiation Index $= \log$ [no. foci $\cdot$ liver^{-1} $\cdot$ mmole^{-1}]
Promotion Index $= V_f/V_c \cdot$ mmole^{-1} $\cdot$ wk^{-1}

Where V_f is the total volume occupied by EAF in the liver of animals treated with the test agent and V_c is the total volume of EAF in the control animals, which have only been initiated. The initiation index is determined following promotion for at least 6 months to demonstrate the progeny of all initiated cells. The promotion index is usually determined after 6 months of treatment with the promoting agent, but other time intervals could be used as well.

Some representative initiation and promotion indices are listed in Table 3. As shown, the initiation potency, as well as the promoting potency, varies with the dose of the same compound, possibly due to a lesser toxicity at the lower levels where the compounds are more efficient in their action.

It is also interesting that the initiation and promotion potencies of a single compound may be relatively quite different. DEN is a potent initiator but a relatively poor promoting agent. 1-Hydroxysafrole is a poor initiating agent but is much more effective as a promoter. Both of these agents are recognized as complete carcinogens on the basis of their effects in vivo. However, the peroxisomal proliferating agent, Wy-14,643, like TCDD, is not mutagenic or DNA-damaging (Wassom et al. 1977; Reddy et al. 1983) but is carcinogenic. These agents, like PB, are effective promoting agents. Boberg et al. (1987) have shown a similar relationship for the complete carcinogen, 1-hydroxysafrole, but in this case a low level of initiation is very apparent.

As discussed above, TCDD is a very potent promoting agent, perhaps the most potent yet reported, but it lacks measurable initiating action. Conversely, butylated hydroxyanisole is a weak promoting agent in comparison with PB (Goldsworthy and Pitot 1985b). Thus, in multistage hepatocarcinogenesis in the rat, it is possible to identify the stage(s) at which a carcinogenic agent acts and to estimate the relative potency of its effect as an initiator and/or promoting agent. As yet no studies have identified agents acting solely at the stage of progression, although complete carcinogens, by definition, must possess such an action.

CONCLUSIONS

Multistage hepatocarcinogenesis is an established model system in the rat. Although many of its features are analogous to multistage epidermal carcinogenesis in the mouse (Pitot 1980), recent investigations, some of which have been reviewed herein, have shown some disparity in the two systems which may be more apparent than real.

As in hepatocarcinogenesis, the alteration of initiation by chemicals as shown is also found in epidermal carcinogenesis (Berry et al. 1979). Identification of very early lesions resulting from initiation is possible in hepatocarcinogenesis but is rarely, if ever, found in the earliest stages of chemical carcinogenesis in mouse skin. However, the reversibility of EAF in all known model systems of multistage hepatocarcinogenesis is analogous to the reversibility of papillomas during the promotion stage of epidermal carcinogenesis (Boutwell 1964; Slaga 1983). Not clearly shown in the latter system is the retention of the potential of papilloma production as shown by the reapplication of the promoting agent after disappearance of the lesions. In multistage hepatocarcinogenesis, such a potential for EAF is quantitatively retained. Finally, the stage of progression as proposed in this model of hepatocarcinogenesis may be analogous to effects seen during epidermal carcinogenesis from the use of a second initiation step following the standard initiation and promotion protocol (Hennings et al. 1985). Chronic application of promoters in multistage epidermal and hepatocarcinogenesis may result in advancement of an occasional clone to irreversible malignancy, i.e., the stage of progression. However, the administration of a second complete carcinogen following (Scherer et al. 1984; Hennings et al. 1985), or even during, an initiation/ promotion regimen (Solt et al. 1977), markedly enhances the establishment of the stage of progression in both of these model systems. Therefore, it is possible that multistage hepatocarcinogenesis as described herein and the stages of initiation, promotion, and progression, as well as their characteristics (Table 1), may have analogies in other systems of multistage carcinogenesis.

ACKNOWLEDGMENTS

The studies described in this paper were supported in part by grants from the National Cancer Institute (CA-07175 and CA-22484) and by a contract from the National Toxicology Program (NO1-ES-3-5024). Dr. Hendrich is a postdoctoral trainee of the National Cancer Institute in nutritional oncology (CA-09451). Dr. Beer is a postdoctoral trainee of the National Cancer Institute in chemical carcinogenesis (CA-07652).

REFERENCES

Barrett, J.C. 1980. A preneoplastic stage in the spontaneous neoplastic transformation of Syrian hamster embryo cells in culture. *Cancer Res.* **40:** 91.

Berry, D.L., T.J. Slaga, J. DiGiovanni, and M.R. Juchau. 1979. Studies with chlorinated dibenzo-p-dioxins, polybrominated biphenyls, and polychlorinated biphenyls in a two-stage system of mouse skin tumorigenesis: Potent anticarcinogenic effects. *N.Y. Acad. Sci.* **320:** 405.

Boberg, E.W. 1986. "Studies on the Metabolic Activation and Deactivation and Hepato-carcinogenicity of 1,-Hydroxysafrole and 3,-Hydroxysafrole." Ph.D. thesis, University of Wisconsin, Madison.

Boberg, E.W., A. Liem, E.C. Miller, and J.A. Miller. 1987. Inhibition by penta-chlorophenol of the initiating and promoting activities of 1'-hydroxysafrole for the formation of enzyme-altered foci and tumors in rat liver. *Carcinogenesis* (in press).

Boutwell, R.K. 1964. Some biological aspects of skin carcinogenesis. *Prog. Exp. Tumor Res.* **4:** 207.

Bursch, W., B. Lauer, I. Timmerman-Trosiener, G. Barthol, J. Schuppler, and R. Schulte-Hermann. 1984. Controlled death (apoptosis) of normal and putative preneoplastic cells in rat liver following withdrawal of tumor promoters. *Carcinogenesis* **5:** 453.

Campbell, H.A., Y.-D. Xu, M.H. Hanigan and H.C. Pitot. 1986. Application of quantitative sterology to the evaluation of phenotypically heterogeneous enzyme-altered foci in the rat liver. *J. Natl. Cancer Inst.* **76:** 751.

Denda, A., P.M. Rao, S. Rajalakshmi, and D.S.R. Sarma. 1986. 5-Acacytidine potentiates initiation induced by carcinogens in rat liver. *Carcinogenesis* **6:** 145.

Enomoto, K. and E. Farber. 1982. Kinetics of phenotypic maturation of remodeling of hyperplastic nodules during liver carcinogenesis. *Cancer Res.* **42:** 2330.

Glauert, H.P., M. Schwarz, and H.C. Pitot. 1986. The phenotypic stability of altered hepatic foci: Effect of the short-term withdrawal of phenobarbital and of the long-term feeding of purified diets after the withdrawal of phenobarbital. *Carcinogenesis* **7:** 117.

Goldsworthy, T.L. and H.C. Pitot. 1985a. The quantitative analysis and stability of histochemical markers of altered hepatic foci in rat liver following initiation by diethylnitrosamine administration and promotion with phenobarbital. *Carcinogenesis* **6:** 1261.

———. 1985b. An approach to the development of a short-term whole-animal bioassay to distinguish initiating agents (incomplete carcinogens), promoting agents, complete carcinogens, and noncarcinogens in rat liver. *J. Toxicol. Environ. Health* **16:** 389.

Greaves, P., E. Irisarri, and A.M. Monro. 1986. Hepatic foci of cellular and enzymatic alteration and nodules in rats treated with clofibrate or diethylnitrosamine followed by phenobarbital: Their rate of onset and their reversibility. *J. Natl. Cancer Inst.* **76:** 475.

Hanigan, M. and H.C. Pitot. 1985. Growth of carcinogen-altered rat hepatocytes in the liver of syngeneic recipients promoted with phenobarbital. *Cancer Res.* **45:** 6063.

Hennings, H., R. Shores, P. Mitchell, E.F. Spangler, and S.H. Yuspa. 1985. Induction of papillomas with a high probability of conversion to malignancy. *Carcinogenesis* **6:** 1607.

Ito, N., M. Tatematsu, K. Nakanishi, R. Hasegawa, T. Takano, K. Imaida, and T. Ogiso. 1980. The effects of various chemicals on the development of hyperplastic liver nodules in hepatectomized rats treated with N-nitrosodiethylamine or N-2-fluorenyl-acetamide. *Gann* **71:** 832.

Kociba, R.J., D.G. Keyes, J.E. Beyer, R.M. Carreon, C.E. Wade, D.A. Dittenber, R.P. Kalnins, L.E. Frauson, C.N. Park, S.D. Barnard, R.A. Hummel, and C.G.

Humiston. 1978. Results of a two-year chronic toxicity and oncogenicity study of 2,3,7,8-tetrachlorodibenzo-p-dioxin in rats. *Toxicol. Appl. Pharmacol.* **46:** 279.

Kunz, H.W., H.A. Tennekes, R.E. Port, M. Schwartz, D. Lorke, and G. Schaude. 1983. Quantitative aspects of chemical carcinogenesis and tumor promotion in liver. *Environ. Health Perspect.* **50:** 113.

Laib, R.J., T. Pellio, U.M. Wunschel, N. Zimmerman, and H.M. Bolt. 1985. The rat liver foci bioassay: II. Investigations on the dose-dependent induction of ATPase-deficient foci by vinyl chloride at very low doses. *Carcinogenesis* **6:** 69.

McCann, J., E. Choi, E. Yamasaki, and B.N. Ames. 1975. Detection of carcinogens as mutagens in the Salmonella/microsome test: Assay of 300 chemicals. *Proc. Natl. Acad. Sci. U.S.A.* **72:** 5135.

Mondal, S., D.W. Brankow, and C. Heidelberger. 1976. Two-stage chemical oncogenesis in cultures of C3H/10T1/2 cells. *Cancer Res.* **36:** 2254.

Moore, M.A., H-J. Hacker, and P. Bannasch. 1983. Phenotypic instability in focal and nodular lesions induced in a short term system and in the rat liver. *Carcinogenesis* **4:** 595.

Peraino, C., R.J.M. Fry, and E. Staffeldt. 1977. Effects of varying the onset and duration of exposure to phenobarbital on its enhancement of 2-acetylaminofluorene-induced hepatic tumorigenesis. *Cancer Res.* **37:** 3623.

Pitot, H.C. 1978. Drugs as promoters of carcinogenesis. In *The induction of drug metabolism,* Symposium Ashford Castle, Ireland, May 24–27, 1978 (ed. R.W. Estabrook and E. Lindenlaub), p. 471. F.K. Schattauer Verlag, Stuttgart and New York.

Pitot, H.C., L. Barsness, T. Goldsworthy, and T. Kitagawa. 1978. Biochemical characterisation of stages of hepatocarcinogenesis after a single dose of diethylnitrosamine. *Nature* **271:** 456.

Pitot, H.C. 1980. Characteristics of stages of hepatocarcinogenesis. In *Carcinogenesis: Fundamental mechanisms and environmental effects* (ed. B. Pullman et al.), p. 219. D. Reidel, Boston, Massachusetts.

Pitot, H.C. and A.E. Sirica. 1980. The stages of initiation and promotion in hepatocarcinogenesis. *Biochim. Biophys. Acta* **605:** 191.

Pitot, H.C., T. Goldsworthy, H.A. Campbell, and A. Poland. 1980. Quantitative evaluation of the promotion by 2,3,7,8-tetrachlorodibenzo-p-dioxin of hepatocarcinogenesis from diethylnitrosamine. *Cancer Res.* **40:** 3616.

Pitot, H.C. 1986. *Fundamentals of oncology.* Marcel Dekker, New York.

Popp, J.A., B.H. Scortichini, and L.K. Garvey. 1985. Quantitative evaluation of hepatic foci of cellular alteration occurring spontaneously in Fischer-344 rats. *Fundam. Appl. Toxicol.* **5:** 314.

Reddy, J.K., D.G. Scarpelli, V. Subbarao, and N.D. Lalwani. 1983. Chemical carcinogens without mutagenic activity: Peroxisome proliferators as a prototype. *Toxicol. Pathol.* **11:** 0192.

Rossi, L., M. Ravera, G. Repetti, and L. Santi. 1977. Long-term administration of DDT or phenobarbital-Na in Wistar rats. *Int. J. Cancer* **19:** 179.

Scherer, E. and P. Emmelot. 1975. Kinetics of induction and growth of precancerous liver-cell foci, and liver tumour formation by diethylnitrosamine in the rat. *Eur. J. Cancer* **11:** 689.

Scherer, E., A.W. Feringa, and P. Emmelot. 1984. Initiation-promotion-initiation. Induction of neoplastic foci within islands of precancerous liver cells in the rat. *Models, Mech. Etiol. Tumor Prom.* **56:** 57.

Schulte-Hermann, R., I. Timmermann-Trosiener, and J. Schuppler. 1983. Promotion of spontaneous preneoplastic cells in rat liver as a possible explanation of tumor production by nonmutagenic compounds. *Cancer Res.* **43:** 839.

Schulte-Hermann, R. 1985. Tumor promotion in the liver. *Arch. Toxicol.* **57:** 147.

Schwarz, M., P. Bannasch, and W. Kunz. 1983. The effect of pre- and post-treatment with phenobarbital on the extent of γ-glutamyltranspeptidase positive foci induced in rat liver by N-nitrosomorpholine. *Cancer Lett.* **21:** 17.

Scribner, J.D. and R. Süss. 1978. Tumor initiation and promotion. *Int. Rev. Exp. Pathol.* **18:** 137.

Slaga, T.J. 1983. Overview of tumor promotion in animals. *Environ. Health Perspect.* **50:** 3.

Solt, D.B., A. Medline, and E. Farber. 1977. Rapid emergence of carcinogen-induced hyperplastic lesions in a new model for the sequential analysis of liver carcinogenesis. *Am. J. Pathol.* **88:** 595.

Takahashi, S., B. Lombardi, and H. Shinozuka. 1982. Progression of carcinogen-induced foci of γ-glutamyltranspeptidase-positive hepatocytes to hepatomas in rats fed a choline-deficient diet. *Int. J. Cancer* **29:** 445.

Takahashi, S., D. Nakae, Y. Yokose, Y. Emi, A. Denda, S. Makami, T. Ohnishi, and Y. Konishi. 1984. Enhancement of DEN initiation of liver carcinogenesis by inhibitors of NAD$^+$ ADP ribosyltransferase in rats. *Carcinogenesis* **5:** 901.

Tatematsu, M., Y. Nagamine, and E. Farber. 1983. Redifferentiation as a basis for remodeling of carcinogen-induced hepatocyte nodules to normal appearing liver. *Cancer Res.* **43:** 5049.

Wassom, J.S., J.E. Huff, and N. Loprieno. 1977/1978. A review of the genetic toxicology of chlorinated dibenzo-p-dioxins. *Mutat. Res.* **47:** 141.

Williams, G.M. 1984. Modulation of chemical carcinogenesis by xenobiotics. *Fundam. Appl. Toxicol.* **4:** 325.

Williams, G.M. and K. Furuya. 1984. Distinction between liver neoplasm promoting and syncarcinogenic effects demonstrated by exposure to phenobarbital or diethylnitrosamine either before or after N-2-fluorenylacetamide. *Carcinogenesis* **5:** 171.

Yuspa, S.H., H. Hennings, and U. Lichte. 1981. Initiator and promoter induced specific changes in epidermal function and biological potential. *J. Supramol. Struct. Cell. Biochem.* **17:** 245.

COMMENTS

TENNANT: In the case of phenobarbital, there is at least reasonable evidence of mutagenicity in *Salmonella*. Clearly, what is important is that the effects of phenobarbital are reversible in the whole animal; so, either by virtue of its pharmacokinetics or whatever, it is not inducing irreversible effects, at least measurable in the whole animal. Would you care to try to distinguish this important property? Is it possible to have substances for which there is at least evidence of mutagenicity or genotoxicity but which do not appear to play a major role in the effect of the chemical in vivo?

PITOT: With this system, it is possible to quantitate the initiation and promotion potencies of a single compound. For example, carcinogens such as the peroxisome proliferating agents have low initiating activity in this system, but they are good promoting agents. Another compound, hydroxysafrole, which forms a covalent adduct with DNA, is a relatively poor initiating agent but is a very effective promoting agent. Thus, for chemicals that exhibit carcinogenic effects in this system, the initiating and promoting potential for any single compound may be determined. Phenobarbital shows no initiating capabilities in this system. Earlier studies from Ames' laboratory showed no mutagenic action of phenobarbital in *Salmonella*. It has some clastogenic activity in *Saccharomyces*. I think you are quite right that as long as an agent shows a biological effect in the whole animal, such results, which are at apparent variances with short-term tests, are biologically more relevant.

WILLIAMS: I think there is additional evidence that phenobarbital is not producing genetic alteration under these conditions. Both Bannasch's group and ours have done the reverse sequence experiments in which phenobarbital is given before the initiating agent. Under those conditions, unlike when two genotoxic carcinogens are given in sequence, there is no summation at all when phenobarbital is given first, in contrast to what might have happened had it any significant DNA reactivity. The fact that phenobarbital, after an interval of cessation, then recalls foci that have essentially the same phenotype as they did when first enhanced by phenobarbital also suggests that the phenobarbital isn't producing any new genetic change resulting in a different spectrum of phenotypes. Do you agree with that?

PITOT: Sure.

TRUMP: But the peroxisome proliferators are carcinogenic alone. They are complete carcinogens.

PITOT: Phenobarbital fed for 2 years to rats resulted in a low percentage of hepatocellular carcinoma.

TRUMP: Okay, but it is not nearly as potent.

PITOT: On a molar basis, phenobarbital is a more potent promoting agent than some of the peroxisome proliferators.

TRUMP: They are much more potent, are they not?

PITOT: No, those that we have studied are not more potent than phenobarbital as promoting agents. Some may be a little better than phenobarbital, but more studies are necessary to prove this. Dioxin is by far the most potent promoting agent in this system by several orders of magnitude.

SWENBERG: It depends on which peroxisomal agent you are talking about.

PITOT: That's true.

SWENBERG: DEHP is very weak, but Wy-14,643 is very potent, causing a 100% incidence of liver tumors.

SIVAK: In your on/off/on experiment, my recollection is that, almost without exception, the numbers of foci later were more than the numbers earlier.

PITOT: Statistically, there is not a significant difference.

SIVAK: You get a trend. For every set it was larger, and it makes one a little suspicious that something is going on.

PITOT: It may be that we didn't wait long enough for complete expression of the initiated foci in the first part of the experiment. We didn't have an adequate control for that. An adequate control would have allowed us to go out to 5 months instead of 4 months with the phenobarbital alone.

YAMASAKI: I wonder whether you can really say there is a threshold, because if you do it with logarithmic scale, you need 10 or 100 times more animals to show any effect. I don't know how you are really measuring threshold. Also, biologically and theoretically, why do you think there is a threshold in promotion?

PITOT: If promotion is reversible, there must be a threshold.

YAMASAKI: I think that is different because you are talking about frequency threshold and not dose threshold.

PITOT: As with any reversible process below some concentration (threshold) of the inciting agent, the process, e.g., tumor promotion, will not take place. But with an irreversible process, there is no way that one can prove or disprove the presence of a threshold by statistical methods, although an apparent threshold has been described for many agents.

SARMA: Phenobarbital, when given for a long time, actually inhibits liver cell proliferation rather than inducing cell proliferation.

PITOT: Initially, however, phenobarbital does increase hepatocyte proliferation.

SARMA: My second point concerns your on/off experiments. We did a similar experiment using other liver tumor promoters and essentially we saw the same picture. But we had a problem. In some models of liver carcinogenesis, when the promoter is off, there is remodeling or regression. Under these conditions, one nodule can look like three or four little foci. When the promoter is back, there can be three or four nodules, even though they originally came from one nodule. This complicates quantitation. Did you see something like this in your experiments?

PITOT: We have seen remodeling, but only in the Solt-Farber model. In the model we have used, one does not get a significant amount of remodeling. It is seen occasionally. However, 30 days after withdrawal from phenobarbital, there is no remodeling whatsoever.

SWENBERG: The selection pressure in the Solt-Farber model is so much greater than in a phenobarbital system that I don't know whether they are really comparable.

ROE: You indicated that the process which you termed promotion took an initiated cell through to the stage of being a tumor. You said that promotion is reversible. Does that mean that the tumor is reversible?

PITOT: By tumor, do you mean neoplasm?

ROE: That's a whole new ball park. Another question concerns species. You are using a rat model and not a mouse model. Is what you say also true for the mouse and is it true both for the high spontaneous liver tumor mouse and for the low spontaneous tumor mouse? Where does the high spontaneous liver tumor incidence mouse fit into this system?

PITOT: Your question poses an interesting problem, but some recent data from one of my colleagues, Norman Drinkwater, indicate that the mouse has a very high level of endogenous promotion. The nature of this promoting action is not clear, although endogenous hormones likely play a role. Thus, one could argue that because of this, although there are a few spontaneously initiated foci in both species, in the mouse, because of a high endogenous promoting capability, more spontaneous tumors are seen than in the rat. We are hopeful, therefore, of finding oncogene alterations in the rat, as have been reported in some adenomas and in almost all hepatic carcinomas in the mouse. It may be that in the rat the reason such alterations have not been generally seen is related to the less effective endogenous promotion. Furthermore, in the mouse, foci and early nodular lesions in the liver are generally not reversible. This, too, may be related to the more effective endogenous promoting environment of the mouse. These are largely theoretical concepts, but they do tend to reconcile the apparent differences between hepatocarcinogenesis in the two species.

Bladder Tumor Promotion

SAMUEL M. COHEN, LEON B. ELLWEIN, AND SONNY L. JOHANSSON
Department of Pathology and Microbiology and the
Eppley Institute for Research on Cancer and Allied Diseases
University of Nebraska Medical Center
Omaha, Nebraska 68105

OVERVIEW

Models of experimental urinary bladder carcinogenesis have been developed similar to the initation-promotion model originally described in mouse skin. Initiation has usually been induced by administration of short courses of known urinary bladder carcinogens. Numerous promoting substances have been identified and have been subdivided into three classes of compounds. The first class represents the sodium salts of moderate to weak acids and includes such substances as sodium saccharin, sodium ascorbate, and sodium o-phenylphenate. The second class represents chemicals that result in urinary calculi and includes such substances as biphenyl and uracil. The third class represents other substances and includes antioxidants, such as butylated hydroxyanisole, and amino acids, such as isoleucine and leucine. Bladder tumor promoters are generally nonmutagenic in most in vitro assays, do not interact covalently with DNA, and induce increased cell proliferation of the bladder epithelium. They usually require administration at very high levels in the diet for long periods of time. Urinary ions, such as sodium, potassium, calcium, and pH, appear to be critical in the expression of biological activity of several of these compounds, particularly those of the first class of promoters. In addition, urine appears to contain a growth factor or factors active as urothelial mitogens which by themselves enhance urinary bladder carcinogenesis. A mathematical model of the carcinogenic process which emphasizes the importance of cell proliferation in the carcinogenic process is presented.

INTRODUCTION

Urinary bladder carcinogenesis has been associated with chemicals since the original description in 1895, by Rehn, of an increased incidence of human bladder cancer in the aniline dye industry in Germany (Cohen 1985). Several aromatic amines have been identified as human bladder carcinogens since that time, including 2-naphthylamine, benzidine, and 4-aminobiphenyl. Although the specific chemical in cigarette smoke which is related to bladder cancer is not known, cigarette smoking is the major etiologic factor in human bladder cancer in the western hemisphere. Several chemically induced models have been developed in dogs and rodents to understand the carcinogenic process better. The most commonly used carcinogens include N-butyl-N-(4-hydroxybutyl)nitrosamine (BBN), adminis-

Banbury Report 25: Nongenotoxic Mechanisms in Carcinogenesis
© Cold Spring Harbor Laboratory. 0-87969-225-1/87. $1.00 + .00

tered in the drinking water, N-[4-(5-nitro-2-furyl)-2-thiazolyl]formamide (FANFT), administered in the diet, and N-methyl-N-nitrosourea (MNU), administered directly into the bladder. These chemicals behave as classical carcinogens. If administered at sufficient dose and period of time, they induce essentially an 100% incidence of bladder cancer in mice or rats, they are metabolically activated to reactive electrophiles, and they bind covalently to DNA (Cohen 1985). If they are administered for short periods of time at relatively low doses, a low incidence of tumors is observed. However, if two or more of these chemicals are administered at these low doses, a significantly increased incidence of tumors results, indicating a synergistic effect. In addition, if these chemicals are administered at low doses sequentially, a similar increase in bladder tumor incidence is observed. However, these studies involve the application of multiple agents that are known complete carcinogens.

More recently, multiagent models have been developed in the rat urinary bladder which are similar to the two-stage model of carcinogenesis originally described in the mouse skin and referred to as the initiation-promotion model of carcinogenesis (Cohen 1985). A suggestion that this model was applicable to the urinary bladder came from studies utilizing the mouse pellet-implantation technique in which the chemical was administered systematically and a pellet was inserted into the bladder. However, it was not until the mid-1970s that a more typical sequence of events was demonstrated by Hicks and her colleagues (Hicks et al. 1973). In her experiments she utilized initiation by intravesical installation of MNU followed by the oral administration of sodium saccharin or sodium cyclamate as promoting substances. Subsequent experiments with the BBN, FANFT, and MNU models have confimed that observation and indicate close similarity between the rat bladder model and the mouse skin model (Cohen 1985). Initiation is irreversible, and promotion requires extended time of administration.

Urinary Bladder Promoters

Numerous substances have been identified as promoters for the urinary bladder in the rat model, and they typically have properties now commonly associated with promoting substances. They generally induce a low level of increased cell proliferation in the urothelium, they are not metabolically activated to reactive electrophiles, they are generally nonmutagenic in in vitro assays, and they do not react directly with DNA (Ashby 1985; Cohen 1985).

Recently, Fukushima et al. (1986a) have subdivided the various promoting substances into three categories. The first includes the sodium salts of several known moderate to weak acids and includes the substances listed in Table 1. The most extensively studied of these compounds are sodium saccharin (Cohen 1985) and sodium ascorbate (Imaida et al. 1984). In contrast to the carcinogenic effect of the sodium salts of these compounds, the calcium salts and the parent acid forms

Table 1
Urinary Bladder Promoters

1. Sodium salts of moderate to weak acids
   sodium saccharin
   sodium ascorbate
   sodium o-phenylphenate
   sodium bicarbonate
   sodium citrate
   monosodium aspartate
   sodium erythorbate
2. Calculus-inducing chemicals
   biphenyl
   uracil
3. Others
   antioxidants
   butylated hydroxyanisole
   butylated hydroxytoluene
   ethoxyquin
   amino acids
   L-leucine
   L-isoleucine
   tryptophan
   others
   allopurinol
   phenobarbital (?)

generally are without promoting activity (Fukushima et al. 1984, 1985, 1986b; Imaida et al. 1984; Kurata et al. 1985; Shirai et al. 1985; Hasegawa and Cohen 1986). Several of these substances include the sodium salts of common biological chemicals, such as sodium bicarbonate, sodium citrate, and monosodium aspartate. The second category of promoting substances consists of agents that act by inducing the appearance of urinary calculi and includes substances such as biphenyl and uracil (Fukushima et al. 1986b). The third category consists of other substances, such as a variety of antioxidants (Fukushima et al. 1984; Imaida et al. 1984), several amino acids (Cohen et al. 1979; Nishio et al. 1986), and other unrelated substances, including allopurinol (Fukushima et al. 1983) and possibly phenobarbital (Wang et al. 1983). With all of these substances a large dose is required, generally greater than 1% of the diet, and they must be administered for relatively long periods of time for the induction of papillomas or carcinomas.

A feature of most of these substances is that their administration, even without prior initiation, results in an increase in the rate of cell proliferation of the bladder epithelium as well as the appearance of a mild hyperplasia. The urinary bladder is generally a mitotically quiescent tissue with a labeling index, following a 1-hour pulse of [^{3}H]thymidine, in the range of less than 0.1%. The administration of these various promoting substances results in an increase in the labeling index of five- to tenfold. This increase in cell proliferation can be quantified either by determination of the labeling index utilizing autoradiography or by observation with light and scanning electron microscopy. There is generally a dose-response for these agents as mitogens or as promoters (Cohen 1985), and high doses are usually required. Administration of lower doses appears to result in no biological response in the bladder epithelium.

For several of the substances in the first class of tumor promoters, the sodium salt is active, whereas other salts and the acid form are relatively or completely inactive. For example, sodium ascorbate is a strong promoting agent in rats (Imaida et al. 1984), whereas ascorbic acid is not (Fukushima et al. 1984). Similar levels of ascorbate are present in the urine following administration of either form. Similarly, sodium saccharin is a promoting agent in the rat urinary bladder, whereas acid saccharin appears to be without promoting activity (West et al. 1983). Utilizing a short-term screen for induction of mitogenic activity, we have demonstrated that different salts of sodium saccharin have a different biological response despite similar concentrations of saccharin in the urine (Hasegawa and Cohen 1986). Sodium saccharin had the greatest activity (Table 2), potassium saccharin was significantly less active than the sodium salt but was significantly more active than the control, and calcium saccharin and acid saccharin resulted in labeling indices not significantly different from that of the control. The urinary concentrations of the saccharin ion following the administration of each of these agents were similar, but there was a dramatic difference in the level of several ions in the urine following the administration of these different salts. Following administration of sodium saccharin and potassium saccharin, there was also a greatly increased urinary volume secondary to an increased consumption of water. The sodium or potassium concentration is relatively high following administration of sodium saccharin or potassium saccharin, respectively, whereas the calcium concentration is approximately at control levels following the administration of these salts. The urinary pH is similar to, or slightly above, the control level with these two salts. In contrast, following the administration

Table 2
Effect of Different Salts of Saccharin on the Mitogenic Response of the Rat Urothelium

Form of saccharin[a]	Labeling index (%)	Urinary saccharin concentration[b] (mmoles/ml)	pH	Urinary concentration[b]	
				Na$^+$ (mEq/l)	Ca^{++} (mg/dl)
Sodium saccharin	0.55 ± 0.20[c]	0.17 ± 0.04	7.2	291 ± 19[d]	24.8 ± 9.6
Potassium saccharin	0.18 ± 0.09[d,e]	0.14 ± 0.04	6.8	153 ± 39	23.9 ± 1.8
Calcium saccharin	0.12 ± 0.11	0.14 ± 0.03	5.7	158 ± 24	41.2 ± 0.5[d]
Acid saccharin	0.07 ± 0.04	0.19 ± 0.02	5.5	139 ± 45	51.6 ± 6.7[d]
Control	0.06 ± 0.04	0	7.1	158 ± 14	34.5 ± 5.8

[a] All forms were administered as 5% of the diet for 10 weeks.
[b] Measured after 4 weeks of administration.
[c] $p < 0.01$ compared to control by Student's t test.
[d] $p < 0.05$ compared to control by Student's t test.
[e] $p < 0.05$ compared to sodium saccharin by Student's t test.

of either calcium saccharin or acid saccharin, urinary calcium is greatly elevated compared to control levels, and urinary pH is significantly less with either of these two chemicals in the diet. It is unclear at this time what role these different urinary ions have in the promoting capacity of these substances. However, it should be noted that in all instances where the sodium salt is active and the acid form is inactive, the urinary level of sodium is elevated in rats fed the sodium salts, the urinary pH is at control or elevated levels, and the urinary calcium is at control levels. In contrast, the acid form results in a normal to elevated calcium and a lower pH.

Not any one of these factors by themselves appears to explain the promoting activity of these substances adequately. The concentration of the administered promoting anion is similar in the promoting and nonpromoting situation. For example, the level of ascorbate or saccharin is similar following the administration of either the sodium salt or the acid form. Utilizing nuclear magnetic resonance (NMR), extensive analysis of saccharin and the interaction of a variety of ions on the ionic structure of the molecule indicate that there is no change in the chemical form of saccharin under a variety of conditions (D.S. Williamson et al., unpubl.). However, an elevated sodium concentration in the urine by itself also does not have promoting activity. For example, sodium hippurate is similar to sodium saccharin and sodium ascorbate with respect to urinary excretion of sodium concentration and administered anion, but, in contrast to sodium ascorbate and sodium saccharin, the urinary pH following sodium hippurate administration is significantly lower. Also, administration of high concentrations of sodium chloride in the diet is without promoting activity (Fukushima et al. 1986b). Interestingly, supporting evidence for the requirement of an elevated urinary pH is the promoting activity of sodium bicarbonate itself (Shirai et al. 1985). Increased urinary volume by itself also does not have mitogenic activity. Administration of furosemide results in an enormous increase in urinary volume but does not result in an increased labeling index of the bladder epithelium, at least following up to 10 weeks of administration (R. Hasegawa and S.M. Cohen, unpubl.).

It appears that several urinary ions and other factors are critical to the promoting activity of the sodium salts of these substances and that all must be at a critical level or biological activity will be greatly diminished or lost. Since the urinary concentration of these different ions can be greatly influenced by the feeding of different laboratory diets, one would suspect that these different diets could result in markedly different biological responses to these different promoting substances. Preliminary evidence with short-term mitogenic assays supports this conclusion, but long-term promotion studies are not yet available to evaluate this hypothesis.

Role of Urine

In addition to acting as a carrier of carcinogens and having marked variations of several ions, the urine appears to play a direct mitogenic role in bladder carcinogenesis. Oyasu and his collegues (Babaya et al. 1983) have demonstrated that normal rat urine contains substances that have enhancing activity in a heterotopic bladder model he has developed. These substances appear to have growth-factor-like activity but are not epidermal growth factor or other known growth factors in the urine. It is completely unknown what the effect of other exogenously administered promoting substances have on the levels or expression of these normal urinary factors. Nevertheless, these growth factors and the different ions in the urine strongly suggest that endogenous and exogenous factors play a role in the carcinogenic process in the bladder.

DISCUSSION

It has become apparent that the carcinogenic process is complicated and affected by numerous variables. In an attempt to manage this complexity and provide the basis for theoretical considerations and planning for further experiments, we have developed a mathematical model of the carcinogenic process utilizing the urinary bladder system (Greenfield et al. 1984). This is based on a two-stage process illustrated in Figure 1. Several assumptions are made concerning the carcinogenic process in this model. The process is assumed to occur with two critical events. The first we have termed initiation, and the second we have labeled transformation. It must be emphasized that this second event results in the development of a cell which will become a malignant tumor, not a benign lesion such as a papilloma. It is assumed that each of these two events is irreversible and that the events occur in the stem cell or stem cell equivalent of the tissue. It is also assumed that each of these events can occur only while the cell is in the active process of the cell cycle, not while the cell is at rest (G_0), and that each of these events is probabilistic in nature. Thus, even under normal circumstances there is a probability, although it is very low, that a normal cell will become initiated during cell division and that an initiated cell can become transformed. Since the rates of these two probabilities are exceedingly low, it is highly unlikely during the normal life span of an animal that bladder cancer will develop. Since we are assuming that either of these two events can only occur during cell division, the two critical parameters become the number of cells present and the number of times each of these cells undergoes mitosis. Thus, the likelihood of a normal stem cell becoming initiated is proportional to the number of normal stem cells, the number of times the normal stem cells undergo mitosis, and the probability that these normal stem cells have of becoming initiated each time they undergo mitosis. Similarly, the likelihood of an initiated stem cell becoming transformed is related to the number of initiated stem cells, the number of times the initiated stem cells undergo mitosis, and the probability that during a cell division one of these initiated stem cells will become transformed. Validation of this model was performed utilizing multiple time periods and multiple times of administration of FANFT. FANFT is known to cause a marked hyperplasia (increased cell

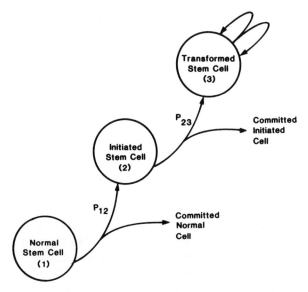

Figure 1

Diagrammatic representation of two-stage carcinogenesis used for mathematical modeling. P_{12} (also referred to as P_I) represents the probability of a cell progressing from state *1* (normal) to state *2* (initiated) during a cell division. P_{23} (also referred to as P_T) represents the probability of a cell progressing from state *2* (initiated) to state *3* (transformed) during a cell division.

number) and increased labeling index, and the model suggests that it potently increases the probability of initiation. However, the probability of transformation did not appear to be affected. Similarly, sodium saccharin induces urothelial hyperplasia and an increase in labeling index, although to a lesser extent than FANFT. In contrast to FANFT, however, in our modeling, sodium saccharin was found not to affect the probability of initiation, essentially what one would expect for a promoting substance, but it also did not have any effect on the transformation probability. Thus, the promoting activity of sodium saccharin can be entirely explained by its hyperplastic and mitogenic properties.

This model places considerable importance on the role of cell number and mitotic rate. For substances such as sodium saccharin, which do not appear to act by direct effect on DNA, these appear to be the critical parameters. This modeling can be applied to substances such as sodium saccharin which, when administered beginning at the time of weaning, did not induce tumors, but which induced a significant incidence of tumors when administered over what has been referred to as two generations (Schoenig et al. 1985). These studies involve the administration of the test agent to the mother during gestation and lactation and then subsequently to the offspring after weaning. If our hypothesis, determined from our modeling, that sodium saccharin acts only by an effect on cell proliferation, is correct, we would predict that sodium saccharin, administered beginning either at the time of birth or at the time of conception, would result in similar incidences of tumors. This is because the in utero fetal bladder is a rapidly proliferating tissue with a labeling index, following a 1-hour pulse of [^{3}H]thymidine, of 10–20% (S.M. Cohen, unpubl.). Thus, it can be assumed that it is dividing as rapidly as possible and that substances such as sodium saccharin will not accelerate this mitotic rate. Recently, a large bioassay was completed which demonstrated that the incidence of bladder tumors was similar whether the administration was begun at the time of birth or at the time of conception (Schoenig et al. 1985).

These results suggest that compounds such as sodium saccharin, which apparently operate by nongenotoxic mechanisms, have their effects in urinary bladder carcinogenesis by enhancing cell proliferation, possibly by nonspecific toxicity to the urothelium and consequent regeneration. We have developed a model that also implies that the carcinogenic process can occur without genotoxicity in a one-generation model. This model involves the ulceration of the bladder epithelium by a variety of mechanisms, followed by the administration of sodium saccharin as a promoting substance. We have utilized ulceration by application of a frozen rod to the serosal surface of the bladder or by intraperitoneal injection of the cyclophosphamide (Cohen et al. 1982). By these means, the bladder epithelium is ulcerated and there is a consequent regenerative hyperplasia which includes nodular and papillary formation but is reversible (Murasaki and Cohen 1983). The bladder epithelium returns to normal within 3–4 weeks of the application of the inciting agent. We have recently demonstrated that the ulceration process with consequent regeneration is the initiating event and that sodium saccharin is behaving only as a promoter (Hasegawa et al. 1985). Thus, the beginning of sodium saccharin administration can occur as long as 18 weeks after the initiating event (Table 3). We have examined the urine during and after the ulcerating procedure and have found that there is no bacterial contamination and no nitrosation, and we can find no evidence for a mutagen being induced as detectable by the Ames assay (Hasegawa et al. 1984). It is unclear what mechanism is involved with initiation by ulceration, but one must keep in mind that the regenerative hyperplasia immediately following ulceration has similar tissue kinetics as seen in the in utero fetal bladder epithelium.

CONCLUSION

Urinary bladder carcinogenesis has been divided into two phases, and numerous substances have been identified that have enhancing activity for bladder carcinogenesis. Several of these substances are normal constituents of the diet. In addition, mitogenic substances present in the normal urine can also enhance

Table 3
Initiation of Bladder Carcinogenesis by Freeze Ulceration

Group	Treatment[a]	Number of rats	Number of rats with bladder carcinoma
1	U→S	36	11(31)[c]
2	U→C(2)[b]→S	36	6(17)
3	U→C(4) →S	40	12(30)
4	U→C(6) →S	36	7(19)
5	U→C(8) →S	39	9(23)
6	S	39	0
7	U→C	39	1(3)
8	C	39	0

[a] U, freeze ulceration; S, sodium saccharin, 5% of the diet; C, control diet

[b] Numbers in parentheses represent weeks of feeding control diet between the time of ulceration and the beginning of sodium saccharin treatment.

[c] Numbers in parentheses represent percentages of effective number of rats in the group with carcinoma.

the carcinogenic process in the bladder. Cell proliferation appears to be critical to the carcinogenic process in the urinary bladder as it is in other tissues. It would appear that a common theme and mechanism for promoting substances is their ability to increase cell proliferation in the target tissue. This can occur by means of a specific receptor on the cell membrane, such as for the phorbol esters, or by nonspecific changes in various intracellular constituents involved in cell proliferation. Some of these factors have been identified and include oncogene products, growth factors or their receptors, intracellular transducing factors, and intracellular ions such as pH, sodium, and calcium.

ACKNOWLEDGMENTS

We gratefully acknowledge the dedicated assistance of several students, fellows, and technologists who have participated in the studies in our laboratory. We also thank Jan Leemkuil and Julie Caniglia for assistance in preparing the manuscript. Studies included in this paper and performed in our laboratory were supported by grants from the State of Nebraska, the National Cancer Institute (CA-32513, CA-28015), and the International Life Sciences Institute-Nutrition Foundation.

REFERENCES

Ashby, J. 1985. The genotoxicity of sodium saccharin and sodium chloride in relation to their cancer-promoting properties. *Food Chem. Toxicol.* **23:** 507.

Babaya, K., K. Izumi, L. Ozono, Y. Miyata, A. Morikawa, J.S. Chmiel, and R. Oyasu. 1983. Capability of urinary components to enhance ornithine decarboxylase activity and promote urothelial tumorigenicity. *Cancer Res.* **43:** 1774.

Cohen, S.M. 1985. Multi-stage carcinogenesis in the urinary bladder. *Food Chem. Toxicol.* **23:** 521.

Cohen, S.M., M. Arai, J.B. Jacobs, and G.H. Friedell. 1979. Promoting effect of saccharin and DL-tryptophan in urinary bladder carcinogenesis. *Cancer Res.* **39:** 1207.

Cohen, S.M., G. Murasaki, S. Fukushima, and R.E. Greenfield. 1982. Effect of regenerative hyperplasia on the urinary bladder: Carcinogenicity of sodium saccharin and N-[4-(5-nitro-2-furyl)-2-thiazolyl]formamide. *Cancer Res.* **42:** 65.

Fukushima, S., A. Hagiwara, T. Ogiso, M. Shibata, and N. Ito. 1983. Promoting effects of various chemicals in rat urinary bladder carcinogenesis initiated by N-nitroso-n-butyl-(4-hydroxybutyl)amine. *Food Chem. Toxicol.* **21:** 59.

Fukushima, S., Y. Kurata, M.-A. Shibata, E. Ikawa, and N. Ito. 1984. Promotion by ascorbic acid, sodium erythorbate and ethoxyquin of neoplastic lesions in rats initiated with N-butyl-N-(4-hydroxybutyl)nitrosamine. *Cancer Lett.* **23:** 29.

Fukushima, S., Y. Kurata, T. Ogiso, M. Okuda, Y. Miyata, and N. Ito. 1985. Pathological analysis of the carcinogenicity of sodium o-phenylphenate and o-phenylphenol. *Oncology* **42:** 304.

Fukushima, S., T. Shirai, and M. Hirose. 1986. Modification of bladder carcinogenesis. *U.S.-Japan Cooperative Cancer Res. Prog.* Nagoya, Japan.

Fukushima, S., W. Thamavit, Y. Kurata, and N. Ito. 1986. Sodium citrate: A promoter of bladder carcinogenesis. *Jpn. J. Cancer Res.* **77:** 1.

Greenfield, R.E., L.B. Ellwein, and S.M. Cohen. 1984. A general probabilistic model of carcinogenesis: Analysis of experimental urinary bladder cancer. *Carcinogenesis* **5:** 437.

Hasegawa, R. and S.M. Cohen. 1986. The effect of different salts of saccharin on the rat urinary bladder. *Cancer Lett.* **30:** 261.

Hasegawa, R., R.E. Greenfield, G. Murasaki, T. Suzuki, and S.M. Cohen. 1985. Initiation of urinary bladder carcinogenesis in rats by freeze ulceration with sodium saccharin promotion. *Cancer Res.* **45:** 1469.

Hasegawa, R., M.K. St.John, M. Cano, P. Issenberg, D.A. Klein, B.A. Walker, J.W. Jones, R.C. Schnell, B.A. Merrick, M.H. Davies, D.T. McMillan, and S.M. Cohen. 1984. Bladder freeze ulceration and sodium saccharin feeding in the rat: Examination for urinary nitrosamines, mutagens and bacteria, and effects on hepatic microsomal enzymes. *Food Chem. Toxicol.* **22:** 935.

Hicks, R.M., J.St.J. Wakefield, and J. Chowaniec. 1973. Co-carcinogenic action of saccharin in the chemical induction of bladder cancer. *Nature* **243:** 347.

Imaida, K., S. Fukushima, T. Shirai, T. Masui, T. Ogiso, and N. Ito. 1984. Promoting activity of butylated hydroxyanisole, butylated hydroxytoluene and sodium L-ascorbate on forestomach and urinary bladder carcinogenesis initiated with methylnitrosourea in F344 male rats. *Gann* **75:** 769.

Kurata, Y., S. Fukushima, T. Ogiso, A. Hatano, and N. Ito. 1985. Promoting effects of the CA^{++} or Na^+ salts of ascorbic acid, aspartic acid and citric acid on BBN bladder carcinogenesis. *44th Ann. Mtg. Japanese Cancer Assoc.*

Murasaki, G. and S.M. Cohen. 1983. Effect of sodium saccharin on urinary bladder epithelial regenerative hyperplasia following freeze ulceration. *Cancer Res.* **43:** 1820.

Nishio, Y., T. Kakizoe, M. Ohtani, S. Sato, T. Sugimura, and S. Fukushima. 1986.

L-isoleucine and L-leucine: Tumor promoters of bladder cancer in rats. *Science* **231:** 843.

Schoenig, G.P., E.I. Goldenthal, R.G. Geil, C.H. Frith, W.R. Richter, and F.W. Carlborg. 1985. Evaluation of the dose response and *in utero* exposure to saccharin in the rat. *Food Chem. Toxicol.* **23:** 475.

Shirai, T., S. Fukushima, M. Shibata, and N. Ito. 1985. The role of Na^+ concentration and urinary pH in promotion of urinary bladder carcinogenesis in rats. *Proc. Am. Assoc. Cancer Res.* **26:** 131.

Wang, C.Y., C.D. Garner, and M. Hirose. 1983. Effect of phenobarbital on the carcinogenesis of N-[4-(5-nitro-2-furyl)-2-thiazolyl]formamide in rats. *Cancer Lett.* **19:** 305.

West, R.W., D.T. Beranek, F.F. Kadlubar, W.G. Sheldon, D.W. Gaylor, R. Cox, J.A. Roszell, and C.C. Irving. 1983. Dose-dependent effects of dietary saccharin on promotion of urinary bladder carcinogenesis and on urothelial DNA adducts after initiation with N-methylnitrosourea. *Adv. Bladder Cancer Res.* **A17:** 87.

COMMENTS

ANDERSON: When you talk about the foci as sites of cell sloughing, what is the evidence that the cells are really lost and the bladder is not just splitting to allow an expansion in its surface area as the volume is expanding and all the rest of the things are happening?

COHEN: If the cells are sloughing, we should be able to find them in the urine; and if you look in the urine, you do see cells there.

ANDERSON: But there are always cells in the urine. Is there a marked increase? Can you actually detect more than you can in a control urine?

COHEN: We are beginning to look quantitatively now.

ANDERSON: We have looked and we could not detect anything.

COHEN: It is very difficult because of the number of cells.

ANDERSON: You said that the lesions you are measuring are nonreversible. How do you do a reversibility study when you are calling them carcinoma? You said they are not reversible.

COHEN: In the first experiment that we did with initiation/promotion, the animals had bladder tumors by the end of 18 months. We kept some of those animals alive for 6 months beyond that point and they still had their tumors.

SLAGA: What kind of mechanism are you thinking about when you use the frozen rod on the bladder? A reversible or irreversible effect? How can you lead to an irreversible event that way?

COHEN: I think there is one of two possibilities: (1) that we are generating something during that process that is causing initiation, or (2) that there is enough cell turnover that, similar to the saccharin two-generation experiment, we are spontaneously generating a few initiated cells.

SLAGA: In the first part, though, are you talking about some chemical change because of the cold?

COHEN: Possibly generating some mutagen or something. We have looked very hard immediately at the time of ulceration and for several hours and days after ulceration for mutagens in the urine, and we can't find any, at least using the Ames assay. We have looked for the possibility of nitrosation occurring to determine if we are generating nitrosamines or nitrosamides. No nitrosation is occurring under those circumstances. We have also looked for bacterial contamination as a source of a compound that might do something bad to the bladder, and there is no bacterial contamination. We have modeled it also, and very much like the two-generation experiment with saccharin, we can generate a few initiated cells just by having a spontaneous rate of approximately 10^{-6} because we have such an enormous amount of cell turnover occurring following ulceration. Essentially, every cell in the bladder undergoes mitosis every day for about 3–5 days after that and then gradually decreases.

SLAGA: Do you think that the skin system with TPA always giving a low level of tumors could be comparable?

COHEN: Yes. One thing I would like to mention is that we did try ulcerating the skin by a couple of different mechanisms and then painting TPA on the ulcers. Initiation on the skin did not occur.

PITOT: Does ulceration of the heterotropic bladder in the absence of urine lead to neoplasm?

COHEN: I don't know if that has been examined.

SWENBERG: What is the evidence that you do in fact have focal hyperplasia at sites devoid of surface epithelium?

COHEN: If you take the scanning EM specimen and turn it sideways, cut it transversely, and look by transmission EM, those foci are anywhere from three to five cell layers thick.

SWENBERG: Have you done labeling experiments? Is it localized there or is it generalized?

COHEN: We have not done the labeling.

SWENBERG: That is necessary, though, isn't it?

COHEN: To prove it, yes.

WILLIAMS: I noticed, that you and others seemed to have a certain amount of reluctance about using the word genotoxic. It is true that in 1983 an IARC report recommended against the use of that word. I think it is fair to say that that advice went largely unheeded. At a recent IARC meeting on short- and long-term tests for carcinogenicity in December 1985, I believe that the overwhelming opinion was that the word genotoxic has its place in the vocabulary. The crucial question, however, is what do we mean by genotoxic. Of course, in the early developments in the distinction between genotoxic and nongenotoxic agents, data from short-term tests played the primary, if not the exclusive, role in distinguishing or helping to distinguish these two classes of agents. I think we have now moved well beyond that level of analysis. That has resulted, in part, from the fact that we now recognize that many of the short-term tests have significant artifacts that yield false-positive results—I believe phenobarbital is an example of one—that really have no relevance to what the chemical is doing in vivo in the target organ under the condition in which it is producing tumors. Another example where this dichotomy became evident was with quercetin, a polyphenolic compound that is highly mutagenic in the Ames *Salmonella* test, but totally devoid of carcinogenicity. So, even now, and I think increasingly in the future, we are going to see more and more application of in vivo methods of assessing genotoxicity or the lack thereof—techniques like the P^{32} postlabeling, and so on, which now begin to provide very important evidence that agents which are nongenotoxic in short-term tests also do not form adducts in the target organ under the conditions in which they are eliciting tumors.

COHEN: Yes, I agree, especially for compounds such as saccharin and bicarbonate, aspartate and citrate, I think that there is more than adequate evidence, at least in the short-term assays, that these are nongenotoxic, at least as defined by those short-term assays, and probably will not be genotoxic, in the sense that they directly affect DNA in the target tissue, as well.

Cell Injury, Ion Regulation, and Tumor Promotion

BENJAMIN F. TRUMP*† AND IRENE K. BEREZESKY*
*Department of Pathology
University of Maryland School of Medicine
Baltimore, Maryland 21201
†Maryland Institute for Emergency Medical Services Systems
Baltimore, Maryland 21201

OVERVIEW

Investigations carried out in our laboratory over the years have concerned the many processes involved in both acute and chronic cell injury, including neoplasia. We have focused on the characterization of the effects of a variety of cell injuries on a number of cell types with the ultimate goals of (1) finding the final common pathways which lead the cell beyond the stage of reversibility to irreversibility and ultimately to cell death and (2) developing interventions that could modify the course of the reaction to injury and/or promote recovery. Our data have shown not only that membrane phenomena play a major role, but also that deregulation of ions, particularly Na^+, H^+, and Ca^{++}, play an important, if not decisive, role in many cellular phenomena, including tumor promotion. The interactions among these membrane phenomena (including those of the plasma membrane, the endoplasmic reticulum [ER], and the mitochondria), ionic balance, and the cytoskeleton are particularly interesting. Therefore, although much more experimentation is needed for clarification, we have recently advanced a hypothesis proposing that (1) ion deregulation does indeed play a key role in all types of cell injury and (2) not only are a wide variety of pathological processes coupled with such mechanisms, but also many diverse disease states, including neoplasia, may have one, or perhaps only a few, common denominators.

INTRODUCTION

This paper analyzes the relationships between cell injury and carcinogenesis, focusing on the role of ion regulation. The regulation of intracellular ions is a fundamental property of living cells. Although considerable deregulation of ion content and volume can be compensated, severe deregulation can lead to a variety of intracellular catastrophies including cell swelling, organelle volume changes, initiation of cell division, and, if continued, the onset of cell death. Moreover, a balance between intra- and extracellular ions can convert a quiescent cell into one that undergoes either cell division or terminal differentiation. It has been shown, for example, that in transplantable neoplasms, as compared with their normal counterparts, there are remarkably consistent increases in sodium and chlorine concentra-

Banbury Report 25: Nongenotoxic Mechanisms in Carcinogenesis
© Cold Spring Harbor Laboratory. 0-87969-225-1/87. $1.00 + .00

tions (Cameron and Smith 1983). Although both sodium and chlorine are elevated in dividing cells, the magnitude is less than that in the tumor cells. Therefore, an understanding of these relationships must enter into any consideration of control of cell proliferation and differentiation; moreover, all of these phenomena are subject to modulation by interventions that control plasma membrane permeability and intracellular buffering of ionized sodium, hydrogen, and calcium. Recently, considerable attention has been directed toward the role of "second" messengers in the cell (Berridge and Irvine 1984). Although excitable cells, such as neurons and muscle, have provided much information concerning the basic physiologic processes involved in this regulation, it has only recently been recognized that these phenomena regulate a variety of diverse biologic phenomena, ranging from fertilization (Epel 1980) to death (Trump et al. 1980b, 1984). How this precisely relates to cell division, tumor promotion, cell death, and carcinogenesis still eludes exact characterization. At the present time, however, there are sufficient clues to permit the development of hypotheses that may lead to critical new experiments (Trump et al. 1980a, 1981; Trump and Berezesky 1984, 1985a,b, 1987).

The term cell injury refers to the events that occur in cells following any perturbation of homeostasis. Such events within and among cells represent the basis of disease and can be understood in terms of morphologic, physiologic, and biochemical analyses (Trump et al. 1980b). It is clear that injuries to cells can be lethal or sublethal and that they can be characterized in great detail. Such characterizations have been the subject of many studies and reviews, with analyses of these characterizations leading to the formulation of ideas concerning mechanisms. It has become evident from such studies that plasma membrane function plays a critical role in the life and death of cells, in the initiation of cell division, and probably in the initiation of terminal differentiation.

Recently, considerations of the phospholipase-mediated hydrolysis of cell membrane products has led to the concept that phosphotidylinositol phosphate products and diacylglycerol (DAG) may play important, and sometimes calcium-dependent, roles related to cell division and cell differentiation (Berridge and Irvine 1984). How all of the above considerations relate to tumor promotion is, in part, the subject of this volume. Tumor promotion, although poorly defined in terms of mechanisms, clearly bears important relationships to cell injury and therefore to ion regulation (Trump and Berezesky 1987). In this paper, we briefly discuss some of our current results and relate these to the work of other investigators and to our current hypothesis.

RESULTS

Calcium and Cell Injury

The fact that calcium phosphate precipitates occur in or near dead and dying cells has long been known to pathologists. Terms such as dystrophic calcification have often been used to characterize these precipitates. More recently, we and others have been investigating the hypothesis that deregulation of ionized calcium in the cytosol $[Ca^{++}]_i$ may have an important role in the causation of cell injury and cell death. Concurrently, investigators who are studying physiologic phenomena have drawn attention to the idea that calcium may also be an important mediator in physiologic phenomena. Why calcium should be such a key mediator remains speculative. It is clear, however, that severe deregulation of $[Ca^{++}]_i$ concentration can play an important role in a series of catastrophic cellular events, ranging from cell division to cell death. Current technology has provided much improved methodology for measuring $[Ca^{++}]_i$ at both the morphologic and biochemical levels. Such methodology includes X-ray microanalysis and the use of fluorescent probes. As researchers have learned more about the subject, the intimate relationship between calcium regulation and that of other ions, including sodium, hydrogen, and potassium, has become evident. Furthermore, the role of intra- and extracellular calcium has become quite evident in the control of differentiation and division. A recent example is the work by Banyard and Tellam (1985), who observed increased $[Ca^{++}]_i$ in tumor cells.

Through the years, experiments in our laboratory using proximal tubular epithelium in vivo and in vitro, Ehrlich ascites tumor cells (EATC) (Trump and Berezesky 1984), and an experimental rat myocardial infarction model (Osornio-Vargas et al. 1981) have shown that early ultrastructural changes correlate well with changes in total ion content. In EATC, studies of lethal cell injury produced by direct plasma membrane damage with mercurials (Laiho et al. 1983) or by inhibition of energy metabolism with anoxia in glucose-free solutions or with electron transport inhibitors and inhibitors of glycolysis show that the earliest changes in total ion content include increases of sodium and decreases of potassium followed, at later intervals, by increases of total calcium (Laiho and Trump 1974, 1975). There is moderately good correlation between total calcium content and cell death regardless of the type of injury. In the EATC system, anoxic experiments in calcium-free media result in significant delay of cell killing, whereas treatment of such cells with calcium ionophores accentuates the killing (Trump and Berezesky 1985b). These early ion shifts are accompanied by ultrastructural changes, including the formation of blebs at the cell surface. Similar-appearing blebs can be produced by modifying tubulin with vinblastine or actin with cytochalasin. Experiments with rat kidney slices made ischemic at 0–4°C show an identical pattern of change, but at this temperature the rates are greatly reduced (Trump et al. 1974). The development of methods for the isolation and culture of purified rat or rabbit proximal tubular epithelial cells now permits the use of fluorescent probes to measure $[Ca^{++}]_i$ and pH_i.

When isolated rabbit kidney tubule fragments or proximal tubular epithelial cells are treated with $HgCl_2$ at concentrations of 25–50 μM, cell killing occurs within 60 minutes, preceded by dramatic formation of blebs at the cell surface (Trump et al.

1985). This is associated with a rapid rise in $[Ca^{++}]_i$, as measured with Quin 2 or Fura 2 (Trump and Smith 1986), which does not occur if extracellular calcium $[Ca^{++}]_e$ is eliminated, indicating that much of the rise occurs because of influx from the extracellular medium. Elimination of Ca^{++} from the medium is also associated with lesser degrees of cell killing and modification of bleb formation as mentioned below. Treatment of rabbit tubular epithelial by anoxia also results in a rapid rise in $[Ca^{++}]_i$ (Smith and Trump 1986), to values approximating 1.5 times normal for 40 minutes, at which time aeration results in a return to baseline levels. During this same period of time, pH_i rises from 6.9 to 7.1 and is similarly reversed by reoxygenation (Smith and Trump 1986). When rabbit proximal tubular cells, plated on coverslips, are treated with potassium cyanide (KCN) to inhibit respiration, the changes that occur with time include blebbing and ultrastructural alterations. These changes are also accompanied by striking reorganizations of the cytoskeleton, as measured by immunofluorescence staining of actin (Trump et al. 1985). The role of influx of $[Ca^{++}]_e$ on killing in energy-depleted cells is also under study. In contrast to EATC and $HgCl_2$-treated kidney cells, variation of medium calcium from less than 0.05 mM to 3.0 mM results in protection (Sato et al. 1982). In fact, the rate of killing is, if anything, greater in the low-$[Ca^{++}]_e$ case. On the other hand, when both respiration and glycolysis are blocked with KCN and iodoacetic acid, a marked delay in cell killing is noted if Ca^{++} is eliminated from the suspending medium. Significant differences in survival occur even at 3 hours, although by 6 hours relatively little difference is seen.

A similar progression of total ion content, as measured by X-ray microanalysis, is seen in ischemic rat myocardium where an early increase in sodium and a decrease in potassium content are followed by an increase in total calcium after the point of no return (Osornio-Vargas et al. 1981). In this case, much of the increased calcium is sequestered in the form of hydroxyapatite within the mitochondria.

Bleb Formation

The formation of blebs at the cell surface has been noted for some years as a common early reaction to injury; moreover, such bleb formation typically occurs at the time of cell division. Characterization of this phenomenon has therefore attracted attention, since it is an early reaction to injury including tumor promoters. These blebs represent protrusions of the cytosol which are surrounded by the plasma membrane at the free surface of epithelial cells in vivo and on all sides of cells maintained in suspension. Their function is presently unknown. Recent data from our laboratory indicate that blebs contain increased concentrations of calcium and may contain redistributed calmodulin. It is clear that drug-induced modulation of microtubules or actin can reproduce many aspects of these blebs, and it is also evident that similar topological changes can occur in the phenomenon that has been termed apoptosis. The formation of blebs seems to be related, at least with some injuries including $HgCl_2$ treatment of renal tubular epithelium, to the influx of calcium from the extracellular space—in the sense that they can be prevented by reduction of calcium in the extracellular suspending medium. Also, similar-appearing blebs are rapidly induced by A23187 in the presence, but not in the absence, of calcium in the suspending medium.

Phospholipase Activation and Its Relation to Cell Injury

The activity of cellular phospholipase plays an important role in physiologic and pathologic phenomena, an example being the role of phospholipase C in the cellular events that are mediated through the phosphotidylinositol (PI) pathway. Furthermore, it is well known that microbial agents that result in cell death sometimes operate through the elaboration of phospholipases. Progress in this area has been relatively slow and somewhat speculative because of difficulties of intracellular localization and measurement of phospholipase activation. At the same time, many lines of evidence indicate that phospholipase activity must be involved in the events that lead to cell death, including effects of inhibitors. Although there may be more than one final common pathway that leads to cell killing, activation of phospholipase seems to be an important, if not major, pathway, since the effects of modifying phospholipids in the plasma membrane and organelle membranes are obvious (Smith et al. 1980). Modification of plasma membrane phospholipid and consequent changes in permeability seem to be a key to several types of cell death that occur in vivo.

Calcium and Cellular Differentiation

Studies by Yuspa (1984) and Hennings et al. (1980) have clearly shown that modulations of $[Ca^{++}]_e$ can significantly affect the rates of cell division and/or terminal differentiation in cultured epidermal cells. Rather similar results have been obtained in bronchial epithelial cultures by Lechner (1984). In brief, the data suggest that in these epithelia, low levels of calcium are associated with cell division, whereas more physiologic levels are associated with terminal differentiation. Although this represents a normal response in the skin, it represents an abnormal response in the bronchial epithelium in that, in vivo, the latter maintains a columnar differentiation in spite of serum calcium concentrations of approximately 1 mM. In the bronchus, Lechner (1984) observed that serum is synergistic with $[Ca^{++}]_e$, and in the skin, Yuspa (1984) observed that carcinogen treatment may alter the response in that carcinogen-treated cells lack the terminal differentiation response. Squamous differentiation in columnar epithelia, such as the mucous cells of the bronchus, is characterized by clonal growth inhibition, irreversible inhibition of DNA synthesis, an increase in extracellular plasminogen activator activity, an increase in calcium ionophore-induced cross-linked envelope formation, and an increased cell area. It has been shown by Masui and colleagues (1986) that transforming growth factor-β (TGF-β) is the most likely serum-derived factor responsible for inducing normal human bronchial epithelial cells to undergo terminal differentiation. It is probably significant that this group observed a differential effect of TGF-β on normal cell lines as opposed to tumor cell lines, and that epinephrine antagonized the induced inhibition of DNA synthesis and squamous differentiation independently of altered cyclic AMP levels. The lack of induced differentiation in carcinoma cells may provide a significant growth advantage. A variety of putative tumor promoters, including TPA and formaldehyde, also include terminal differentiation in normal cell lines as opposed to lung carcinoma cell lines (Willey et al. 1984; Saladino et al. 1985).

The mechanism of calcium-induced differentiation control is at present unknown. As shown in Figure 1, it might represent, in part, changes involving the PI pathway, including DAG and inositoltriphosphate (InsP$_3$) through the Na$^+$/H$^+$ carrier. In any event, the changes probably involve a control point that differs in normal and initiated carcinogen-treated cells. At the present time, there are no data on intracellular ion content, especially [Ca^{++}]$_i$, following such treatments. As mentioned below, it is of parallel interest to note that terminal differentiation in the form of keratinizing squamous metaplasia occurs as one part of the regenerative cycle in hamster tracheal epithelium.

Sodium-Proton Exchange

The phenomenon of Na$^+$/H$^+$ exchange is being extensively characterized in a variety of dividing and nondividing cell systems, having been emphasized by earlier studies on ion movements at the time of fertilization. This amiloride-sensitivepathway is active in a variety of transporting and nontransporting epithelia and is associated with cytoplasmic alkalinization. Recently developed fluorescent probes have significantly facilitated the study of this phenomenon. The method by which such alkalinization mediates cell division or other types of cell changes is not known. It is, however, quite clear that alkalinization of the cytoplasm also predisposes cells to lethal injury following several models of toxic injury (Penttila and Trump 1974). The Na$^+$/H$^+$ carrier appears to be activated by protein kinase C (Nishizuka 1984), which, in turn, is modulated by phorbol esters directly and by several growth factors indirectly through the PI pathway (Castagna et al. 1982; Burns and Rozengurt 1983; Moolenaar et al. 1984a,b, 1986; Rozengurt et al. 1984). Cytoplasmic alkalinization may also have differential effects on initiated cells versus normal cells, promoting cell division in the former and terminal differentiation in the latter.

DISCUSSION

Figure 1 indicates several possibilities of interaction between events that occur in acute cell injury and those that occur in growth regulation, i.e., the relationship between cell injury and carcinogenesis. As mentioned elsewhere in this volume,

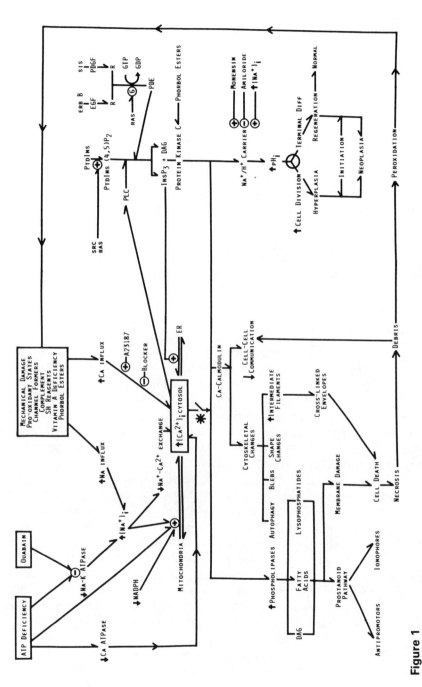

Figure 1

Flowchart illustrating our hypothesis of the many phenomena that occur following ion deregulation, specifically $[Ca^+]_i$, $[Na]_i$, and pH_i and the relationships with cell injury, normal regeneration, and neoplasia. (See text for discussion.)

many complete carcinogens at carcinogenic doses are associated with acute cell injury, often including necrosis and regeneration prior to the development of preneoplastic lesions. Furthermore, rapid developments have been occurring which link oncogene products to intracellular messengers, including $[Ca^{++}]_i$, products of the PI pathway, and Na^+/H^+ exchange, all of which are, in turn, interactive as indicated in the hypothesis. Studies with a series of putative tumor promoters or growth factors in bronchial epithelium have revealed differential effects on division versus terminal differentiation, some of which may be mediated through protein kinase C, in the case of phorbol esters, and then through the Na^+/H^+ carrier. The differential effects are indicated by a switch in the flowchart (Fig. 1); the nature of these effects is currently unknown, but they seem to differ in normal and neoplastic cells. It is our hypothesis that the early stimuli for regeneration, e.g., after renal tubular necrosis of hepatocellular necrosis, relate to sublethal injury in the bordering cells, which may be activated to enter the mitotic cycle via sublethal ion deregulation. Subsequently, these cells respond to differentiation signals, regaining normal internal ion regulation. The apparently critical role of pH_i in this entire scheme is of great recent interest, as alkalinization can, in several cell systems, reproduce many of the effects of growth factors.

SUMMARY

Our hypothesis correlating ion regulation with the many cell effects and responses related to tumor promotion that ensue is summarized in the flowchart of Figure 1. Important highlights include the fact that deregulation of $[Ca^{++}]_i$ is a common early event following lethal cell injury. At least in some cases, modifications of that increase, e.g., by eliminating calcium influx from the extracellular space, can affect the course of the injury delaying or preventing cell death. Since, in some cells, Na^+/Ca^{++} exchange may be an important deregulating mechanism, intervention designed to prevent either calcium or sodium entry may prove to be useful. We know less at the present time about exchanges between intracellular compartments, but we do know that some experiments fail to show protection through elimination of calcium from the medium. It is also possible that in the near future we will find that this is because calcium redistribution is an important factor. Many of the events that occur in acute cell injury seem to be the direct result of calcium activation. Such events include activation of phospholipases A and C, formation of blebs and cytoskeletal changes, and, in the case of many epithelial cells, the formation of cross-linked envelopes. Elevation of $[Ca^{++}]_i$ may have different effects in normal cells as compared to tumor cells; such certainly seems to be the case in normal human bronchial epithelium as compared to tumor cell lines. This is indicated in Figure 1 by the switch under $[Ca^{++}]_i$.

The right side of the flowchart shows some possible interactions of growth factors and oncogene products, as they may interact with the PI pathway, and shows how they may mediate elevations of $[Ca^{++}]_i$ as indicated by the effects of $InsP_3$ on the calcium with the ER. In some cases, tumor promoters directly activate protein kinase C and these pathways converge again at the Na^+-H^+ carrier and the alkalinization steps. Other intervention points are also possible, including amiloride or amiloride-like compounds, modifiers of sodium entry, and modifiers of calmodulin.

It thus seems clear that the details of ion regulation in cell injury represent a fertile field for detailed investigation. Our work strongly indicates pivotal roles for both calcium and sodium in cell killing as well as in tumorigenesis, particularly tumor promotion. An understanding of these phenomena holds the promise of bringing together a variety of information on signal transduction, gene regulation, cytoskeletal function, and membrane transport in a diversity of normal and abnormal cell process.

ACKNOWLEDGMENTS

We are very grateful to our colleagues for their contributions to this work. We especially thank R.E. Bulger, M.W. Kahng, K.U. Laiho, W.J. Mergner, A. Penttila, P.C. Phelps, A.L. Regec, M.W. Smith, and T. Sato. We are also indebted to our Publications Division, Department of Pathology, University of Maryland School of Medicine, without whom this paper would not be possible. These studies were supported by National Institutes of Health grants AM-15440 and NO1-CP-15738. This is contribution no. 2271 from the Cellular Pathobiology Laboratory.

REFERENCES

Banyard, M.R.C. and R.L. Tellam. 1985. The free cytoplasmic calcium concentration of tumorigenic and non-tumorigenic human somatic cell hybrids. *Br. J. Cancer* **51:** 761.

Berridge, M.J. and R.F. Irvine. 1984. Inositol triphosphate, a novel second messenger in cellular signal transduction. *Nature* **312:** 315.

Burns, C.P. and E. Rozengurt. 1983. Extracellular Na^+ and initiation of DNA synthesis: Role of intracellular pH and K^+. *J. Cell Biol.* **98:** 1082.

Cameron, I.L. and N.K.R. Smith. 1983. The ionic regulation of cell reproduction in normal and tumor cells. *Surv. Synth. Pathol. Res.* **2:** 206.

Castagna, M., Y. Takai, K. Kaibuchi, K. Sand, U. Kikkawa, and Y. Nishizuka. 1982. Direct activation of calcium-activated phospholipid-dependent protein kinase by tumor-promoting phorbol esters. *J. Biol. Chem.* **257:** 7847.

Epel, D. 1980. Ionic triggers in the fertilization of sea urchin eggs. *Ann. N.Y. Acad. Sci.* **339:** 74.

Hennings, H., D. Michaels, C. Cheng, K. Steinert, K. Holbrook, and S.H. Yuspa. 1980. Calcium regulation of growth and differentiation of mouse epidermal cells in culture. *Cell* **19:** 245.

Laiho, K.U. and B.F. Trump. 1974. Relationship of ion, water, and cell volume changes in cellular injury of Ehrlich ascites tumor cells. *Lab. Invest.* **31:** 207.

———. 1975. Mitochondrial changes, ion and water shifts in the cellular injury of Ehrlich ascites tumor cells. *Beitr. Pathol.* **155:** 237.

Laiho, K.U., I.K. Berezesky, and B.F. Trump. 1983. The role of calcium in cell injury. Studies in Ehrlich ascites tumor cells following injury with anoxia and organic mercurials. *Surv. Synth. Pathol. Res.* **2:** 170.

Lechner, J.F. 1984. Interdependent regulation of epithelial cell replication by nutrients, hormones, growth factors, and cell density. *Fed. Proc.* **43:** 116.

Masui, T., L.M. Wakefield, J.F. Lechner, M.A. LaVeck, M.B. Sporn, and C.C. Harris. 1986. Type β transforming growth factor: A differentiation-inducing serum factor for normal human bronchial epithelial cells. *Proc. Natl. Acad. Sci. U.S.A.* **83:** 2438.

Moolenaar, W.H., L.C.J. Tertoolen, and S.W. de Laat. 1984a. Phorbol ester and diacylglycerol mimic growth factors in raising cytoplasmic pH. *Nature* **312:** 371.

———. 1984b. Growth factors immediately raise cytoplasmic free Ca^{2+} in human fibroblasts. *J. Biol. Chem.* **259:** 8066.

———. 1986. The epidermal growth factor-induced calcium signal in A431 cells. *J. Biol. Chem.* **261:** 279.

Nishizuka, Y. 1984. The role of protein kinase C in cell surface signal transduction and tumor production. *Nature* **308:** 693.

Osornio-Vargas, A.R., I.K. Berezesky, and B.F. Trump. 1981. Progression of ion movements during acute myocardial infarction in the rat. An x-ray microanalysis study. *Scanning Electron Microsc.* **2:** 463.

Penttila, A. and B.F. Trump. 1974. Extracellular acidosis protects Ehrlich ascites tumor cells and rat renal cortex against anoxic injury. *Science* **185:** 277.

Rozengurt, E., A. Rodriguez-Pena, M. Coombs, and J. Sinnett-Smith. 1984. Diacylglycerol stimulates DNA synthesis and cell division in mouse 3T3 cells: Role of Ca^{2+}-sensitive phospholipid-dependent protein kinase. *Proc. Natl. Acad. Sci. U.S.A.* **81:** 5748.

Saladino, A.J., J.C. Willey, J.F. Lechner, R.C. Grafstrom, M. Laveck, and C.C. Harris. 1985. Effects of formaldehyde, acetaldehyde, benzoyl peroxide, and hydrogen peroxide on cultured normal human bronchial epithelial cells. *Cancer Res.* **45:** 2522.

Sato, T., I.K. Berezesky, and B.F. Trump. 1982. The role of extracellular (EC) calcium on isolated rat proximal tubule cells. *J. Cell Biol.* **93:** 466a.

Smith, M.W. and B.F. Trump. 1986. Use of intracellular fluorescent markers for measuring effect of hypoxia on cytosolic calcium and pH in rabbit renal tubular cells. *Fed. Proc.* **45:** 1528.

Smith, M.W., Y. Collan, M.W. Kahng, and B.F. Trump. 1980. Changes in mitochondrial lipids of rat kidney during ischemia. *Biochim. Biophys. Acta* **618:** 192.

Trump, B.F. and I.K. Berezesky. 1984. The role of sodium and calcium regulation in toxic cell injury. In *Drug metabolism and drug toxicity* (ed. J.R. Mitchell and M.G. Horning), p. 261. Raven Press, New York.

———. 1985a. The role of calcium in cell injury and repair: A hypothesis. *Surv. Synth. Pathol. Res.* **4:** 248.

———. 1985b. Cellular ion regulation and disease. A hypothesis. In *Current topics in membranes and transport* (ed. A.E. Shamoo), vol. 25, p. 279. Academic Press, New York.

———. 1987. The role of ion regulation in respiratory carcinogenesis. In *Current problems in tumour pathology. Lung carcinomas* (ed. E.M. McDowell), vol. 3, p. 162. Churchill Livingstone, Edinburgh, Scotland.

Trump, B.F. and M.W. Smith. 1986. FURA-2 measurement of cytosolic calcium in $HgCl_2$-treated rabbit renal tubular cells. *Fed. Proc.* **45:** 1726.

Trump, B.F., J.M. Strum, and R.E. Bulger. 1974. Studies on the pathogenesis of ischemic cell injury. I. Relation between ion and water shifts and cell ultrastructure in rat kidney slices during swelling at 0–4°C. *Virchows Arch. Abt. B Zellpathol.* **16:** 1.

Trump, B.F., I.K. Berezesky, K.U. Laiho, A.R. Osornio, W.J. Mergner, and M.W. Smith. 1980a. The role of calcium in cell injury. A review. *Scanning Electron Microsc.* **2:** 437.

Trump, B.F., E.M. McDowell, and A.U. Arstila. 1980b. Cellular reaction to injury. In *Principles of pathobiology* (ed. R.B. Hill, Jr. et al.), 3rd ed., p. 20. Oxford University Press, New York.

Trump, B.F., I.K. Berezesky, and P.C. Phelps. 1981. Sodium and calcium regulation and the role of the cytoskeleton in the pathogenesis of disease: A review and hypothesis. *Scanning Electron Microsc.* **2:** 435.

Trump, B.F., I.S. Ambudkar, P.C. Phelps, M.W. Smith, and A.L. Regec. 1985. Cell membrane injury and intracellular calcium regulation in renal tubular epithelial cells. *J. Cell Biol.* **101:** 62a.

Trump, B.F., I.K. Berezesky, T. Sato, K.U. Laiho, P.C. Phelps, and N. DeClaris. 1984. Cell calcium, cell injury and cell death. *Environ. Health Perspect.* **57:** 281.

Willey, J.C., C.E. Moser, J.F. Lechner, and C.C. Harris. 1984. Differential effects of 12-0-tetradecanoylphorbol-13-acetate on cultured normal and neoplastic human bronchial epithelial cells. *Cancer Res.* **44:** 5124.

Yuspa, S.H. 1984. Mechanisms of initiation and promotion in mouse epidermis. *Int. Agency Res. Cancer Sci. Publ.* **56:** 191.

COMMENTS

GHOSHAL: When you add more calcium, you get more cell killing, which, in turn, causes compensatory cell proliferation and tumor promotion. We have different experiences when we do it in vivo. While it is known that choline-deficient (CD) diet causes initiation, and promotion in the liver cells, when liver cells are initiated with a carcinogen and then promoted by CD diet, a certain number of foci or nodules of a certain size are obtained. When the carcinogen-initiated rats were promoted by the same CD diet but with extra calcium added to it, both the number and size of the nodules were reduced.

TRUMP: Is this modified calcium in the diet?

GHOSHAL: Yes, it is. The number and size of foci reduced with the calcium-added diet; and also when the cell proliferation is reduced one-tenth, cell killing is reduced. Here calcium is inhibiting. On the other hand, in your in vitro system, you find that even calcium is killing the cells.

TRUMP: Let me clarify that point because it correlates very well with the in vitro situation, as far as we know it, in both the skin and the bronchus. If you assume that the diet mainly affects the extracellular calcium in the bowel lumen, then the results would be the same as those found in vitro. If the extracellular calcium is 1 mM or 2 mM, Yuspa clearly showed that keratinocytes would differentiate as they normally do; whereas if he reduced the calcium to very low levels, they would continue to divide. So, extracellular calcium at 1 mM or 2 mM seems, in several epithelia, to suppress division and cause differentiation. The intracellular calcium may have the opposite effect. Increased intracellular calcium and alkalinization occur at mitosis and probably following treatment with several growth factors. There, it may cause cell division in some cases and terminal differentiation in others, depending on the rules of the cell in question. Therefore, increased outside calcium and increased intracellular ionized calcium can have opposite effects. For example, if you lower outside calcium, cells dissociate. We usually use that to dissociate epithelia; whereas, if you raise calcium inside the cell, they also dissociate.

GHOSHAL: So, in the in vivo situation, what would be the role of extracellular calcium?

TRUMP: We are controlling in vitro specifically in a very defined situation, a discrete situation in a dish, where you can set the calcium at whatever you want. You really can't do that experiment in vivo because the animal will go into tetany and you really can't do that analogous thing. But, in any case, raising extracellular calcium in vitro is associated with terminal differentiation and cessation of division.

DI GIOVANNI: On what cells did you do the cross-linked envelope assays?

TRUMP: Those experiments were done on normal human bronchial epithelium and a series of human carcinoma cell lines, a couple of adenocarcinomas, a mucoepidermoid and a squamous carcinoma. Also, I should like to mention the recent work of Masui in Harris' laboratory—essentially the same effect of TPA is shown by transforming growth factor-β. In that system, it again induces differentiation, suppresses division, in normal cells as opposed to the cell lines. How that relates to intracellular ion ratios is under study.

DI GIOVANNI: Does benzoyl peroxide induce differentiation in mouse epidermal cells? It is my understanding that Yuspa at the National Institutes of Health has shown that it does not induce differentiation in mouse epidermal cells. Does it actually have the same effect?

SLAGA: It doesn't have the same magnitude effect that TPA has. It will do it a little bit; but it is not overwhelming.

DI GIOVANNI: In your system, benzoyl peroxide was quite effective.

TRUMP: It was very effective.

DI GIOVANNI: I wonder then if there is a significant difference between the human and the mouse systems.

TRUMP: I don't know.

SLAGA: Could be.

TRUMP: Did you ever do that in vitro with epidermal cultures?

DI GIOVANNI: The data I'm referring to come from Yuspa's laboratory.

TRUMP: With benzoyl peroxide? It could be a big one. Again, the bronchus is different from the bladder, the liver, and the skin because, in the case of bronchus, we have only one layer of epithelium normally. We have a cell that cannot divide, the ciliated cell; we have the mucous cell which can and does readily divide in wound repair; we have a basal cell whose function is totally mysterious; and then we have these endocrine cells which apparently can divide. The bronchial epithelium has a very low rate of cell turnover normally, unless you injure it. Then the labeling indexes go sky high in the mucous cells and a little bit in the basal cells, and then it covers the wound. You get involved with epidermoid metaplasia, much of which sloughs, and then in some way it reconstructs back to normal.

ROE: Coming back to the in vivo situation, I will give evidence for two target sites in the rat to the fact that either increased calcium absorption and/or hypercalcemia are associated with increased tumor incidence, the adrenal medulla, and the interstitial cells of the testis.

TRUMP: Does it have the occurrence of hormonally associated phemonena simultaneously?

ROE: Yes. I shall also be saying that you cannot do a clean experiment in an overfed rat; they are full of hormonal abnormalities.

WILLIAMS: I have two points, one just a little further to this interesting report on the effect of exogenous calcium. Lipkin of the Sloan-Kettering Institute has also found that if he increases the amount of calcium in the diet to patients that have hyperproliferative states of the intestinal epithelium, which place them at higher risk of adenoma and colon cancer formation, that the proliferative index is reduced closer to the normal level. The exact mechanism for this has not been elucidated, but since it is known that luminal bile acids will raise the proliferative index in the intestinal mucosa, he has hypothesized that the calcium may be forming insoluble complexes with bile acids or free fatty acids. This may have relevance to liver carcinogenesis because there is some evidence that bile acids have a promoting effect in liver.

TRUMP: I know that paper. Did he actually think that by increasing the diet he was changing the calcium concentration in which these cells were bathed? Because, after all, with the intestinal epithelium, you can potentially change the extracellular luminal calcium concentration.

WILLIAMS: The amount of calcium in the fecal stream is considered to be important. I don't know whether serum calcium levels were changed.

TRUMP: At least on the luminal side of those cells, you could make them see more calcium.

WILLIAMS: There is another aspect to this. I think you made a point about the difference between tumor cells and normal cells in regulating calcium. That reminded me of studies that were done by Whitfield in Ottawa, which we have also confirmed, although there are exceptions. When the calcium content in culture medium was reduced from 1.8 mM to 0.0035 mM, then normal liver cells ceased proliferation, whereas transformed liver cells continued to proliferate. Whitfield had reported this originally for some other cell types. There are, however, a number of discrepancies which may relate to individual phenotypic abnormalities in different tumor cells; but I think it does indicate that there is something about certain tumor cells that makes them less dependent upon the extracellular calcium levels.

TRUMP: And we still do not know the mechanism of that extracellular-calcium-mediated effect. It is still not clear whether that is really changing inside or whether the effect is totally outside. The rules seem to be the opposite; epidermal cells seem to have the opposite rules of normal hepatocytes.

ANDERSON: I wonder if that could have anything to do with whether the tissue has an active circulation or not when the epithelial cells depend upon diffusion.

TRUMP: As compared to, say, a liver cell?

ANDERSON: Yes.

TRUMP: Like a skin, dependent?

ANDERSON: Right. The rate at which it can exchange.

TRUMP: Leighton in Philadelphia has data suggesting that the gradients in that type of epithelium are involved—gradients of everything, pH, oxygen, and probably calcium.

Session 2:
Forced Cell Proliferation

Orotic Acid, a Novel Liver Tumor Promoter: Studies on Its Mechanism of Action

EZIO LACONI, SHANTHI VASUDEVAN, PREMA M. RAO, SRINIVASAN
RAJALAKSHMI, AND DITTAKAVI S.R. SARMA
Department of Pathology
University of Toronto
Toronto, Ontario M5S 1A8, Canada

OVERVIEW

Xenobiotics are used to perturb homeostasis of DNA and/or membranes with a view to understanding the carcinogenic process. Recently, we tried a different approach to disturb homeostasis of DNA and/or membranes, viz. metabolic manipulations, and to study their influence on different phases of the carcinogenic process. Nucleotide pools offered a unique possibility in the sense that they can exert a two-pronged attack on both DNA and membranes. By being precursors of nucleic acid synthesis and carriers of sugars in the cell, imbalances can upset homeostasis in DNA and in glycosylation of proteins and lipids, including that of membranes. When orotic acid, a pyrimidine nucleotide precursor, is fed, it induces nucleotide pool imbalance and changes in DNA and in membrane glycosylation, and it promotes carcinogenesis in the liver. The significance of this approach lies in the prospect that, since nucleotide pools are normal cellular components, it may be one way to promote carcinogenesis in a wide variety of organs. Perhaps a consideration of greater significance is that nucleotide pools change under several nutritional, metabolic, and pathological conditions.

INTRODUCTION

One of our approaches to understand the carcinogenic process is to identify those metabolic events which, when disturbed, influence the pathogenesis of cancer development. Nucleotide pools appear to be an important cellular factor that can influence the carcinogenic process. As nucleic acid pools are precursors of nucleic acid synthesis and carriers of sugars in the cell, an imbalance can perturb the normal homeostasis of both DNA and membranes, the two targets often implicated in the carcinogenic process (Fig. 1).

When orotic acid (OA), a precursor of pyrimidine nucleotide biosynthesis, is fed to rats, it results in increased uridine nucleotides (nucleotide pool imbalance) (Handschumacher et al. 1960; Rajalakshmi et al. 1961; Marchetti et al. 1964), induces alterations in DNA (Rao et al. 1985a) and in membrane glycosylation (Martin et al. 1982), and promotes carcinogenesis in the liver (Columbano et al.

Banbury Report 25: Nongenotoxic Mechanisms in Carcinogenesis
© Cold Spring Harbor Laboratory. 0-87969-225-1/87. $1.00 + .00

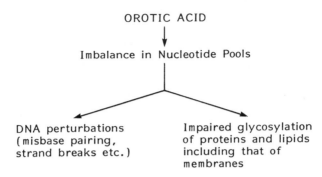

OROTIC ACID

Imbalance in Nucleotide Pools

DNA perturbations
(misbase pairing,
strand breaks etc.)

Impaired glycosylation
of proteins and lipids
including that of
membranes

Figure 1
Schematic representation of the two-pronged attack on DNA and membranes by an imbalance in nucleotide pools.

1982; Rao et al. 1983, 1984; Laurier et al. 1984) and in the intestine (Rao et al. 1986). The significance of these observations is far-reaching largely because nucleotide pools are normal cellular components and the pool sizes change under several physiological and pathological conditions. The creation of an imbalance in nucleotide pools may be one common mechanism by which carcinogenesis can be promoted in a wide variety of organs. In view of these considerations, it became important to determine (1) the type of nucleotide pool imbalance that can promote carcinogenesis and (2) the mechanism by which such an imbalance exerts promoting effects.

RESULTS

In the present study, the promoting ability of a regimen was assayed by monitoring the number and size of gamma glutamyl transferase (GGT)-positive foci and nodules in the liver of initiated rats following exposure to the promoting regimen.

Our earlier studies indicated that OA is a liver tumor promoter (Columbano et al. 1982; Rao et al. 1983, 1984; Laurier et al. 1984) and did not induce initiated hepatocytes (E. Laconi and D.S.R. Sarma, unpubl.). Attempts to understand the mechanism by which OA promotes liver carcinogenesis revealed that OA must be metabolized to form uridine nucleotides before it can exert its promoting effect (Rao et al. 1985b). The next series of experiments was designed to determine whether the promoting ability is unique to the imbalance in nucleotide pools created by the increase in uridine nucleotides or whether any other type of imbalance in nucleotide pools can also exert the promoting effect. Male Fischer 344 (F344) rats (150 g) initiated with a single necrogenic dose of diethylnitrosamine (DEN) (200 mg/kg,i.p.) and exposed for 10 weeks to diets containing 0.3% adenine, 1% adenosine, 1% guanosine, 1% cytidine, or 1% uridine did not develop any GGT-positive foci/nodules. Our earlier studies indicated that thymidine exerted a weak but significant promotional effect in the liver (Rao et al. 1984). These results suggested that only certain types of nucleotide pool imbalances, especially those created by feeding OA and, to a limited extent, those created by thymidine, can promote carcinogenesis in the rat liver.

The next question concerned the mechanism by which OA or the resulting nucleotide pool imbalance promotes liver carcinogenesis. The obvious consideration would be whether OA, like many other tumor promoters, induces liver cell proliferation. Interestingly, feeding OA for 3 days, 5 weeks, or 10 weeks did not induce liver cell proliferation, monitored as labeled hepatocytes, following implantation of an osmotic minipump containing [^{3}H]thymidine for 2–5 days. The next question would then be whether OA inhibits normal liver cell proliferation while permitting the initiated hepatocytes to respond to cell proliferative stimuli and to grow to form hepatic nodules as seen in the resistant-hepatocyte model (Solt and Farber 1976; Cayama et al. 1978). Again, OA did not inhibit liver cell proliferation following partial hepatectomy and did not even delay chain elongation of the newly made DNA (J. Pegg et al., unpubl.). These observations should be treated cautiously because even a slight inhibition of normal cell proliferation may become significant over a period of time. This line of argument becomes more meaningful, especially when we consider that OA takes a long time (approx. 5–10 weeks) to exert its promoting effects.

The next series of experiments was designed to determine whether OA is mitogenic to GGT-positive foci. To study this aspect, GGT-positive foci were initiated with a single necrogenic dose of DEN (200 mg/kg, i.p.) and promoted with a diet deficient in choline (Sells et al. 1979). After developing the foci, the rats were exposed to a 1% OA diet for 3 days, and the labeling index was monitored in both foci and the surrounding liver. Results presented in Table 1 clearly indicate that exposure to OA for 3 days did not result in any increased labeling index either in GGT-positive foci/nodules or in the surrounding liver. In a similar type of experiment when the foci were exposed to other liver tumor promoters, such as phenobarbital, hexachlorocyclohexane, nafenopin, and certain steroid compounds, enhanced cell proliferation in GGT-positive foci was observed (Schulte-Hermann et al. 1981).

DISCUSSION

The results of this study revealed that only a particular type of imbalance in the nucleotide pools, such as the one created in the liver by feeding OA, can promote liver carcinogenesis in the rat. The mechanism by which OA promotes liver carcinogenesis does not appear to be related to any ability of OA to induce liver cell proliferation nor to any capacity to inhibit the uninitiated hepatocytes while permitting the initiated hepatocytes to respond to growth stimuli to form hepatic

Table 1
Influence of Orotic Acid on Hepatocyte Proliferation in Hepatic Nodules and in Surrounding Liver

| | Labeling index in | |
Treatment	nodules	surrounding liver
Basal diet	5.0 ± 1.14	0.44 ± 0.05
1% Orotic acid diet	6.5 ± 2.39	0.70 ± 0.25

Male F344 rats (150 g) were initiated with a single necrogenic dose of diethylnitrosamine (200 mg/kg, i.p). A week later the rats were exposed to a diet deficient in choline. Ten weeks thereafter the rats were transferred to a basal diet (diet no. 101, Dyets, Inc. Bethlehem, PA). Ten days later the rats were divided into two groups of three animals each. One group continued to receive the basal diet while the other received the basal diet containing 1% OA. Starting from day 3, each rat received four injections of [^{3}H]thymidine (100 μCi/rat, i.p.) 8 hours apart. The rats were killed 1 hour after the last injection. Livers were processed for autoradiography; 3000–5000 hepatocytes were counted per slide and the labeling index was expressed as percentage of labeled cells per total cells counted. Values are the average of three rats ± S.E.

nodules. These observations are quite significant because a wide variety of tumor promoters induce hyperplasia in the target organ. For example, liver tumor promoters such as phenobarbital, α-hexachlorocyclohexane, nafenopin, steroid compounds (Schulte-Hermann et al. 1981), and a choline-deficient diet (Boss et al. 1976; Abanobi et al. 1982; Ghoshal 1982) induce hyperplasia in the liver; and the skin tumor promoters, including the active phorbol esters, induce hyperplasia in skin. In addition, phenobarbital, nafenopin, α-hexachlorocyclohexane, and the steroid promoters induce hyperplasia to a greater extent in the hepatic nodules, compared to that in the surrounding liver (Schulte-Hermann et al. 1981). However, the situation with OA appears to be different because it does not induce cell proliferative response either in the normal liver or in GGT-positive foci/nodules. These results are intriguing and prompted us to speculate the following: Initiated hepatocytes acquire new properties, including increased growth potential, as they progress to form hepatic nodules. This progressive acquisition can be achieved by repeated number of cell cycles. Since initiated hepatocytes are changing during promotion/progression, cell proliferation, in addition to amplifying the number of cells, must be contributing some qualitative change in the initiated cell, namely, genomic changes such as regulation of gene expression and gene rearrangements. Perhaps tumor promoters also induce similar changes in the initiated cell and thereby reduce the number of cell cycles required for the initiated hepatocyte to reach a point in the sequence of events that occur during promotion and progression. If a particular tumor promoter is an inducer of cell proliferation, then it will further reduce the time taken for the initiated hepatocytes to reach a point in the sequence.

This line of argument suggests that (1) tumor promoters need not be inducers of cell proliferation and (2) proliferation alone can exert the promoting effect. Thus, there may be three types of tumor promoters: those that do not induce cell proliferation but have the capacity to induce certain critical changes in the initiated cells, those that predominantly induce cell proliferation, and those that not only can induce cell proliferation, but also can induce critical changes in initiated cells. Identification of these different classes of tumor promoters and studies on the mechanism of their action may help us to understand the promotion phase of the carcinogenic process better.

SUMMARY AND CONCLUSION

OA, a precursor of pyrimidine nucleotide biosynthesis, is an excellent promoter of liver carcinogenesis. OA needs to be metabolized to form uridine nucleotides and create an imbalance in nucleotide pools for it to exert its promoting effect in rat liver. Adenine, adenosine, guanosine, cytidine, and uridine, however, could not exert any promoting effect. These results suggest that only a particular type of imbalance in nucleotide pools, such as the one created by feeding OA, appears to exert liver tumor promotion. Attempts to understand the mechanism of liver tumor promotion by OA revealed that OA, unlike a wide variety of liver tumor promoters, is not a direct mitogen for either the normal liver or the GGT-positive foci/nodules. It was speculated that cell proliferation, in addition to amplifying the initiated hepatocytes, also contributes some qualitative changes because of which initiated hepatocytes progressively acquire new properties, including increasing growth potential. Tumor promoters can contribute these changes and reduce the number of cell cycles required for the initiated hepatocytes to reach a point in the sequence of events that occur during tumor promotion. Thus, tumor promoters need not be inducers of cell proliferation.

ACKNOWLEDGMENTS

We wish to thank Lori Cutler for her excellent secretarial help. The study was supported in part by U.S. Public Health Service grants CA-37077 and CA-23958 from the National Cancer Institute and from the National Cancer Institute, Canada. E.L. was supported by Associazione Italiana per la Ricerca sul Cancro.

REFERENCES

Abanobi, S.E., B. Lombardi, and H. Shinozuka. 1982. Stimulation of DNA synthesis and cell proliferation in the liver of rats fed a choline-devoid diet and their suppression by phenobarbital. *Cancer Res.* **42:** 412.

Boss, J.M., E. Rosenmann, and G. Zajicek. 1976. Alpha-fetoprotein and liver cell proliferation in rats fed choline-deficient diet. *Z. Ernaehrungswiss* **15:** 211.

Cayama, E., H. Tsuda, D.S.R. Sarma, and E. Farber. 1978. Initiation of chemical carcinogenesis requires cell proliferation. *Nature* **275:** 60.

Columbano, A., G.M. Ledda, P.M. Rao, S. Rajalakshmi, and D.S.R. Sarma. 1982. Dietary orotic acid, a new selective growth stimulus for carcinogen altered hepatocytes in rat. *Cancer Lett.* **16:** 191.

Ghoshal, A.K. 1982. Choline-lipotrope deficient (CLD) diet as a mitogenic substitute for partial hepatectomy (PH) in the induction of resistant hepatocytes by carcinogens as a short term in vivo test. *Proc. Am. Assoc. Cancer Res.* **23:** 96.

Handschumacher, R.E., W.A. Creasey, J.J. Jaffe, C.A. Pasternak, and L. Hankin. 1960. Biochemical and nutritional studies on the induction of fatty liver by dietary orotic acid. *Proc. Natl. Acad. Sci. U.S.A.* **46:** 178.

Laurier, C., M. Tatematsu, P.M. Rao, S. Rajalakshmi, and D.S.R. Sarma. 1984. Promotion by orotic acid of liver carcinogenesis in rats initiated by 1,2-dimethylhydrazine. *Cancer Res.* **44:** 2186.

Marchetti, M., P. Puddu, and C.M. Caldarera. 1964. Metabolic aspects of orotic acid fatty liver: Nucleotide control mechanisms of lipid metabolism. *Biochem. J.* **92:** 46.

Martin, A., M-C. Biol, A. Raisonnier, R. Infante, P. Louisot, and M. Richard. 1982. Impaired glycosylation in liver microsomes of orotic acid fed rats. *Biochim. Biophys. Acta* **718:** 85.

Rajalakshmi, S., D.S.R. Sarma, and P.S. Sarma. 1961. Studies on orotic acid fatty liver. *Biochem. J.* **80:** 375.

Rao, P.M., E. Laconi, S. Vasudevan, S. Rajalakshmi, and D.S.R. Sarma. 1986. Orotic acid, a liver tumor promoter, also promotes carcinogenesis of the intestine. *Proc. Am. Assoc. Cancer Res.* **27:** 142.

Rao, P.M., Y. Nagamine, M.W. Roomi, S. Rajalakshmi, and D.S.R. Sarma. 1984. Orotic acid, a new promoter for experimental liver carcinogenesis. *Toxicol. Pathol.* **12:** 173.

Rao, P.M., S. Rajalakshmi, A. Alam, D.S.R. Sarma, M. Pala, and S. Parodi. 1985a. Orotic acid, a promoter of liver carcinogenesis, induces DNA damage in rat liver. *Carcinogenesis* **6:** 765.

Rao, P.M., S. Rajalakshmi, and D.S.R. Sarma. 1985b. Modulation of the promoting effect of orotic acid (OA) by adenine in rat liver. *Proc. Am. Assoc. Cancer Res.* **26:** 199.

Rao, P.M., Y. Nagamine, R-K. Ho, M.W. Roomi, C. Laurier, S. Rajalakshmi, and D.S.R. Sarma. 1983. Dietary orotic acid enhances the incidence of γ-glutamyltransferase positive foci in rat liver induced by chemical carcinogens. *Carcinogenesis* **4:** 1541.

Schulte-Hermann, R., G. Ohde, J. Schuppler, and I. Timmermann-Trosiener. 1981. Enhanced proliferation of putative preneoplastic cells in rat liver following treatment with the tumor promoters phenobarbital, hexachlorocyclohexane, steroid compounds and nafenopin. *Cancer Res.* **41:** 2556.

Sells, M.A., S.L. Katyal, S. Sell, H. Shinozuka, and B. Lombardi. 1979. Induction of foci of altered, γ-glutamyl transpeptidase positive hepatocytes in carcinogen treated rats fed a choline deficient diet. *Br. J. Cancer* **40:** 274.

Solt, D.B. and E. Farber. 1976. New principle for the analysis of chemical carcinogenesis. *Nature* **263:** 701.

Role of Stimulation of Liver Growth by Chemicals in Hepatocarcinogenesis

ROLF SCHULTE-HERMANN, WOLFRAM PARZEFALL, AND WILFRIED BURSCH
Institute für Tumorbiologie-Krebsforschung
A-1090 Vienna, Austria

OVERVIEW

Numerous nongenotoxic drugs, hormones, and environmental pollutants may produce liver cancer in rodents. These findings are of considerable concern with respect to human health. Many nongenotoxic hepatocarcinogens promote tumor development from preexistent preneoplastic lesions in rodent liver. In this paper, we review briefly the process of adaptive growth triggered by these agents in normal liver, as well as the role of cell proliferation and cell death by apoptosis for the regulation of cell number. Subsequently, we compare these effects in normal liver with similar changes in putative preneoplastic foci. We also present a hypothesis explaining the growth of foci during tumor promotion.

INTRODUCTION

Numerous compounds have been found that produce liver tumors in long-term animal experiments, although they do not exhibit detectable genotoxic activity. Examples are presented in Table 1; as indicated, these compounds include important drugs, hormones, and environmental pollutants.

The role played by these agents in human hepatocarcinogenesis is difficult to estimate. Long-term use of contraceptive steroids in rare cases may result in the appearance of tumors in human liver. Such tumors usually seem to be benign, and in some instances they regressed after withdrawal of the steroids (Popper 1979; Kerlin et al. 1983). Phenobarbital (PB) and other antiepileptic drugs alone did not lead to a detectable increase in the number of liver cancers. However, a slight excess of liver tumors (8 among 8000 patients) was noted in persons pretreated with the carcinogenic drug thorotrast (Clemmesen and Hjalgrim-Jensen 1978). This suggests the possibility of a tumor-promoting effect of PB in human liver. No evidence is available to support a carcinogenic or promoting effect of organochlorine compounds in human liver, but in view of the almost ubiquitous occurrence of these compounds in our environment and foodstuffs, any such effect—unless very strong—would be difficult to detect.

Studies on the mechanisms of action of nongenotoxic carcinogens should provide information useful to assess health risks posed by these compounds. As a possible clue to these mechanisms, it is very important to note that many of these compounds

Banbury Report 25: Nongenotoxic Mechanisms in Carcinogenesis
© Cold Spring Harbor Laboratory. 0-87969-225-1/87. $1.00 + .00

Table 1
Some Nongenotoxic Hepatocarcinogens and Their Acute Hepatic Effects

	Induction of		
Prototype	monooxygenases	other	growth
Phenobarbital, DDT, HCH, HCB, some PCBs and PBBs	P-450-PB		+
TCDD, some PCBs	P-450-MC		+
Cyproterone acetate, progesterone	P-450-PCN		+
Estradiol esters, ethinylestradiol	—	clotting factors, angiotensinogen, etc.	+
Clofibrate, nafenopin, diethylhexylphthalate	P-450-Clof.	peroxisomal enzymes	+

Reference: Schulte-Hermann 1985. *Abbreviations*: HCH, hexachlorohexane; HCB, hexachlorobenzene; PCB, polychlorinated biphenyls; PBB, polybrominated biphenyls.

have been found to promote tumor development and/or to induce growth and multiplication of putative preneoplastic foci in rat liver (Table 1) (Schulte-Hermann 1985). Since preneoplastic lesions seem to occur spontaneously quite frequently in the liver of untreated rodents, the hypothesis has been raised that tumor formation by nongenotoxic agents, as shown in Table 1, may result from promotion of spontaneous preneoplastic lesions (Schulte-Hermann and Parzefall 1982; Schulte-Hermann et al. 1983; Ward 1983).

Studies on liver tumor promotion would thus appear pertinent. Farber and co-workers have raised the hypothesis that preneoplastic lesions in the liver are resistant to cytotoxic effects and therefore may have a growth advantage during long-term treatment with cytotoxic promoters (Solt and Farber 1976; Farber and Cameron 1980). However, the agents listed in Table 1 exhibit little if any cytotoxicity in the liver (with the exception of TCDD and other ligands of the TCDD receptor). Instead they induce what appears to be adaptive growth and enzyme changes in the liver (Table 1). We have investigated for several years the possible relationship of these adaptive changes to tumor promotion. We summarize below some crucial experiments and recent concepts. All experiments reported here were performed with female Wistar rats.

RESULTS AND DISCUSSION

Liver Growth

Administration of many nongenotoxic hepatocarcinogens to experimental animals results in liver enlargement. This enlargement reflects an ordered growth, usually by hypertrophy and/or hyperplasia. Studies with model compounds from most of the compound groups listed in Table 1 provided the following evidence for the occurrence of hyperplasia: increases of hepatic DNA content, of hepatic DNA synthesis (assayed biochemically and autoradiographically), and of mitotic activity. Cell ploidy was not enhanced in rat liver but was enhanced in mouse liver. Multiplication of hepatocytes is the dominant cause of liver hyperplasia, but sinus wall cells participate in the growth process (Schulte-Hermann 1974, 1979a; Schulte-Hermann et al. 1980a,b; Bursch and Schulte-Hermann 1983; Ochs et al. 1986).

Some of these observations are illustrated in Figure 1, using cyproterone acetate (CPA) as an example. It should be noted that even though the growth stimulus is

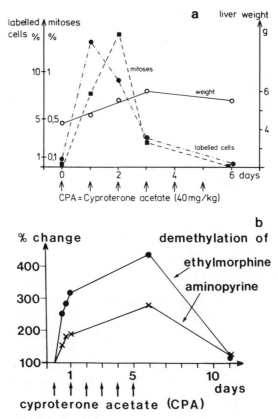

Figure 1

Effects of daily doses of 40 mg/kg cyproterone acetate on rat liver size and cell proliferation (*a*) and on hepatic monooxygenases (*b*). DNA synthesis was measured by autoradiography after [³H]thymidine injection, and the percentage of labeled hepatocytes is indicated. Activity of monooxygenases was assayed with isolated microsomes using the demethylation of ethylmorphine and aminopyrine as test reactions.

administered daily, cell proliferation is only transiently enhanced, and liver size and DNA content do not increase steadily but apparently reach a new steady state at an enhanced level (Fig. 1a). Obviously, growth control in the liver is not knocked out by CPA; the same is true for the other compounds considered. Rather, it is in focal lesions that mechanisms controlling homeostasis of cell number fail during long-term treatment. Liver growth as described here is apparently different from growth occurring during fetal development or during regeneration (Schulte-Hermann 1979b), because it is associated with excessive increases in specific hepatic functions such as drug metabolism (Fig. 1b), peroxisomal fatty acid β-oxidation, or others (Table 1).

Both growth and increased synthesis of enzymes probably represent adaptive responses to enhanced functional load imposed on the liver by metabolism of exogenous lipophilic agents, by the blocking of metabolic pathways that utilize fatty acids, by hormone effects, and so on (Schulte-Hermann 1974, 1979a). To cope with such functional loads, the liver offers a limited number of adaptive strategies or programs (Schulte-Hermann 1979a). In addition to controlling the synthesis of specific enzymes, these programs seem to contain as an optional component a signal that triggers hepatocyte proliferation. In fact, in the mature hepatocyte, replication and differentiation (adaptation) are not mutually exclusive. Thus, after PB treatment, synthesis of drug-metabolizing enzymes and of nuclear DNA occurs in the same subpopulation of hepatocytes in the pericentral area (Schulte-Hermann et al. 1984a). In conclusion, the group of (nongenotoxic) carcinogens represented by the examples in Table 1 are hormones or compounds with hormone-like effects. They trigger the expression of (adaptive) gene programs in the liver.

Involution of the Enlarged and Hyperfunctional Liver

Liver enlargement and increased enzyme activity readily disappear once the inducing compound is withdrawn and eliminated from the body (Fig. 1) (Schulte-Hermann 1974, 1979a). At least with some agents of relatively short biological persistence such as CPA, part of the enhanced DNA content disappears as well in a matter of a few days (Fig. 2) (Levine et al. 1977; Bursch et al. 1984, 1985). This rapid elimination of DNA appears to be due to a particular type of cell death, recently termed apoptosis (Wyllie et al. 1980) and known to occur at certain stages of embryological development or during involution of endocrine-dependent organs. The following findings on cell death during involution of adaptive liver growth seem pertinent:

1. The incidence of apoptosis is highest during the period of rapid elimination of DNA (Fig. 2).
2. The occurrence of apoptosis can be prevented by application of various inducers of liver growth (i.e., nongenotoxic hepatocarcinogens) (Fig. 3). This observation is important because it discriminates apoptosis from damage-induced cell

death such as that occurring after application of CCl₄. It strongly suggests that cell death by apoptosis has a function in the control of tissue cell number.

3. When the functional load of the liver is reduced by other measures, e.g., by starvation, involution of the organ is likewise associated with apoptosis of hepatocytes (W. Bursch, unpubl.).

4. Apoptosis appears to be a short-lived phenomenon lasting less than 4 hours (Fig. 3) (Bursch et al. 1985). This explains why apoptotic counts are relatively low even at times of massive elimination of DNA (see Fig. 2).

5. Apoptosis does not appear to hit cells randomly. Rather, "old" cells that did not replicate during liver growth are eliminated preferentially (Bursch et al. 1985). The basis of this selectivity is not known.

These findings strongly suggest that cell death by apoptosis is an important regulator of cell number in adult liver. Our current concept is depicted in Figure 4. We believe that cells in a resting liver (G_0) have two options to leave G_0: replication and death. Application of a growth stimulus (or cell deficit) will stimulate replication and inhibit death and thereby create and maintain tissue hyperplasia. The reverse is true when the growth stimulus is removed.

Effects of Tumor Promoters on Liver Foci

Putative preneoplastic foci are known to exhibit a number of phenotypic alterations from normal liver. We have recently pointed out that many of these alterations are also found in normal liver after treatment with PB or other liver tumor promoters,

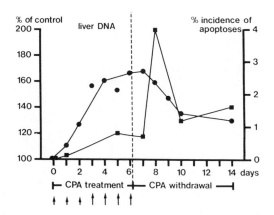

Figure 2

Liver DNA and apoptoses during and after treatment with CPA at doses of 100 mg/kg (short arrows) and 130 mg/kg (long arrows). The increase of total liver DNA is expressed in percentage of untreated and solvent-treated controls. The incidence of apoptosis indicates the number of apoptotic bodies found per 100 intact hepatocytes in histological sections.

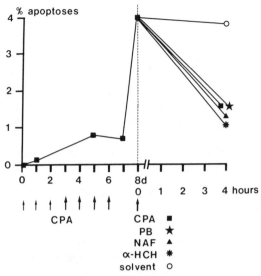

Figure 3

Prevention of apoptoses by treatment with various stimuli of liver growth. The experimental schedule until day 8 was identical to that described in Fig. 2. Then, one of the following compounds was administered in aqueous suspension at a dose of 130 mg/kg of body weight: CPA, PB, nafenopin (NAF), and α- hexachlorocyclohexane (α-HCH).

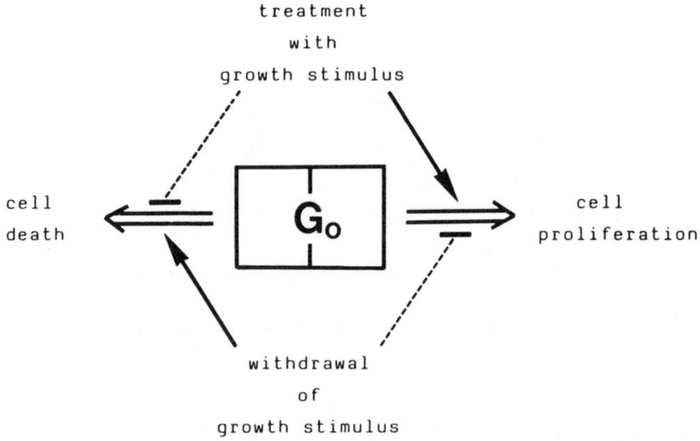

Figure 4

Schematic representation suggesting the interactions between liver growth stimuli and cell proliferation or cell death (apoptosis). (→) Stimulation; (----) inhibition.

although they are usually less pronounced than in foci (Table 2). We have therefore raised the hypothesis that focal hepatocytes are in a new state of differentiation in which they seem to be overspecialized for efficient performance of drug metabolism and proliferation (Fig. 5) (Schulte-Hermann 1985). In this context, an important difference between focal and neoplastic nodules must be emphasized. In contrast to the latter lesions, foci occasionally express cytochrome $P-450_b$ even without treatment and strongly express it after PB administration. Even carcinomas, when obtained after long-term promotion with PB, exhibited high monooxygenase activities (Schulte-Hermann et al. 1984a,b).

Much of the heterogeneity of focal phenotypes (Pitot et al. 1978) may result from incomplete expression of the adaptive gene program. PB treatment leads to more complete and more intense expression of the program (Pitot et al. 1978). This is also illustrated in Figure 6 (top) by the appearance of many more foci with distinct borders. Likewise, an inhibitory effect of PB on phenotypic remodeling of foci was described previously (Watanabe and Williams 1978). Furthermore, the large increase in numbers of foci during PB administration results from induction of phenotypic markers in "remodeled" foci, rather than from the formation of new foci from single initiated cells (Schulte-Hermann et al. 1982, 1984a, 1986).

Foci also show an accelerated increase in size during promoter treatment (Schulte-Hermann et al. 1982; Schulte-Hermann 1985). This would fit well into the concept that foci can overexpress adaptive responses to PB (including adaptive cell proliferation). However, control of the growth of foci turned out to be more complicated than originally thought. First, we found that foci have an enhanced

Table 2

Similarities between Responses of Normal Liver to PB or Related Promoters and the Phenotypic Alterations in Putative Preneoplastic Foci

Promoter	Changes in normal liver	Changes in liver foci
Cytochrome P-450-PB	+	+
Epoxide hydratase	+	+
Glucuronyl transferases	+	+
GSH transferase B	+	+
Gamma glutamyl transpeptidase	+	+
Glucose-6-phosphatase	−	−
Glucose-6-*P*-dehydrogenase	+	+
Pyruvate kinase L	−	−
DNA synthesis, mitosis	+	+
Ribonuclease	−	−
Deoxyribonuclease	−	−
Smooth endoplasmic reticulum	+	+

References: Schulte-Hermann 1985. + indicates increase; − indicates decrease.

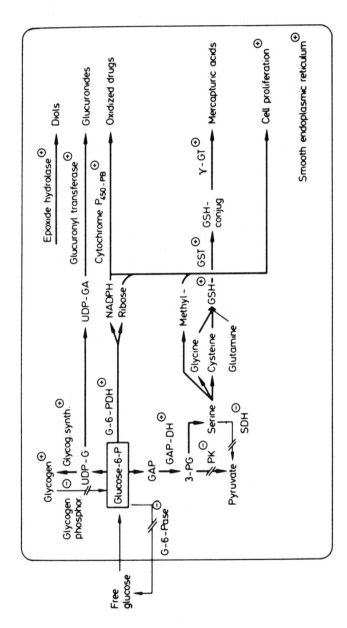

Figure 5

Metabolic pathways in preneoplastic hepatocytes: overspecialization for drug metabolism and cell proliferation (hypothesis). Phenotypic alterations found so far in putative preneoplastic cells of rat liver are indicated by + (increase) and −(decrease) with respect to normal hepatocytes. Favored pathways are shown by thick arrows; inhibited pathways are shown by thin arrows with interruptions. As a result of the alterations shown, less free glucose should be released into the circulation and less glucose should undergo glycolysis; therefore, more glucose would be available for synthesis of substrates for drug metabolism and macromolecules during cell replication. (Glycogen phosphor.) Glycogen phosphorylase; (G-6-Pase) glucose-6-phosphatase; (Glycog. synth.) glycogen synthetase; (UDP-G) uridine diphosphate glucose; (UDP-GA) uridine diphosphate glucuronic acid; (GAP) glycerol aldehyde phosphate; (GAP-DH) GAP dehydrogenase; (3-PG) 3-phosphoglycerate; (PK) pyruvate kinase; (SDH) serine dehydrogenase; (G-6-PDH) glucose-6-phosphate dehydrogenase; (GST) GSH transferase; (GSH conjug.) GSH conjugates; (γ-GT) gamma glutamyl transferase. (Reprinted, with permission, from Schulte-Hermann 1985.)

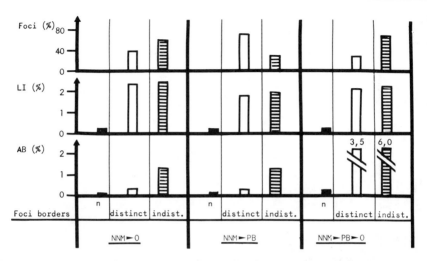

Figure 6

Effect of long-term treatment with PB and of PB withdrawal on remodeling, DNA synthesis, and apoptoses in foci. Foci were induced by a single dose of 250 mg/kg *N*-nitrosomorpholine (NNM). Subsequently, rats received either basal diet (NNM → O) or a diet containing PB for 28 weeks; concentrations were adjusted to provide daily doses of 50 mg/kg b.w. of PB (NNM → PB). (NNM → PB → O) PB withdrawn for 6 weeks after 28 weeks of treatment. (n) Normal (surrounding) liver; foci were classified as having distinct borders (as an index for nonremodeling state) or indistinct borders (as indicating a state of remodeling or incomplete phenotypic expression). (*Top*) Percentage of foci with distinct/indistinct borders; (*center*) DNA synthesis (LI = labeling index, labeled hepatocytes per 100 hepatocytes); (*bottom*) apoptotic bodies per 100 intact hepatocytes. (Data from I. Timmermann-Trosiener and R. Schulte-Hermann, in prep.)

basal rate of proliferative activity (Fig. 6, center), which is further increased by single doses of various tumor promoters (Schulte-Hermann et al. 1981). However, as in normal liver (see above), this increase is only a transient one, and during continuous PB treatment, proliferation rates in foci are not higher than they are without promotion (Fig. 6, center), despite a considerable difference in focal growth rates (Schulte-Hermann et al. 1982). This prompted us to study quantitatively cell death and remodeling in foci.

Cell Death in Foci during Promotion and Remodeling (Involution)

We have studied the occurrence and incidence of signs of cell death in foci (Bursch et al. 1984). A representative result is shown in Figure 7. As indicated, the incidence of apoptotic bodies (ABs) is severalfold higher than in normal resting liver (cf. Fig. 2); PB treatment resulted in a moderate decrease, withdrawal of PB resulted in an excessive increase, and readministration of PB again resulted in a decrease of ABs. Thus, these effects resemble those of CPA in noninitiated liver

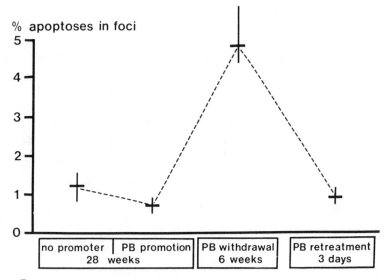

Figure 7

Incidence of cell death (apoptosis) in foci during and after PB treatment. Experimental conditions and explanations are given in Fig. 6. Vertical bars indicate 95% confidence limits.

(cf. Figs. 2 and 3). These findings suggest that (1) cell death (apoptosis) in foci is of a similar regulatory nature as in normal liver, (2) cell death is much more frequent in foci than in normal liver (i.e., focal cells seem to have a shorter life span than normal hepatocytes), and (3) PB treatment seems to prolong the life span of focal hepatocytes.

With respect to the growth deficit noted in foci without promotion, we assume that a relatively high rate of cell death at least partially counterbalances the enhanced proliferative activity. In addition, remodeling of focal cells to the normal phenotype may also be a (negative) determinant of focal growth (see below).

What does the enhanced occurrence of cell death in foci mean? As mentioned above, without promoter treatment many foci express their program of phenotypic alterations only incompletely. Incomplete expression is also found after withdrawal of the promoters (Fig. 6), and this phenomenon is known as remodeling. Tatematsu et al. (1983) have suggested redifferentiation to normal-appearing liver as the basis of remodeling after AAF treatment is stopped. If we understand the induction of the altered phenotype by a promoter like PB as overexpression of the adaptive program, then remodeling after PB withdrawal should be regarded as de-adaptation and involution as described above for noninitiated liver. We have therefore checked whether apoptosis would be associated with remodeling phenomena, and this appears to be the case (Fig. 6., bottom). Although no difference in cell proliferation

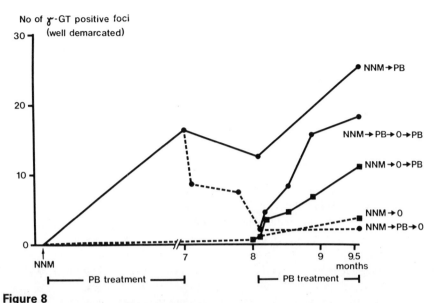

Figure 8

Effect of withdrawal and retreatment with PB on the incidence of GGT-positive foci. For experimental details, see Fig. 6. Foci numbers are given per square centimeter of section area. (●) Rats treated with PB for the first 7 months; (■) rats not treated with PB during the first 7 months; (——) treated rats; (----) rats not treated. (Data from U. Gerbracht et al., in prep.)

was apparent, ABs were clearly more abundant in foci with indistinct borders than in their sharply demarcated counterparts. Thus, apoptosis in foci, to some extent, seems to be associated with incomplete phenotypic expression or remodeling and may reflect an involution phenomenon similar to that in normal liver when the functional load resulting in expression of certain gene programs is reduced. Thus, the observed inhibition of cell death in foci by PB may reflect a "normal" regulatory event that is quantitatively out of balance with cell proliferation.

Is Liver Tumor Promotion Reversible?

Do remodeling and high rates of cell death after withdrawal of PB indicate that the promotion of focal growth is reversible? A preliminary answer to this question is shown in Figure 8. In this experiment, when PB was withdrawn after promoting treatment for 7 months, the number of well-demarcated gamma glutamyl transpeptidase (GGT)-positive foci dropped sharply. Similar observations were reported previously (Schulte-Hermann et al. 1982; Glauert et al. 1986). After 4 weeks on basal diet, PB treatment was reinitiated. This resulted in a rapid emergence of foci; their number was clearly higher than in the animals that received no PB for the first 7 months, but only from 8 months onward. Similar results were obtained when the total area occupied by GGT-positive foci was calculated. These results suggest that the incidence of cell death during PB withdrawal was not sufficient to eliminate physically most of the foci at 7 months. Rather, most of the foci detectable lost only their distinct phenotypic appearance and readily reexpressed it upon retreatment with the promoter. The question as to reversibility may thus get two answers: The induction of phenotypic alterations in foci by a tumor promoter may be readily reversible; the induction of cell multiplication in foci does not appear to be reversible, at least not in the present observation period of 4 weeks.

CONCLUSION AND SUMMARY

Nongenotoxic hepatocarcinogens (see Table 1), with the possible exception of hypolipidemics and phthalates, promote the development of liver tumors. During short-term treatment, they induce the expression of gene programs in normal liver which consist of functional changes and growth. Growth occurs through hypertrophy and hyperplasia. All changes are self-limited and reversible; hyperplasia can regress through apoptosis, a specific form of cell death regulated by the presence or absence of hepatic growth stimuli.

Foci of putative preneoplastic hepatocytes seem to express such gene programs, although incompletely, even without inducer. Promoters such as PB trigger responses in foci that are qualitatively similar to those in normal liver, but quantitatively more pronounced (overexpression).

Both cell types show transient increases in proliferation. The crucial difference lies in the quantity of cell replication, which is severalfold higher in foci than in normal liver. Without promoting treatment, this enhanced proliferation is counterbalanced in most foci by cell death (apoptosis) and remodeling; promoters inhibit the latter two processes and thereby stimulate the growth of foci.

REFERENCES

Bursch, W. and R. Schulte-Hermann. 1983. Synchronization of hepatic DNA synthesis by scheduled feeding and lighting in mice treated with the chemical inducer of liver growth α-hexachlorocyclohexane. *Cell Tissue Kinet.* **16:** 125.

Bursch, W., H.S. Taper, B. Lauer, and R. Schulte-Hermann. 1985. Quantitative histological and histochemical studies on the occurrence and stages of controlled cell death (apoptosis) during regression of rat liver hyperplasia. *Virchows Arch. B Cell Pathol.* **50:** 153.

Bursch, W., B. Lauer, I. Timmermann-Trosiener, G. Barthel, J. Schuppler, and R. Schulte-Hermann. 1984. Controlled death (apoptosis) of normal and putative preneoplastic cells in rat liver following withdrawal of tumor promoters. *Carcinogenesis* **5:** 453.

Clemmesen, J. and S. Hjalgrim-Jensen. 1978. Is phenobarbital carcinogenic? A follow-up of 8078 epileptics. *Ecotoxicol. Environ. Saf.* **1:** 457.

Farber, E. and R. Cameron. 1980. The sequential analysis of cancer development. *Adv. Cancer Res.* **31:** 125.

Glauert, H.P., M. Schwarz, and H.C. Pitot. 1986. The phenotypic stability of altered hepatic foci: Effect of the short-term withdrawal of phenobarbital and of the long-term feeding of purified diets after the withdrawal of phenobarbital. *Carcinogenesis* **7:** 117.

Kerlin, P., G.L. Davies, D.B. McGill, L.H. Weiland, M.A. Adson, and P.F. Sheedy. 1983. Hepatic adenoma and focal nodular hyperplasia: Clinical, pathologic, and radiologic features. *Gastroenterology* **84:** 994.

Levine, W.G., M.G. Ord, and L.A. Stocken. 1977. Some biochemical changes associated with nafenopin-induced liver growth in the rat. *Biochem. Pharmacol.* **26:** 939.

Ochs, H., B. Düsterberg, P. Günzel, and R. Schulte-Hermann. 1986. Effect of tumor promoting contraceptive steroids on growth and drug metabolizing enzymes in rat liver. *Cancer Res.* **46:** 1224.

Pitot, H.C., L. Barsness, T. Goldsworthy, and T. Kitagawa. 1978. Biochemical characterisation of stages of hepatocarcinogenesis after a single dose of diethyl-nitrosamine. *Nature* **271:** 456.

Popper, H. 1979. Hepatic cancers in man: Quantitative perspectives. *Environ Res.* **19:** 482.

Schulte-Hermann, R. 1974. Induction of liver growth by xenobiotic compounds and other stimuli. *Crit. Rev. Toxicol.* **3:** 97.

———. 1979a. Reactions of the liver to injury: Adaptation. In *Toxic injury of the liver* (ed. E. Farber and M. M. Fisher), part A, p. 385. Marcel Dekker, New York.

———. 1979b. Adaptive liver growth induced by xenobiotic compounds: Its nature and mechanism. *Arch. Toxicol. Suppl.* **2:** 113.

———. 1985. Tumor promotion in the liver. *Arch. Toxicol.* **57:** 147.

Schulte-Hermann, R. and W. Parzefall. 1981. Failure to discriminate initiation from promotion of liver tumors in a long-term study with the phenobarbital-type inducer α- hexachlorocyclohexane and the role of sustained stimulation of hepatic growth and monooxygenases. *Cancer Res.* **41:** 4140.

Schulte-Hermann, R., I. Timmermann-Trosiener, and J. Schuppler. 1982. Response of liver foci in rats to hepatic tumor promoters. *Toxicol. Pathol.* **10:** 63.

———. 1983. Promotion of spontaneous preneoplastic cells in rat liver as a possible explanation of tumor production by nonmutagenic compounds. *Cancer Res.* **43:** 839.

———. 1984a. Aberrant expression of adaptation to phenobarbital may cause selective growth of foci of altered cells in rat liver. *Int. Agency Res. Cancer Sci. Publ.* **56:** 67.

———. 1986. Facilitated expression of adaptive responses to phenobarbital in putative prestages of liver cancer. *Carcinogenesis* **7:** 1651.

Schulte-Hermann, R., N. Roome, I. Timmermann-Trosiener, and J. Schuppler. 1984b. Immunocytochemical demonstration of a phenobarbital-inducible cytochrome P450 in putative preneoplastic foci of rat liver. *Carcinogenesis* **5:** 149.

Schulte-Hermann, R., G. Ohde, J. Schuppler, and I. Timmermann-Trosiener. 1981. Enhanced proliferation of putative preneoplastic cells in rat liver following treatment with the tumor promoters phenobarbital, hexachlorocyclohexane, steroid compounds, and nafenopin. *Cancer Res.* **41:** 2556.

Schulte-Hermann, R., V. Hoffmann, W. Parzefall, M. Kallenbach, A. Gerhardt, and J. Schuppler. 1980a. Adaptive responses of rat liver to the gestagen and anti-androgen cyproterone acetate and other inducers. II. Induction of growth. *Chem. Biol. Interact.* **31:** 287.

Schulte-Hermann, R., V. Hoffmann, and H. Landgraf. 1980b. Adaptive responses of rat liver to the gestagen and anti-androgen cyproterone acetate and other inducers. III. Cytological changes. *Chem. Biol. Interact.* **31:** 301.

Solt, D. and E. Farber. 1976. New principle for the analysis of chemical carcinogenesis. *Nature* **263:** 701.

Tatematsu, M., Y. Nagamine, and E. Farber. 1983. Redifferentiation as a basis for remodeling of carcinogen-induced hepatocyte nodules to normal appearing liver. *Cancer Res.* **43:** 5049.

Ward, J.M. 1983. Increased susceptibility of livers of aged F344/NCr rats to the effects of phenobarbital on the incidence, morphology, and histochemistry of hepatocellular foci and neoplasms. *J. Natl. Cancer Inst.* **71:** 815.

Watanabe, K. and G.M. Williams. 1978. Enhancement of rat hepatocellular altered foci by the liver tumor promoter phenobarbital: Evidence that foci are precursors of neoplasms and that the promoter acts on carcinogen-induced lesions. *J. Natl. Cancer Inst.* **61:** 1311.

Wyllie, A.H., J.F.R. Kerr, and A.R. Currie. 1980. Cell death: The significance of apoptosis. *Int. Rev. Cytol.* **68:** 251.

COMMENTS

PITOT: Since there are different phenotypes in the foci, have you ever looked to see if there is a difference in the labeling index in the foci of different phenotypes?

PARZEFALL: We have only looked at the phenotype of GGT-positive cells and not at what the labeling indexes are in other phenotypic expressions; so I cannot tell you.

PITOT: You haven't done that for the apoptoses either?

PARZEFALL: No, we haven't.

ROE: Are the microscopic appearances of apoptosis just single-cell death, or may one see multicellular areas of necrosis?

PARZEFALL: It seems to be a type of single-cell death. I can show you later some morphologic pictures which I did not want to show in this talk.

GHOSHAL: In your first slide, where you showed the GGT-positive focus, you showed the P-450 and other changes were returning. It seemed to me the focus is remodeling; does it come back?

PARZEFALL: Yes, that is our impression, that foci without addition of a promoter seem to be in a type of remodeling state, and therefore we have indicated here that this may equal a remodeling.

GHOSHAL: In the remodeling focus, the behavior is expected to be like normal cells, surrounding cells.

PARZEFALL: Right. But, when you apply the promoter, then you find no remodeling, which was here indicated as antiremodeling; and then, you find also that cell death is prevented.

GHOSHAL: If you want to see the effect of your promotion on the focus, then you have to study the foci that persist and not those that are remodeling.

PARZEFALL: How should we then distinguish between remodeling and nonremodeling foci? As long as we do not have the promoter, then might any focus be in a position to remodel?

GHOSHAL: All the foci are not remodeling because some go to cancer. It has been shown that there are nodules inside the nodules and cancer inside the nodules. You have to show the effect of your promoter on the persistent nodules, not on those remodeling ones.

PARZEFALL: I think that the foci produced by the selection regimen under AAF seem to have somewhat different properties. I have shown that the phenotype seems to remodel. You remember, we withdraw the phenobarbital and the incidence of foci which are GGT-positive drops almost down to control levels. Then we observe remodeling.

GHOSHAL: What about the apoptotic one? Does it come back to normalcy, or does it stay there or go out?

PARZEFALL: No, it stays high. We had measured the apoptotic incidence six weeks after phenobarbital was withdrawn, and it still was at a very high rate.

MAGEE: I may be the only one here who does not know, but can you tell me what exactly remodeling means?

PARZEFALL: It was defined in the paper of Tatematsu and Farber. We think that the expression of the phenotype is not stable, but it is able to regress.

MAGEE: So, does it differ then from just regression of papillomas?

SLAGA: Same thing.

PITOT: Remodeling might be considered biochemical metaplasia.

WILLIAMS: When you say remodeling now, is it in the sense that you believe it is accomplished by the loss of the cells from the foci due to death? That is very different than a phenotypic reversion.

PARZEFALL: We believe that both things occur, that cell death does not account for the full reversion of foci, and that what is thought to be remodeling is only a loss of a phenotypic marker in a given cell which is readily reexpressed after readdition of a promoter. So cell death and phenotypic remodeling may be two different mechanisms of regression.

WILLIAMS: Basically a change in phenotype.

PARZEFALL: Right.

Role of Cytotoxicity in the Carcinogenic Process

RICHARD H. REITZ
Mammalian and Environmental Toxicology Laboratory
Dow Chemical Company
Midland, Michigan 48640

OVERVIEW

It is now well documented that many materials that are capable of increasing the rates of tumor expression in animal bioassays apparently do so without reacting directly with DNA. These materials are called nongenotoxic carcinogens and are fundamentally different from agents that influence tumor expression through direct interaction with DNA (genotoxic carcinogens). A mathematical model that incorporates descriptions of metabolic activation, homeostatic control of critical macromolecules, saturable DNA repair systems, and rates of cell division influenced by chemical treatment has been developed, and this model was employed to demonstrate the ways in which nongenotoxic effects may influence the carcinogenic process in animals.

INTRODUCTION

There are many possible mechanisms through which interaction of chemicals and nongenetic components of the cell could influence the tumorigenic process, and several of these have been the subject of extensive research programs. This discussion focuses on one such mechanism: forced regeneration following cytotoxicity induced through chemical exposure.

Cytotoxicity (and compensatory cellular division) frequently occur in chronic animal studies because of the practice of giving animals a "maximum tolerated dose" in an effort to increase the likelihood that potential carcinogenicity will be detected. Berman et al. (1978) and Maher et al. (1979) have clearly shown that rapidly dividing cells are more sensitive to the action of transforming and/or mutagenic chemicals than are nondividing cells. Consequently, induction of cytotoxicity in target organs may have a profound "cocarcinogenic" effect with low levels of endogenous carcinogens. Since the animals used in bioassays have an appreciable rate of tumor development in the absence of any chemical treatment (e.g., lung and liver tumors in the B6C3F$_1$ mouse; leukemia and testicular cancer in the F344 rat), nongenotoxic carcinogens could increase the tumor yield without themselves "initiating" any new tumors.

In our laboratory, we have had experience with two chemicals that seem to fit the definition of nongenotoxic carcinogens acting through cytotoxic mechanisms: chloroform and sodium orthophenylphenol (SOPP).

Banbury Report 25: Nongenotoxic Mechanisms in Carcinogenesis
© Cold Spring Harbor Laboratory. 0-87969-225-1/87. $1.00 + .00

Chloroform

This material was found to produce tumors of the liver and kidney when high, cytotoxic doses were administered to rodents (National Cancer Institute 1976). However, although chloroform has been exhaustively studied in short-term tests, it appears to be almost completely devoid of direct genotoxic activity (Simon et al. 1977; Bridges et al. 1981; Brookes and Preston 1981). Furthermore, in vivo studies with [^{14}C]chloroform failed to demonstrate significant binding of chloroform to DNA, and carcinogenic doses of chloroform failed to induce DNA repair in vivo (Reitz et al. 1982). However, when carcinogenic doses of chloroform were administered to B6C3F$_1$ mice, microscopic examination and [^{3}H]thymidine uptake studies revealed cytotoxicity in liver and kidney tissues (Reitz et al. 1982).

Sodium Orthophenylphenol

Hiraga and Fujii (1981) reported that F344 rats consuming diets supplemented with high levels of SOPP developed tumors of the urinary tract, especially bladder tumors. However, like chloroform, this material did not show significant genotoxicity in various short-term tests and failed to show DNA binding in vivo (Yoshida et al. 1980; Reitz et al. 1983). Subsequently, SOPP was demonstrated to induce cytotoxicity in bladder epithelial cells at tumorigenic doses (Reitz et al. 1984).

To visualize the effects such agents may have on the tumorigenic process, a computer model derived from the work of Gehring and Blau (1977) and Reitz and Watanabe (1985) was developed. This model contains a series of simultaneous differential equations that were evaluated with ACSL (Mitchell and Gauthier Associates, Concord, Massachusetts). This program is available in a variety of configurations, including one that runs on the IBM personal computer, and all simulations shown in this paper were performed on an IBM-AT with 512K of memory and a 80287 math coprocessor.

RESULTS

Definition of the Model

A diagrammatic representation of the computer model is shown in Figure 1. This model assumes that the chemical requires metabolic activation before reaction with cellular components, but it could be modified to deal with directly reactive chemicals. A chemical enters the body in this simulation by first-order absorption (ka) from the gastrointestinal tract, and the amount of parent chemical inside the body at any time is given as AI. Other types of exposure could be simulated (e.g., inhalation of the chemical or dermal exposure) by substitution of appropriate equations here. Once the chemical has entered the body, it is either eliminated from

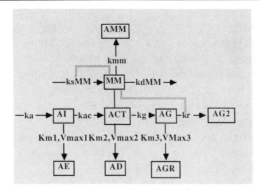

Figure 1

Diagram of the computer model used to simulate the effects of cytotoxicity on the carcinogenic process. (ka) Absorption rate constant; (kac) rate of metabolic activation; (kg) rate of binding to genetic material; (ksMM) variable rate of synthesis of MM; (kdMM) rate of degradation of MM; (kmm) rate of binding to MM; (AI, AE, ACT, AD, AMM, AG) amount of chemical absorbed, eliminated, activated, detoxified, bound to MM, and bound to genetic material, respectively; (AGR) amount of AG repaired by DNA repair systems; (AG2) DNA damage consolidated by replication; (MM) concentration of the critical macromolecule necessary for cell survival.

the body (AE) or activated to a reactive species (ACT). The activated chemical may then follow one of four routes: (1) It may be detoxified to give AD; (2) it may react with critical macromolecules (MM) to form macromolecular adducts (AMM); (3) it may react with noncritical, nongenetic molecules (not shown in Fig. 1 because of space limitations); or (4) it may react with genetic material to form AG. The adduct with genetic material (AG) may itself undergo DNA repair to yield repaired genetic material (AGR), or it may undergo replication before repair to give AG2.

It is assumed in the model that replication of genetic material containing unrepaired adducts may cause permanent alteration of the information within the cell (i.e., mutation) by causing misreading during formation of the complementary strands during cell division. Other possible mechanisms for modulating DNA activity (e.g., DNA methylation) are not considered here.

In this model, the rates of elimination (Km1, Vmax1), detoxification (Km2, Vmax2), and DNA repair (Km3, Vmax3) were simulated as capacity-limited processes described by Michaelis-Menten kinetics. The rate of reaction of ACT with MM (kmm) was described as a second-order process dependent on the concentration of both ACT and MM, and the rate of reaction of ACT with genetic material (kg) or nongenetic material (kng) was described as a pseudo-first-order process, since it appeared likely that the extent of reaction would be small (i.e., the concentration of unreacted molecules would remain essentially constant throughout the exposure).

This model is similar to that presented by Gehring and Blau (1977) but includes two additional features:

1. The depletion of macromolecules (MM) through reaction with activated chemical (ACT) is governed by a homeostatic mechanism such as those known to control levels of cellular components in nature. This causes the first-order rate constant for resynthesis of MM (ksMM) to increase to a predetermined maximum as the concentration of MM within the cell diminishes. (The first-order rate constant for degradation of MM, kdMM, is not affected by the concentration of MM).

2. The rate of cellular division (kr) is linked to the concentration of MM within the cell. It is assumed that cells in the model are dependent upon MM for some critical function. When MM is depleted in the model, some of the cells begin to die and are replaced by division of the survivors. It is assumed that the sensitivity of the cells to MM depletion follows a normal distribution, and an approximation for digital computers (Hastings 1955) was used to calculate the total number of cells affected in the model.

The equations that define these aspects of the model may be found in the program source code (see Fig. 5) under the headings Control of MM Synthesis and Control of Replication Rate, respectively.

It must be emphasized that the parameters employed in the model were chosen for purposes of illustration only. No attempt was made to include actual experimental data for any specific compound, since the objective was only to demonstrate the general types of effects that nongenotoxic agents might produce in vivo. However, sophisticated models of carcinogenesis have already been presented in the literature (Greenfield et al. 1984), and there is reason to believe that similar models could be developed for chloroform and SOPP if experimental data on the levels of glutathione and macromolecular binding, and rates of metabolism and cell division, were available. Development of such models is currently under way in our laboratory.

Time Course Data

Simulated values of the amount of chemical eliminated unchanged from the body, the amount of activated metabolite detoxified within the body, and the amount of activated metabolite escaping detoxification and binding to other macromolecules (including genetic material) are shown in Figure 2 for initial "doses" between 1 and 1000. The doses are in arbitrary units and were chosen to cover the region where nonlinearities in elimination, detoxification, and DNA repair exist.

In each case, the simulated data were normalized by dividing the parameters by D0, the administered dose, and then renormalized by dividing by the value of that parameter when the initial dose was equal to 1. Thus, if all the processes were linearly related to the administered dose, each of these lines would be parallel to the X-axis and would have a value of 1 throughout the entire range. As the dose increases from 1 to 100, the elimination of chemical (AE) becomes saturated,

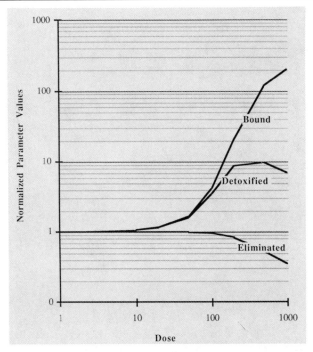

Figure 2
Simulated amounts of chemical eliminated, detoxified, or bound to some sort of macromolecule as a function of administered dose. The values have been normalized so that if all the processes modeled were linear, the lines would have a value of 1 throughout the dose range.

resulting in a larger percentage of the chemical being available for metabolic activation. This causes the proportion of the dose that is processed by the detoxification process (AD) to rise until that process also becomes saturated (at doses above 100). Saturation of detoxification results in a disproportionate level of chemical being bound to critical macromolecules, noncritical macromolecules, and genetic material (Fig. 2).

The homeostatic mechanism controlling MM synthesis in this model prevents significant depletion of MM following doses of 1, 10, or 100 units (simulated data not shown). However, saturation of detoxification and elimination mechanisms following a dose of 1000 results in a transient depletion of the critical macromolecule (MM) that cannot be balanced by the compensatory rise in MM synthesis (Fig. 3). As a result of the fall in concentration of the critical macromolecule, a certain percentage of the cells die and are subsequently replaced by cellular regeneration. The replication rate in the target organ for the next 24 hours is thus a function of the normal distribution curve relating cell death to loss of MM. In this model, it was

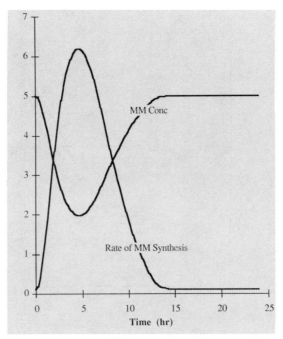

Figure 3

Simulated time course for the concentration of the critical macromolecule necessary for cell survival (MM) and the variable rate of its resynthesis after an administered dose of 1000 arbitrary units.

assumed that there were endogenous processes that provided a low background of alterations to DNA. Consequently, even for a nongenotoxic agent (kg = 0 in the model), an increase in kr would cause an increase in the number of genetic alterations that had been consolidated by replication (AG2, nongenotoxic) during the day on which the animal was dosed (Fig. 4). This means that a series of cytotoxic doses of a nongenotoxic agent could produce the same effect (an increase in the level of AG2) as a series of doses of a weakly genotoxic agent.

The model can be also be used to simulate the dose-response curve for an agent that is both cytotoxic and genotoxic by setting kg to some value greater than zero. Levels of DNA adducts formed with kg = 1.0 (equivalent to a potent genotoxin) after a series of doses from 1 to 1000 are also shown in Figure 4 (AG2, genotoxic).

With the constants used in this model, the simulated values of AG2 formed after a dose of 1000 units are almost seven orders of magnitude higher than would be predicted from linear extrapolation of AG2 levels at a dose of 1. This dramatic increase results from the fact that cellular replication has increased at the very time that DNA repair mechanisms are saturated and hence less efficient in removing DNA damage.

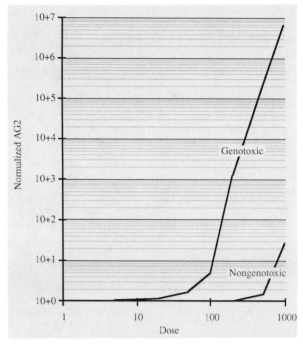

Figure 4

Simulated values of the amount of replicated genetic lesions (AG2) for nongenotoxic (kg = 0) and genotoxic (kg = 1) agents as a function of dose.

SUMMARY

The computer model presented here is, of course, completely hypothetical, since none of the constants employed are related to real experimental data. Nevertheless, the components of the model are taken from real-life situations. Many elimination, detoxification, and DNA repair processes are known to be capacity-limited; the concentrations of critical components of the cell are usually tightly regulated by feedback control mechanisms; and populations of cells exposed to toxic agents (e.g., bacteria and disinfectant agents) probably do have normally distributed sensitivities. Given these general assumptions, the model demonstrates one possible way in which a cytotoxic agent might influence the tumorigenic process without any direct effect on DNA. We hope that development of models such as these may provide some guidance in assessing the risk associated with the exposure of humans to nongenotoxic carcinogens.

A software package available from Mitchell and Gauthier Associates (Concord, Massachusetts) was used to process the computer model simulating the effects of cytotoxicity on the carcinogenic process. The source code for this model is presented in Figure 5.

```
PROGRAM BANBURY.CSL


INITIAL      $'This section defines the constants used in the Model'

CONSTANT    D0 = 1.0        $'Initial Dose Value (arbitrary units)'
CONSTANT    kab = 0.4       $'Absorption Rate Constant'
CONSTANT    Km1 = 0.5       $'Km for Elim of Parent'
CONSTANT    Vm1 = 2.5       $'Vmax for Elim of Parent'
CONSTANT    Km2 = 0.1       $'Km for Detox of ACT'
CONSTANT    Vm2 = 0.5       $'Vmax for Detox of ACT'
CONSTANT    Km3 = 0.01      $'Km for DNA Repair'
CONSTANT    Vm3 = 1.0       $'Vmax for DNA Repair'
CONSTANT    kmm = 0.1       $'Rate Constant MM Binding'
CONSTANT    kg = 1.0        $'Rate Constant DNA Binding'
CONSTANT    kac = 1.0       $'Activation rate constant'

CONSTANT    MM0 = 5.0       $'Set Point for MM Synthesis'
CONSTANT    MM2 = 3.1746    $'Midpoint of Cell Death Distribution'
CONSTANT    SIGMA = 0.25    $'Relative width of Distribution'
CONSTANT    ksMax = 10.0    $'Max Rate of synthesis of MM'
CONSTANT    kdMM =  0.1     $'Rate Constant Endog. Destruct of MM'
CONSTANT    ks0  =  0.1     $'Rate Constant Endog. Synthesis of MM'
CONSTANT    kr0  = 1.0E-4   $'Endogenous Cell Division Rate'

            SIGMA2 = SIGMA * MM2   $'Calc SIGMA in Absolute Units'
            LNMM0  = ALOG(MM0)     $'For Log Transformation'

CONSTANT  TSTOP = 24.0     $'End of Simulation         '
CONSTANT  POINTS = 96.0    $'To control number of outputs'
            CINT = TSTOP/POINTS    $'Communication Interval'

END $ ' of INITIAL Section '

DYNAMIC
    TERMT(T .GE. TSTOP)
DERIVATIVE

    ALGORITHM IALG = 2
    NSTEPS    NSTP = 1000


'*************************************************'
'--------- Control of Replication Rate -------'
'*************************************************'


'Approximation for Digital Computers from Hastings (1955)'
   'ND1 is the Input Function (Dist along axis of Norm Dist Curve)'
   'ND2 is the area under the NDist curve up to point (MM0 - MM)'
   'ND2 will always be between 0 and 1 and = fraction affected. '
```

Figure 5

Source code for computer model used to visualize the effects of agents on the tumorigenic process.

```
ND1 = ((MM0 - MM) - MM2) / SIGMA2      $ 'Calc the Input Function'
PARM1 = ABS(ND1)                       $ 'Convert Absolute Value'
PARM2 = 1.0 / (1.0 + 0.2316419*PARM1)
ND3 = 0.3989423 * EXP(-ND1*ND1/2.0)
ND2 = 1.0 - ND3*PARM2*((((1.330274*PARM2 - 1.821256)*PARM2 ...
+ 1.781478)*PARM2 - 0.3565638)*PARM2 + 0.3193815)
NDAREA = RSW(ND1 .LT. 0.0, 1.0-ND2, ND2)
IF( (NDAREA+kr0) .GT. kr ) kr = NDAREA + kr0


'***********************************************'
'--------- Control of MM Synthesis -----------'
'***********************************************'

          ksMM  =  ks0 + ksMax*(MM0 - MM)/MM0

'Model Definition Given Below'

          GUTIN = D0 * EXP(-kab * T) * kab
          RAI = GUTIN  - VM1*AI/(KM1+AI) - AI*kac
          AI  = INTEG(RAI, 0.0)

          RAE = VM1*AI / (KM1 + AI)
          AE  = INTEG(RAE, 0.0)

          RACT = AI*kac - ACT*VM2/(KM2+ACT) - ACT*MM*kmm -ACT*kg
          ACT  = INTEG(RACT, 0.0)

          RAD = ACT*VM2/(KM2+ACT)
          AD  = INTEG(RAD,0.0)

          RAMM = ACT*MM*kmm
          AMM  = INTEG(RAMM, 0.0)

          RAG = ACT*kg - AG*VM3/(KM3+AG)
          AG  = INTEG(RAG, 0.0)

          RAGR = AG*VM3/(KM3+AG)
          AGR  = INTEG(RAGR, 0.0)

          RAG2 = AG*kr
          AG2  = INTEG(RAG2, 0.0)

'Log Transformation here for smoother Integration'

          RLNMM  =  ksMM -kdMM -ACT*kmm
          LNMM   =  INTEG(RLNMM, LNMM0)
          LNMMS  =  RSW(LNMM .GT. -75.0, LNMM, -75.0)
                         $'Smallest = e-75'
          MM  =  EXP(LNMMS)

END  $ ' of DERIVATIVE Section '
END  $ ' of DYNAMIC Section    '
END  $ ' of PROGRAM            '
```

Figure 5 (*Continued***)**

REFERENCES

Berman, J.J., C. Tong, and G.M. Williams. 1978. Enhancement of mutagenesis during cell replication of cultured liver epithelial cells. *Cancer Lett.* **4:** 277.

Bridges, B.A., E. Zieger, and D.B. McGregor. 1981. Summary report on the performance of bacterial mutation assays. *Prog. Mutat. Res.* **1:** 49.

Brookes, P. and R.J. Preston. 1981. Summary report on the performance of *in vitro* mammalian assays. *Prog. Mutat. Res.* **1:** 77.

Gehring, P.J. and G.E. Blau. 1977. Mechanisms of carcinogenesis: Dose response. *J. Environ. Pathol. Toxicol.* **1:** 163.

Greenfield, R.E., L.B. Ellwein, and S.M. Cohen. 1984. A general probabilistic model of carcinogenesis: Analysis of experimental urinary bladder cancer. *Carcinogenesis* **5:** 437.

Hastings, C. 1955. In *Approximations for digital computers*, p. 26. Princeton University Press, Princeton, New Jersey.

Hiraga, K. and T. Fujii. 1981. Induction of tumors of the urinary system in F344 rats by dietary administration of sodium o-phenylphenate. *Food Cosmet. Toxicol.* **19:** 303.

Maher, V.M., D.J. Dorney, A.L. Mendrala, B. Konze-Thomas, and J.J. McCormick. 1979. DNA excision repair processes in human cells can eliminate the cytotoxic and mutagenic consequences of ultraviolet irradiation. *Mutat. Res.* **62:** 311.

National Cancer Institute. 1976. *Carcinogenesis bioassay of chloroform.* National Tech. Inform. Service No. PB264018/AS, Washington, D.C.

Reitz, R.H. and P.G. Watanabe. 1985. Mechanistic considerations in the formulation of carcinogenic risk estimations. *Banbury Rep.* **19:** 241.

Reitz, R.H., T.R. Fox, and J.F. Quast. 1982. Mechanistic considerations for carcinogenic risk estimation: Chloroform. *Environ. Health Perspect.* **46:** 163.

Reitz, R.H., T.R. Fox, J.F. Quast, E.A. Hermann, and P.G. Watanabe. 1983. Molecular mechanisms involved in the toxicity of orthophenylphenol and its sodium salt. *Chem. Biol. Interact.* **43:** 99.

————. 1984. Biochemical factors involved in the effects of orthophenylphenol (OPP) and sodium orthophenylphenol (SOPP) on the urinary tract of male F344 rats. *Toxicol. Appl. Pharmacol.* **73:** 345.

Simon, V.F., K. Kauhanen, and R.G. Tardiff. 1977. Mutagenic activity of chemicals identified in the drinking water. In *Proceedings of the 2nd International Meeting of the Environmental Mutagen Society*, Edinburgh, Scotland.

Yoshida, S., M. Masubuchi, and K. Hiraga. 1980. Cytogenetic studies of antimicrobials on cultured cells. *Pesticide Abstr.* **80:** 2624.

COMMENTS

WILLIAMS: Concerning the mechanisms by which increased cell proliferation increases tumorigenesis, I think the kind of experiments that you were talking about (starting with that illustration from the work of McCormick and Maher, where proliferation is stimulated at a short time after the exposure to a genotoxic agent, at which time DNA damage is still present) are, in principle, very different from the kind of study that, for example, Dr. Pitot showed, where there is a single exposure to a carcinogen, which can then be followed after an interval by a promoter which can be removed and then reapplied, causing reappearance of the lesions. Those latter kinds of experiments I would regard as being true promotion experiments. But the other kinds of studies, where cell proliferation is stimulated either at the time of carcinogen damage, or even shortly thereafter while there are persisting adducts, really are more what was originally termed cocarcinogenesis. The mechanism is quite different. If we are going to be discussing mechanisms of nongenotoxic carcinogens, it behooves us to be clear about what kinds of phenomena we are discussing.

REITZ: I'd be happy to call this cocarcinogenesis if you like. The point is, because of the high doses used in the animal bioassays, cocarcinogenesis may be fairly common in these experiments. Incidentally, when a material is both cytotoxic and genotoxic, as many potent alkylating agents are, the model predicts a pronounced synergistic effect between genotoxicity and cytotoxicity at high dose levels.

MAGEE: In connection with what you have just said, wouldn't you expect all genotoxic agents to be cytotoxic if the dose was made big enough?

REITZ: As you know very well, with dimethylnitrosamine you don't have to go very high above the initiating dose before you begin to see very significant liver damage.

SARMA: There are some exceptions, though. Methylnitrosourea doesn't induce liver cell necrosis. You may kill the animal before you see necrosis in the liver.

TRUMP: Yes. That is not the usual case; that was the point that I was trying to make. It is in the usual case with complete carcinogens that you have necrosis, regeneration, and mutagenicity.

SWENBERG: Well, along that line, I think we have to remember that most of these compounds get tested at an MTD. Since cytotoxicity is a high-dose effect, it is probably one of the factors responsible for nonlinearities. By and large, I do not believe these are adequately factored into the regulatory assessment.

The Value of Measuring Cell Replication as a Predictive Index of Tissue-specific Tumorigenic Potential

DAVID J. LOURY, THOMAS L. GOLDSWORTHY, AND
BYRON E. BUTTERWORTH
Chemical Industry Institute of Toxicology
Department of Genetic Toxicology
Research Triangle Park, North Carolina 27709

OVERVIEW

There is increasing concern that some of the chemicals that produce negative results in short-term tests for genotoxicity may represent human carcinogens. At the present time, few short-term assays are available for the detection of nongenotoxic carcinogens. The data presented in this paper demonstrate that many nongenotoxic agents that induce hepatic or renal tumors in laboratory animals also increase replicative DNA synthesis in the appropriate target organ following short-term exposure. Of the 16 inducers of cell replication in the liver surveyed, 15 have exhibited tumorigenic activity in either the rat or mouse liver. Among the five renal carcinogens evaluated, four were found to increase renal DNA synthesis activity. An examination of the parameters influencing the stimulation of replicative DNA synthesis in the liver of male F344 rats revealed the importance of controlling lighting cycles. The data suggest that the quantitation of replicative DNA synthesis as a measure of cell replication activity provides a reasonably accurate indication of the tumorigenic potential of chemical agents possessing little, if any, genotoxic activity. Thus, this method represents an attractive first-step approach to the short-term detection of nongenotoxic carcinogens.

INTRODUCTION

The preliminary screening of new compounds for carcinogenic potential is generally conducted with one or more short-term assays designed to detect genotoxicity. By far the most frequently used primary screening system is the *Salmonella* mutagenicity assay (Ashby 1982). In validation studies, this assay has detected between 63% 92% of the carcinogens tested (Rinkus and Legator 1979); that is, the false-negative rate of the *Salmonella* mutagenicity test varies between 8% and 37%. Many of the carcinogens that fail to induce mutations in the *Salmonella* assay give negative results in many other short-term assays for genotoxicity and are thus classified as nongenotoxic (ICPEMC 1984). This class of carcinogens creates a serious

Banbury Report 25: Nongenotoxic Mechanisms in Carcinogenesis
© Cold Spring Harbor Laboratory. 0-87969-225-1/87. $1.00 + .00

dilemma for screening programs, since very few short-term tests for carcinogenic potential rely on a nongenetic endpoint. Therefore, a considerable need exists to expand our present understanding of the mechanisms involved in the tumorigenic activity of nongenotoxic carcinogens and to develop short-term assays for the detection of this class of compounds.

Current interest in measuring chemically induced cell proliferation as a means of identifying nongenotoxic carcinogens stems from a variety of theoretical consider-ations and experimental observations. Studies have shown that carcinogens have a greater ability to induce tumors if administered when the cells of a target tissue are rapidly dividing (Frei and Harsono 1967; Craddock 1973). The increased synthesis of DNA in replicating tissue apparently facilitates the initiation of chemically induced carcinogenesis by converting chemical-DNA lesions into permanent somatic mutations before they can be repaired. In a similar manner, an elevation in cell proliferation activity may increase the conversion of spontaneously occurring DNA lesions into somatic mutations and accelerate the formation of mutations arising from the normal DNA replication process (Stott et al. 1981). Furthermore, the altered structural configuration of replicating DNA may enhance the initiation of tumorigenesis by facilitating the formation of chemical-DNA adducts (Rajalakshmi et al. 1982).

Besides affecting the initiation stage of carcinogenesis, chemically induced cell replication may also promote the development of neoplastic lesions. For example, the number of preneoplastic foci in the liver of rats treated with benzo(a)pyrene or dimethylhydrazine is dramatically increased when, 3 weeks after treatment, rats are exposed to doses of carbon tetrachloride that stimulate hepatic cell division (Tsudu et al. 1980; Mirsalis et al. 1982). Similarly, the induction of epidermal cell proliferation appears to be an important factor in the second-stage promotion of mouse skin tumors (Slaga 1984). Recent studies have also demonstrated that neoplastic development in the kidney can be promoted by agents that induce tubular regeneration through a nephrotoxic mechanism (Shirai et al. 1984).

Proposed Classification System for Potential Hepatocarcinogens

Previously, we proposed that potential hepatocarcinogens can be divided into three distinct categories (Butterworth et al. 1985). The first category consists of compounds (type I agents) that cause primary genetic damage to the liver in vivo. Such compounds have a high likelihood of being hepatocarcinogens. The second group consists of compounds (type II agents) that lack direct genotoxicity in the liver but induce an adaptive response characterized by an increase in the number of liver cells. This response is referred to here as additive hyperplasia. The third group is made up of compounds (type III agents) that induce hepatic necrosis but exhibit no measurable hepatic genotoxicity when administered to the whole animal. The cell proliferation produced by such agents is referred to here as regenerative hyperplasia. As mentioned above, many nephrotoxic agents also promote the development of renal neoplasms. Nongenotoxic nephrotoxicants may therefore represent a class of potential kidney carcinogens similar in character to type III hepatotoxicants.

Several facile laboratory procedures are available for determining whether chemically induced cell replication in the liver represents a regenerative or an additive response. Identifying features of an additive response are as follows: (1) an increase in the total DNA content of the liver; (2) an increase in liver weight when coupled with an increase in replicative DNA synthesis; (3) no histopathological signs of necrosis; (4) no increase in serum alanine transaminase (ALT/SGPT) activity; and (5) for compounds with a relatively short whole-body half-life, replicative DNA synthesis that is maximal 24 hours after treatment. Regenerative hyperplasia in the liver is characterized by (1) histopathological signs of necrosis, (2) an increase in serum alanine transaminase activity, and (3) replicative DNA synthesis that is generally maximal 48 hours after treatment.

Most of the methods currently used for assessing in vivo cell proliferation activity are based upon the quantitative determination of replicative DNA synthesis (RDS). In the present study, the induction of RDS activity by nongenotoxic compounds was evaluated as a predictive indicator of carcinogenic potential in the liver and kidney. Also, experimental parameters influencing the detection of RDS activity in the liver were examined.

RESULTS

RDS as an Indicator of Carcinogenic Potential

The carcinogenic activity of various nongenotoxic inducers of hepatic and renal cell proliferation are presented in Tables 1 through 3. Chemicals were chosen so as to comprise a number of chemical classes. For the purposes of this report, compounds with little to no in vitro genotoxicity were considered to be nongenotoxic. Ideally, in vivo determinations of genotoxicity in the liver and kidney would have provided a more realistic basis for selecting nongenotoxic compounds. However, at their present stage of development, in vivo assays generally do not afford the same degree of sensitivity as in vitro systems, and the number of compounds examined by these methods is relatively small. Nevertheless, a negative response in an in vitro genotoxicity assay cannot be viewed as irrefutable evidence that a compound lacks genotoxic activity in vivo, as was demonstrated in the case of dinitrotoluene (Mirsalis and Butterworth 1982).

Nongenotoxic agents that cause additive hyperplasia in the liver (type II agents) are presented in Table 1. Phenobarbital is considered the prototype compound of this group, which includes various organochlorine insecticides, the food additive butylated hydroxytoluene (BHT), hypolipidemic drugs, halogenated biphenyl

Table 1
Induction of Liver Tumors by Stimulators of Additive Hyperplasia (Type II Agents) in the Liver

Agent	In vitro genotoxicity	↑ in Replicative DNA synthesis[a]	Liver tumors[b] mouse	Liver tumors[b] rat	References
Phenobarbital	–	+	+	+	IARC (1977); Schulte-Hermann et al. (1982); ICPEMC (1984)
α-HCH[c]	–	+	+	+	Ito et al. (1975, 1976); Shirasu et al. (1976); Schulte-Hermann (1977)
Dieldrin	–	(+)[d]	+	–	IARC (1974); McCann et al. (1975)
Aldrin	–	(+)[d]	+	–	IARC (1974); Rinkus and Legator (1979)
DDT	–	(+)[d]	+	w + [e]	IARC (1974); Rossi et al. (1977); Purchase et al. (1978)
BHT	–	+	–	–	Shulte-Hermann et al. (1971); NCI (1979); ICPEMC (1984)
Nafenopin	–	+	+	+	IARC (1980); Schulte-Hermann et al. (1983a)
DEHP	–	+	+	+	NTP (1983a); Butterworth et al. (1984); Zeiger et al. (1985)
Wy-14,643	–	+[f]	+	+	Reddy et al. (1979); Warren et al. (1980)
PBB	–	+	+	+	IARC (1978); NTP (1983b); Mirsalis et al. (1985)
TCDD	–	+	+	+	Geiger and Neal (1981); NTP (1982); Lutz et al. (1984)
Ethinylestradiol	–	+	–	+	IARC (1979a); Lang and Redmann (1979); Ochs et al. (1986)
TMP	–	+	n.a.[g]	n.a.	Loury et al. (1986)

[a] Replicative DNA synthesis measured in rat liver.
[b] Both hepatocarcinomas and hepatoadenomas are reported as tumors.
[c] Abbreviations: (α-HCH) α-hexachlorocyclohexane; (DDT) dichlorodiphenyltrichloroethane; (BHT) butylated hydroxytoluene; (DEHP) di(2-ethylhexyl)phthalate; (Wy-14,643) [4-chloro-6-(2,3-xylidino)-2-pyrimidinylthio]acetic acid; (PBB) polybrominated biphenyls; (TCDD) 2,3,7,8-tetrachlorodibenzodioxin; (TMP) 2,2,4-trimethylpentane.
[d] Total DNA content of liver increased (Schulte-Hermann 1974).
[e] Both negative and positive tumorigenic results have been reported.
[f] Measured in mouse hepatocytes.
[g] Tumorigenicity data not available (n.a.).

compounds such as polybrominated biphenyls (PBBs), and sex steroids. Reports of increased RDS in the rat liver were found for 10 of the 13 type II compounds listed. The three exceptions, dieldrin, aldrin, and DDT, are considered presumptive inducers of RDS because each increases the total DNA content of the liver. Of the 12 type II compounds for which tumorigenicity was available, 10 compounds caused an increase in liver tumors (both hepatocarcinomas and hepatoadenomas) in the mouse, and 9 compounds (including DDT, which gave negative and positive responses) increased the incidence of liver tumors in the rat.

Only limited data were available concerning the induction of DNA synthesis by cytotoxic mouse and rat liver toxins possessing, at most, weak genotoxic activity in vitro (type III agents; Table 2). Tumorigenic activity in the mouse liver has been observed with all five of the compounds listed, whereas only two of the five compounds were tumorigenic in the rat. In the three cases where RDS data were available for both the mouse and the rat, greater activity was observed in the mouse.

Table 2
Induction of Liver Tumors by Cytotoxic Mouse and Rat Hepatotoxicants Possessing, at Most, Weak Genotoxic Activity In Vitro (Type III Agents)

Agent	In vitro genotoxicity	↑ in Replicative DNA synthesis[a]		Liver tumors[b]		References
		mouse	rat	mouse	rat	
Carbon tetrachloride	−	+ +	+	+ +	+	Weisburger (1977); ICPEMC (1984); Loury et al. (1986)
Chloroform	−	+ +	−	+ +	−	Weisburger (1977); ICPEMC (1984); Pereira et al. (1984)
Trichloroethylene	w + [c]	+ +	+	+	−	Scott et al. (1982); IPCS (1985); Lundberg et al. (1986)
Tetrachloroethylene (perchloroethylene)	w + [c]	+ +	+	+	−	Brem et al. (1974); Truffert et al. (1977); IARC (1979b); Schumann et al. (1980); Hayes et al. (1986)
Tannic acid	−			+	+	IARC (1976); Shimoi et al. (1985)

[a] Replicative DNA synthesis measured in rat liver.
[b] Both hepatocarcinomas and hepatoadenomas are reported as tumors.
[c] (w +) Weak activity in *Salmonella* mutagenicity assay.

The data presented in Table 3 are a compilation of renal RDS responses observed in experiments performed in our laboratory. Kidney tumorigenicity data were available for seven of the nine compounds listed. RDS responses correlated to tumorigenic activity in six out of seven cases, with the one exception being the kidney carcinogen trichloroethylene. It should be noted, however, that trichloroethylene is a weak genotoxicant in vitro and may also have genotoxic activity in vivo (Costa and Ivanetich 1984).

Methods for Measuring RDS

Normally, in vivo RDS activity is determined using either liquid scintillation counting or autoradiographic methods for detecting the incorporation of radiolabeled thymidine into DNA. Although liquid scintillation counting provides a rapid assessment of RDS activity, certain factors may limit the validity of results obtained by this method. For instance, some chemical agents may alter the amount of radioactive label available for incorporation by modulating thymidine pool sizes and rates of phosphorylation (Oberdisse et al. 1970). Scintillometric methods also cannot distinguish repair synthesis (induced by genotoxic agents) from replicative synthesis. Furthermore, experimental errors associated with the administration of radiolabeled thymidine can reduce the precision with which RDS responses are measured. These potential shortcomings can be avoided, however, if RDS activity is determined by quantitative autoradiography. This technique involves the identification and quantitation of cells undergoing RDS (S-phase cells) and is not influenced quantitatively by thymidine availability.

An autoradiographic determination of in vivo RDS activity can be made either from thin tissue slices prepared from animals injected with tritiated thymidine ([^{3}H]thymidine) or from preparations of isolated cells exposed to [^{3}H]thymidine in vitro. Because a relatively high concentration of [^{3}H]thymidine can be delivered to isolated cells, emulsion-exposure times of 1 week or less are generally adequate when in vitro radiolabeling is used. In contrast, tissues radiolabeled in vivo can require up to 6 weeks of emulsion exposure. In our laboratory, in vivo RDS activity is generally assessed by radiolabeling cells in vitro. Following a 4-hour incubation with medium containing 10 μCi/ml [^{3}H]thymidine, cells are fixed and washed thoroughly. Cells are then mounted onto glass microscope slides and dipped in photographic emulsion. After a 1-week exposure in the dark, the emulsion is developed to reveal silver grains (Loury et al. 1986). The percentage of cells in S phase (those with a dense pattern of silver grains over the nucleus) on each slide is determined as a measure of RDS activity. In general, three slides are scored per animal. Because responses are more variable in the liver than in the kidney, the determination of hepatic RDS activity usually requires a group size of five to six animals instead of the three animals per group normally employed for renal RDS determinations.

Table 3
Induction of Renal Tumors by Agents That Increase Replicative DNA
Synthesis in the Kidney

Agent	In vitro genotoxicity	↑ in Replicative DNA synthesis[a] male	female	Kidney tumors[b] male	female	References
Chloroform	−	+ +	+	+ +	+	Weisburger (1977); ICPEMC (1984)
Tetrachloroethylene	−	+		+	−	NTP (1986)
Pentachloroethane	−	+		+	−	NTP (1983c)
Trichloroethylene	w +[c]	−		+	−	NTP (1983d); IPCS (1985)
Unleaded gasoline	w +[d]	+ +	−	+	−	MacFarland (1982); Loury et al. (1987)
2,2,4-Trimethylpentane	−	+ +	−	n.a.[e]	n.a.	Richardson et al. (1986)
Gentamicin			+ +	n.a.	n.a.	Laurent et al. (1984)
Carbon tetrachloride	−	−		−	−	Weisburger (1977); ICPEMC (1984)
Iodoform		−		−	−	Weisburger (1977)

[a] Replicative DNA synthesis measured in rat kidney. Except for the response reported for gentamicin, all DNA synthesis responses were measured in this laboratory.
[b] Epithelial tumors in the rat.
[c] Weakly active in *Salmonella* mutagenicity assay.
[d] Weakly active in hepatocyte/UDS assay.
[e] Tumorigenicity data not available (n.a.).

Parameters Affecting the Measurement of RDS in the Liver

Chemically induced and basal RDS activities in the liver may be affected by a variety of factors. Previously, Schulte-Hermann (1977) demonstrated that the stimulation of hepatic RDS by α-hexachlorocyclohexane (α-HCH) in female Wistar rats is influenced by lighting cycles and food intake. The onset of RDS activity was found to occur invariably 5–8 hours after food was made available to the rats. Lighting cycles did not directly affect RDS, but rather influenced the timing of food consumption. In these experiments, the normal light-dark cycle was inverted (dark phase: 8:00 am to 8:00 pm) and food was available for only the first 5 hours of the dark period.

We have conducted a series of experiments to determine the influence of feeding and lighting cycles on chemically induced RDS activity in the male Fischer 344 (F344) rat. In particular, we wished to know whether peak RDS activity could be measured in these animals during normal working hours without inverting the normal lighting cycle. The RDS response characteristics of the F344 rat were of special interest because of the growing body of information from the National Toxicology Program concerning the induction of liver tumors in this strain of rat.

Hepatic RDS was induced by 2,2,4-trimethylpentane (TMP), a nephrotoxic component of unleaded gasoline that stimulates additive hyperplasia in the liver (Loury et al. 1986). Animals were adapted for 3 days to a light-dark cycle in which the dark period occurred between 9:00 pm and 7:00 am. This lighting schedule represents only a minor deviation from the normally maintained 7:00 am to 7:00 pm light-dark cycle. One group of rats was allowed access to food between 9:30 pm and 7:00 am, and another group received food between 1:30 am and 8:00 am. Following the adaptation period, rats were treated by gavage with a single 500 mg/kg dose of TMP or an equivalent volume of corn oil at 8:00 am. Lighting and feeding cycles were maintained for an additional 24-hour period, after which rats were given intraperitoneal injections of [^{3}H]thymidine 1 hour prior to sacrifice by asphyxiation with carbon dioxide. Livers were perfused with phosphate-buffered saline and excised. Methods described by Schulte-Hermann (1977) were used to isolate hepatic DNA and determine its specific activity.

As illustrated in Figure 1, a peak in thymidine incorporation occurred 26 hours (10:00 am) after treatment with TMP irrespective of feeding times. This response pattern indicates that in male F344 rats, the time of food administration during the dark period does not affect the timing of the TMP-induced RDS response. The effect of lighting cycles on the RDS response to TMP was evaluated by advancing the light-to-dark transition by 3 hours (from 9:00 am to midnight). As illustrated in Figure 2, the rise in DNA synthesis was delayed by 3 hours and thus peaked at 29 hours after treatment. A comparison of Figures 1 and 2 shows that in all cases, RDS activity peaked at 13 hours after the light-to-dark transition of the previous night. Thus, for the sex and strain of rat examined, the light-dark rhythm and not the feeding schedule was the dominant factor influencing the timing of DNA synthesis induced by TMP.

For the routine measurement of RDS in the liver of male F344 rats, it is clear that lighting cycles must be controlled. Experiments utilizing isolated cells should be performed such that [^{3}H]thymidine is administered at approximately 11–12 hours after the light-to-dark transition of the previous night. To accomplish this during normal working hours, a 10:00 pm to 8:00 am dark period may be most satisfactory. Rats require only 3 days to adapt to this schedule if previously maintained on a 7:00 am to 7:00 pm cycle. Furthermore, hepatic RDS activity should be measured at both 24 and 48 hours after treatment to ensure detection of the widest spectrum of compounds.

DISCUSSION

The data presented in this paper provide some insights into the relationship between the induction of DNA synthesis and the tumorigenic potential of nongenotoxic compounds. Hyperplastic responses in the liver and kidney to nongenotoxic agents were compared to carcinogenic responses. With the exception of BHT, each of the agents capable of inducing additive hyperplasia in the liver increased the liver tumor

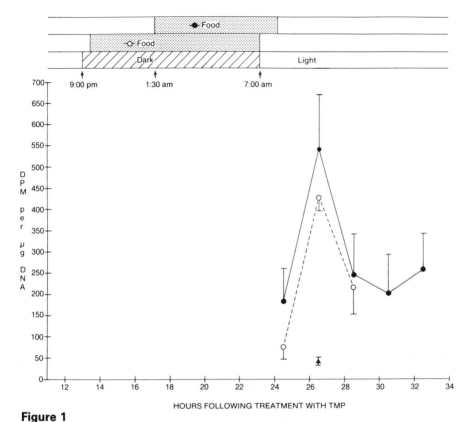

Figure 1

Thymidine incorporation into hepatic DNA of rats exposed to 2,2,4-trimethylpentane (TMP). Rats were preadapted for 3 days to the indicated lighting and feeding cycles. Treated rats (●,○) received 500 mg/kg TMP by gavage at 8:00 am. Control rats (▲) were maintained on a 1:30–8:00 am feeding cycle and received an equivalent volume of corn oil at 8:00 am. Each point is the mean of five animals. All animals were injected with [^{3}H]thymidine 1 hr prior to sacrifice at the indicated times. Error bars represent the standard error of the mean.

incidence in either rats or mice (Table 1). Thus, based on the compounds examined, the measurement of hepatic RDS as an indicator of carcinogenic potential in the liver (either mouse or rat) had a predictive value of 91% (predictive value is defined by Purchase [1982] as the number of positive results from carcinogens divided by the total number of positive results). More specifically, RDS activity induced in the rat liver by type II agents was a predictive indicator of tumorigenic activity in the mouse liver in 83% of the cases examined and predicted tumorigenicity in the rat liver in 75% of all cases. Recently, Purchase (1982) demonstrated that if a relatively large proportion of the compounds examined in a validation study are carcinogens, the performance of a short-term assay will be biased in a favorable direction. Since

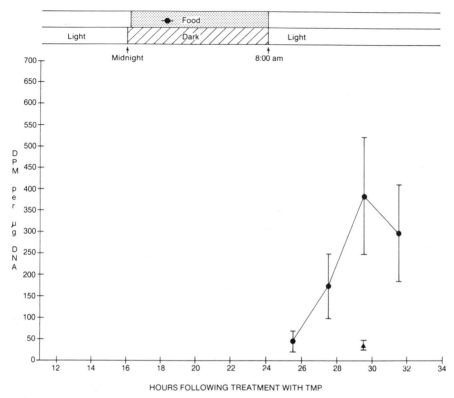

Figure 2

Thymidine incorporation into hepatic DNA of rats exposed to TMP. Rats were preadapted for 3 days to the indicated lighting and feeding cycle. Treated rats (●) received 500 mg/kg TMP by gavage at 8:00 am. See Fig. 1 for description of other conditions.

over 90% of the type II compounds listed in Table 1 were classified as carcinogens, the predictive values reported here are probably somewhat optimistic. Nevertheless, we believe the data indicate that nongenotoxic inducers of additive cell proliferation in the liver have at least a moderately high probability of increasing the hepatic tumor incidence in rats and/or mice following chronic administration.

A limited number of nongenotoxic compounds were examined that induce regenerative hyperplasia in the liver (Table 2). The data suggest the RDS responses to these agents are somewhat species-dependent, with the mouse generally being more sensitive than the rat. Species sensitivity to the induction of liver tumors paralleled hepatotoxicity as measured by RDS. The data presented indicate that when administered over the life span of an animal, type III agents have a modest probability of increasing the hepatic tumor incidence in the animal species in which the activity is measured. It should be noted that many apparently nongenotoxic agents produce liver tumors in the mouse but not in the rat, suggesting that mouse liver cells may, in some way, already be initiated (Ward et al. 1979; Doull et al. 1983). Many long-term bioassay studies are criticized as irrelevant because of the extraordinarily high doses of compound used to induce tumors. Further studies correlating recurrent cytotoxicity to the induction of hepatic tumors may better define the value of measuring cell turnover as a predictive index for carcinogenic potential and may provide a relevant new parameter for determining the "maximum tolerated dose" for long-term exposure.

The relationship between chemically induced RDS activity in the kidney and the induction of renal neoplasia was evaluated. Elevated RDS activity provided an indication of renal carcinogenic potential in the case of chloroform, tetrachloro-ethylene, pentachloroethane, and unleaded gasoline; however, no RDS activity was observed with the renal carcinogen trichloroethylene. Thus, many of the compounds that induce RDS in the kidney appear to be weak renal carcinogens, whereas other agents such as trichloroethylene apparently induce renal neoplasms by a mechanism unrelated to the stimulation of RDS activity in nonneoplastic tissue.

Nongenotoxic inducers of additive hyperplasia in the liver (type II agents) may be tumorigenic by virtue of a mechanism distinct from that involved in the tumorigenic activity of cytotoxic compounds. Although both types of agents increase replicative DNA synthesis in the liver, the response associated with additive hyperplasia is transitory. Once the liver has attained a certain size, a feedback mechanism comes into play that limits cell proliferation and DNA synthesis (Schulte-Hermann and Schmitz 1980). Type II agents produce an increase in cell proliferation within preneoplastic liver foci as well, but this activity also returns to noninduced levels following repeated exposure (Schulte-Hermann et al. 1982, 1983a). Studies have demonstrated that the promotion of liver tumors by type II agents is most effective when administration is continued well beyond the period of elevated cell proliferation (Peraino et al. 1973), suggesting that enhanced RDS activity is not directly coupled to the tumorigenic activity of type II agents. Even though a feedback mechanism exists for limiting RDS activity, apparently not all of the cellular processes stimulated by type II compounds are regulated in a similar manner. For instance, monooxygenase activities are increased and remain increased following continuous exposure to these agents (Ghazal et al. 1964; Schulte-Hermann and Parzefall 1981). It is therefore conceivable that some of the cellular functions associated with cell division and possibly carcinogenesis may remain activated by the continual presence of type II compounds. Recent experimental evidence indicates that the tumorigenic activity of type II compounds may be related to the ability of these agents to promote the neoplastic development of spontane-ously initiated cells (Schulte-Hermann et al. 1983b). Although the precise mecha-nism of this promotion effect is not known, the inhibition of cell death within preneoplastic foci may be one important factor (Bursch et al. 1984).

In this paper, we examined the relationship between the induction of RDS by nongenotoxic carcinogens and the tumorigenic activity of these agents in the liver and kidney. The methods presented here are valuable complements to existing techniques for determining chemically induced hyperplasia. Nongenotoxic agents were found to have a moderately high probability of increasing tumor incidence rates in tissues where RDS activity was induced. We believe that cell proliferation stimulated by chronic exposure to cytotoxic agents may initiate tumorigenesis by accelerating the accumulation of somatic mutations and/or may promote the development of spontaneously induced preneoplastic cells. However, increased cell replication per se does not appear to be directly related to the tumorigenic activity of agents that induce additive hyperplasia in the liver. This conclusion is based on experimental evidence indicating that continuous exposure to such agents is associated with only a transient increase in cell proliferation activity.

REFERENCES

Ashby, J. 1982. Screening chemicals for mutagenicity. In *Mutagenicity, new horizons in genetic toxicology* (ed. J.A. Heddle), p. 1. Academic Press, New York.

Brem, H., A.B. Stein, and H.S. Rosenkranz. 1974. The mutagenicity and DNA modifying effect of haloalkanes. *Cancer Res.* **34**: 2576.

Bursch, W., B. Lauer, I. Timmermann-Trosiener, G. Barthel, J. Schuppler, and R. Schulte-Hermann. 1984. Controlled death (apoptosis) of normal and putative preneoplastic cells in the rat liver following withdrawal of tumor promotors. *Carcinogenesis* **5**: 453.

Butterworth, B.E., D.J. Loury, and T. Smith-Oliver. 1985. The value of measurement of both genotoxicity and forced cell proliferation in assessing the potential carcinogenicity of chemicals. *Proc. Int. Conf. Environ. Mut.* **4**: 214.

Butterworth, B.E., E. Bermudez, T. Smith-Oliver, L. Earle, R. Cattley, J. Martin, J.A. Popp, S. Strom, R. Jirtle, and G. Michalopoulos. 1984. Lack of genotoxic activity of di(2-ethylhexyl)phthalate (DEHP) in rat and human hepatocytes. *Carcinogenesis* **5**: 1329.

Costa, A.K. and K.M. Ivanetich. 1984. Chlorinated ethylenes: Their metabolism and effect on DNA repair in rat hepatocytes. *Carcinogenesis* **5**: 1629.

Craddock, V.M. 1973. Induction of liver tumors in rats by a single treatment with nitroso compounds given after partial hepatectomy. *Nature* **245**: 386.

Doull, J., B.A. Bridges, R. Kroes, L. Golberg, I.C. Munro, O.E. Paynter, H.C. Pitot, R. Squire, G. Williams, and W. Darby. 1983. The relevance of mouse liver hepatomas to human carcinogenic risk. In *A report of the international expert advisory committee to the nutrition foundation*. The Nutrition Foundation, Inc., Washington, D.C.

Frei, J.V. and T. Harsono. 1967. Increased susceptibility to low doses of a carcinogen of epidermal cells in stimulated DNA synthesis. *Cancer Res.* **27**: 1482.

Geiger, L.E. and R.A. Neal. 1981. Mutagenicity testing of 2,3,7,8-tetrachlorodibenzo-p-dioxin in histidine auxotrophs of *Salmonella typhimurium*. *Toxicol. Appl. Pharmacol.* **59**: 125.

Ghazal, A., W. Koransky, J. Portig, H.W. Vohland, and I. Klempau. 1964. Beschleunigung von Entgiftungsreaktionen durch verschiedene Insecticide. *Arch. Exp. Pathol. Pharmakol.* **249**: 1.

Hayes, J.R., L.W. Condie, Jr., and J.F. Borzellica. 1986. The subchronic toxicity of tetrachloroethylene (perchloroethylene) administered in the drinking water of rats. *Fundam. Appl. Toxicol.* **7**: 119.

International Agency for Research on Cancer (IARC). 1974. *Monographs on the evaluation of carcinogenic risk of chemicals to man: Some organochlorine pesticides,* vol. 5. IARC, Lyon, France.

————. 1976. *Monographs on the evaluation of carcinogenic risk of chemicals to man: Some naturally occurring substances,* vol. 10. IARC, Lyon, France.

————. 1977. *Monographs on the evaluation of carcinogenic risk of chemicals to man: Some miscellaneous pharmaceutical substances,* vol. 13. IARC, Lyon, France.

————. 1978. *Monographs on the evaluation of carcinogenic risk of chemicals to man: Polychlorinated biphenyls,* vol. 18. IARC, Lyon, France.

————. 1979a. *Monographs on the evaluation of the carcinogenic risk of chemicals to humans: Sex hormones II,* vol. 21. IARC, Lyon, France.

————. 1979b. *Monographs on the evaluation of carcinogenic risk of chemicals to man: Some halogenated hydrocarbons,* vol. 20. IARC, Lyon, France.

————. 1980. *Monographs on the evaluation of the carcinogenic risk of chemicals to humans: Some pharmaceutical drugs,* vol. 24. IARC, Lyon, France.

International Commission for Protection against Environmental Mutagens and Carcinogens (ICPEMC). 1984. Report of ICPEMC Task Group 5 on the differentiation between genotoxic and non-genotoxic carcinogens. *Mutat. Res.* **133**: 1.

International Programme on Chemical Safety (IPCS). 1985. *Environmental health criteria 50: Trichloroethylene,* p. 69. World Health Organization, Geneva, Switzerland.

Ito, N., H. Nagasaki, H. Aoe, S. Sugihara, Y. Miyata, M. Arai, and T. Shirai. 1975. Development of hepatocellular carcinomas in rats treated with benzene hexachloride. *J. Natl. Cancer Inst.* **54**: 801.

Ito, N., M. Hananouchi, S. Sugihara, T. Shirai, H. Tsuda, S. Fukushima, and H. Nagasaki. 1976. Reversibility and irreversibility of liver tumors in mice induced by the α isomer of 1,2,3,4,5,6-hexachlorocyclohexane. *Cancer Res.* **36**: 2227.

Lang, R. and U. Redmann. 1979. Non-mutagenicity of some sex hormones in the Ames *Salmonella*/microsome mutagenicity test. *Mutat. Res.* **67**: 361.

Laurent, G., G. Toubeau, P. Maldague, M.B. Carlier, J.A. Heuson-Stiennon, and P. Tulkens. 1984. Tubular regeneration in rat kidney cortex during treatment with gentamicin at a low dose. *Arch. Toxicol. Suppl.* **7**: 459.

Loury, D.J., T. Smith-Oliver, and B.E. Butterworth. 1987. Assessment of unscheduled DNA synthesis and cell replication in rat kidney cells exposed *in vitro* or *in vivo* to unleaded gasoline. *Toxicol. Appl. Pharmacol.* **87**: 127.

Loury, D.J., T. Smith-Oliver, S. Strom, R. Jirtle, G. Michalopoulos, and B.E. Butterworth. 1986. Assessment of unscheduled and replicative DNA synthesis in hepatocytes treated *in vivo* and *in vitro* with unleaded gasoline or 2,2,4-trimethylpentane. *Toxicol. Appl. Pharmacol.* **85**: 11.

Lundberg, I., M. Ekdahl, T. Kronevi, V. Lidums, and S. Lundberg. 1986. Relative hepatotoxicity of some industrial solvents after intraperitoneal injection or inhalation exposure in rats. *Environ. Res.* **40**: 411.

Lutz, W.K., M.T. Busser, and P. Sagelsdorff. 1984. Potency of carcinogens derived from covalent DNA binding and stimulation of DNA synthesis in rat liver. *Toxicol. Pathol.* **12:** 106.

MacFarland, H.N. 1982. Chronic gasoline toxicity. In *Proceedings of the Symposium on the Toxicology of Petroleum Hydrocarbons* (ed. H.N. MacFarland et al.), p. 78. American Petroleum Institute, Washington, D.C.

McCann, I., E. Choi, E. Yamasaki, and B.N. Ames. 1975. Detection of carcinogens as mutagens in the *Salmonella*/microsome test. Assay of 300 chemicals. *Proc. Natl. Acad. Sci. U.S.A.* **72:** 5135.

Mirsalis, J.C. and B.E. Butterworth. 1982. Induction of unscheduled DNA synthesis in rat hepatocytes following *in vivo* treatment with dinitrotoluene. *Carcinogenesis* **3:** 241.

Mirsalis, J.C., C.K. Tyson, and B.E. Butterworth. 1982. Detection of genotoxic carcinogens in the *in vivo-in vitro* hepatocyte DNA repair assay. *Environ. Mutagen.* **4:** 553.

Mirsalis, J.C., C.K. Tyson, E.N. Loh, K.L. Steinmetz, J.P. Bakke, C.M. Hamilton, D.K. Spak, and J.W. Spalding. 1985. Induction of hepatic cell proliferation and unscheduled DNA synthesis in mouse hepatocytes following *in vivo* treatment. *Carcinogenesis* **6:** 1521.

National Cancer Institute (NCI). 1979. *Bioassay of butylated hydroxytoluene (BHT) for possible carcinogenicity,* tech. report no. 150. National Institutes of Health, Bethesda, Maryland.

National Toxicology Program (NTP). 1982. *Carcinogenesis bioassay of 2,3,7,8-tetrachlorodibenzo-p-dioxin in osborne-mendel rats and B6C3F1 mice (gavage study),* tech. report no. 209. National Toxicology Program, Research Triangle Park, North Carolina.

————. 1983a. *Carcinogenesis bioassay of di(2-ethylhexyl)phthalate in F-344 rats and B6C3F1 mice (gavage study),* tech. report no. 217. National Toxicology Program, Research Triangle Park, North Carolina.

————. 1983b. *Carcinogenesis studies of polybrominated biphenyl mixture (Firemaster FF-1) in F-344/N rats and B6C3F1 mice (gavage study),* tech. report no. 244. National Toxicology Program, Research Triangle Park, North Carolina.

————. 1983c. *Carcinogenesis bioassay of pentachloroethane in F-344/N rats and B6C3F1 mice (gavage study),* tech. report no. 232. National Toxicology Program, Research Triangle Park, North Carolina.

————. 1983d. *Carcinogenesis bioassay of trichloroethylene in F-344 rats and B6C3F1 mice (gavage study),* tech. report no. 002. National Toxicology Program, Research Triangle Park, North Carolina.

————. 1986. *Carcinogenesis bioassay of tetrachloroethylene (perchloroethylene) in F-344/N rats and B6C3F1 mice (inhalation study),* tech. report no. 311. National Toxicology Program, Research Triangle Park, North Carolina.

Oberdisse, E., C. Hochstrate, and H.J. Merker. 1970. Influence of drugs on induction of enzymes involved in DNA metabolism. *Proc. Int. Congr. Pharmacol.* **4:** 318.

Ochs, H., B. Dusterberg, P. Gunzel, and R. Schulte-Hermann. 1986. Effect of tumor promoting contraceptive steroids on growth and drug metabolizing enzymes in rat liver. *Cancer Res.* **46:** 1224.

Peraino, C., R.J.M. Fry, E. Staffeldt, and W.E. Kisieleski. 1973. Effects of varying the exposure to phenobarbital on its enhancement of 2-acetylaminofluorene-induced hepatic tumorigenesis in the rat. *Cancer Res.* **33:** 27701.

Pereira, M.A., R.E. Savage, C.W. Guion, and P.A. Wernsing. 1984. Effect of chloroform on hepatic and renal DNA synthesis and ornithine decarboxylase activity in mice and rats. *Toxicol. Lett.* **21**: 357.

Purchase, I.F.H. 1982. An appraisal of predictive tests for carcinogenicity. *Mutat. Res.* **99**: 53.

Purchase, I.F.H., E. Longstaff, J. Ashby, J.A. Styles, D. Anderson, P.A. LePevre, and F.R. Westwood. 1978. An evaluation of 6 short-term tests for detecting organic chemical carcinogens. *Br. J. Cancer* **37**: 873.

Rajalakshmi, S., P.M. Rao, and D.S.R. Sarma. 1982. Chemical carcinogenesis: Interactions on carcinogens with nucleic acids. In *Cancer: A comprehensive treatise* (ed. F.F. Becker), p. 335. Plenum Press, New York.

Reddy, J.K., M.S. Rao, D.L. Azarnoff, and S. Sell. 1979. Mitogenic and carcinogenic effects of hypolipidemic peroxisome proliferator, [4-chloro-6-(2,3-xylidino)-2-pyrimidinylthio] acetic acid, in rat and mouse liver. *Cancer Res.* **39**: 152.

Richardson, K.A., J.L. Wilmer, D. Smith-Simpson, and T.R. Skopek. 1986. Assessment of the genotoxic potential of unleaded gasoline and 2,2,4-trimethylpentane in human lymphoblasts *in vitro. Toxicol. Appl. Pharmacol.* **82**: 316.

Rinkus, S.J. and M.S. Legator. 1979. Chemical characterization of 465 known or suspected carcinogens and their correlation with mutagenic activity in the *Salmonella typhimurium* system. *Cancer Res.* **39**: 3289.

Rossi, L., M. Ravera, G. Repetli, and L. Sunti. 1977. Long-term administration of DDT or phenobarbital-Na in Wistar rats. *Int. J. Cancer* **19**: 179.

Schulte-Hermann, R. 1974. Induction of liver growth by xenobiotic compounds and other stimuli. *Crit. Rev. Toxicol.* **3**: 97.

———. 1977. Two-stage control of cell proliferation induced in rat liver by α-hexachlorocyclohexane. *Cancer Res.* **37**: 166.

Schulte-Hermann, R. and W. Parzefall. 1981. Failure to discriminate initiation from promotion of liver tumors in a long-term study with the phenobarbital-type inducer α-hexachlorocyclohexane and the role of sustained stimulation of hepatic growth and monooxygenases. *Cancer Res.* **41**: 4140.

Schulte-Hermann, R. and E. Schmitz. 1980. Feedback inhibition of hepatic DNA synthesis. *Cell Tissue Kinet.* **13**:371.

Schulte-Hermann, R., I. Timmermann-Trosiener, and J. Schuppler. 1982. Response of liver foci in rats to hepatic tumor promoters. *Toxicol. Pathol.* **10**: 63.

———. 1983b. Promotion of spontaneous preneoplastic cells in rat liver as a possible explanation of tumor production by nonmutagenic compounds. *Cancer Res.* **43**: 839.

Schulte-Hermann, R., W. Koransky, C. Leberl, and G. Noack. 1971. Hyperplasia and hypertrophy of the rat liver induced by α-hexachlorocyclohexane and butylhydroxytoluene. Retention of the hyperplasia during involution of the enlarged organ. *Virchows Arch. Abt. B. Zellpathol.* **9**: 125.

Schulte-Hermann, R., J. Schuppler, I. Timmermann-Trosiener, G. Ohde, W. Bursch, and H. Berger. 1983a. The role of growth of normal and preneoplastic cell populations of tumor promotion in rat liver. *Environ. Health Perspect.* **50**: 185.

Schumann, A.M., J.F. Quast, and P.G. Watanabe. 1980. The pharmacokinetics and macromolecular interactions of perchloroethylene in mice and rats as related to oncogenicity. *Toxicol. Appl. Pharmacol.* **55**: 207.

Shimoi, K., Y. Nakamura, I. Tomita, and T. Kada. 1985. Bio-antimutagenic effects of tannic acid on UV and chemically induced mutagenesis in *Escherichia coli* B/r. *Mutat. Res.* **149:** 17.

Shirai, T., M. Ohshima, A. Masuda, S. Tamano, and N. Ito. 1984. Promotion of 2-(ethylnitrosamino)ethanol-induced renal carcinogenesis in rats by nephrotoxic compounds: Positive responses with folic acid, basic lead acetate, and N-(3,5-dichlorophenyl)succinimide but not with 2,3-dibromo-1-propanol phosphate. *J. Natl. Cancer Inst.* **72:** 477.

Shirasu, Y., M. Moriya, K. Kato, A. Furuhashi, and T. Kada. 1976. Mutagenicity screening of pesticides in the microbial system. *Mutat. Res.* **48:** 173.

Slaga, T.J. 1984. Multistage skin tumor promotion and specificity of inhibition. In *Mechanisms of tumor promotion. Tumor promotion and skin carcinogenesis* (ed. T.J. Slaga), vol. 2, p. 189. CRC Press, Boca Raton, Florida.

Stott, W.T., J.F. Quast, and P.G. Watanabe. 1982. The pharmacokinetics and macromolecular interactions of trichloroethylene in mice and rats. *Toxicol. Appl. Pharmacol.* **62:** 137.

Stott, W.T., R.H. Reitz, A.M. Schumann, and P.G. Watanabe. 1981. Genetic and nongenetic events in neoplasia. *Food Cosmet. Toxicol.* **19:** 567.

Truffert, L., C. Girard-Wellon, E. Emmerich, C. Neauport, and J. Ripault. 1977. Early experimental demonstration of the hepatotoxicity of some chlorinated solvents by the study of the synthesis of hepatic DNA. *Arch. Mal. Prof. Med. Trav. Secur. Soc.* **38:** 261.

Tsudu, H., G. Lee, and E. Rarber. 1980. Induction of resistant hepatocytcs as a new principle for a possible short-term *in vivo* test for carcinogens. *Cancer Res.* **40:** 1157.

Ward, J.M., R.A. Griesemer, and E.K. Weisburger. 1979. The mouse liver tumor as an endpoint in carcinogenesis test. *Toxicol. Appl. Pharmacol.* **51:** 389.

Warren, J.R., V.F. Simmon, and J.K. Reddy. 1980. Properties of hypolipidemic peroxisome proliferators in the lymphocyte [^{3}H]thymidine and *Salmonella* mutagenesis assays. *Cancer Res.* **40:** 36.

Weisburger, E.K. 1977. Carcinogenicity studies on halogenated hydrocarbons. *Environ. Health Perspect.* **21:** 7.

Zeiger, E., S. Haworth, K. Mortelmans, and W. Spek. 1985. Mutagenicity testing of di(2-ethylhexyl)phthalate and related chemicals in *Salmonella. Environ. Mutagen.* **7:** 213.

COMMENTS

TRUMP: In the kidney, lead may be an example of the sort of type II agent that you mentioned in the liver. In other words, it is cocarcinogenic very effectively with fluorobiphenylacetamide; it produces mitogenesis in the kidney, but no necrosis.

SARMA: Drs. Columbano and Ledda-Columbano observed that lead induces hyperplasia in the liver as well as in the kidney without inducing necrosis at certain doses.

LOURY: If lead is mitogenic in the kidney without producing necrosis, its effects would be different than most of the compounds that we have tested so far. We can detect a small amount of focal necrosis and regeneration that is undetectable on a histopathological level by using replicative DNA synthesis. Thus, in the kidney, lead may produce a low, histologically undetectable, level of necrosis or may be purely mitogenic, similar to the type II agents in the liver.

DI GIOVANNI: In situations where you are not causing a lot of visible cell death, is there actually an early inhibition in DNA synthesis that precedes the subsequent increase?

LOURY: No, we haven't seen that. We do time course studies, and at 2 hours and 12 hours after treatment we see only normal basal levels of activity. The earliest time that we see this increase is at 24 hours.

DI GIOVANNI: In the mouse skin, for example, compounds like TPA and other tumor promoters cause an early inhibition in DNA synthesis, which may or may not be related to toxic effects. This early inhibition is subsequently followed by regenerative or reactive hyperplasia and increased DNA synthesis.

SARMA: During cell death preceding the regenerative hyperplasia or in the apoptotic phase following mitogenic hyperplasia, is there an oxidative type of damage? In the former case, because of inflammatory cells coming in, there may be an oxidative burst and an oxidative damage. In the latter case, which is characterized by the absence of inflammatory cells, do you have some type of oxidative damage? If there is, then you might have mild genotoxicity built into these systems.

LOURY: That is a possibility, but we cannot measure that effect using these techniques.

DIAMOND: Some of the best agents to force proliferation are viruses. Papilloma-virus and Epstein-Barr virus increase the pool of cells that could be targets for genotoxic and nongenotoxic agents. Also, hepatitis virus induces regenerative hyperplasia. I think it is somewhat of a mistake to consider one class of agents without at least thinking about other classes.

WILLIAMS: How many agents have you tested up to a maximally tolerated dose that do not induce liver cell proliferation? As I think about the capacity of the liver to biotransform xenobiotics, I really wonder whether there are any agents that aren't capable of inflicting some degree of liver cell injury with compensatory proliferation.

LOURY: Numerous agents that are not toxic to the liver do not produce proliferation in that tissue. The vehicles water, corn oil, and DMSO do not.

Non-liver carcinogens such as pyrene do not. The point is that very often carcinogens that are not DNA-reactive do produce a hyperplastic response in the target tissue. The value of the whole-animal approach is that one can examine DNA repair and cell proliferation using doses that are equivalent to what are used in the long-term bioassay. In the case of the kidney, we have observed no increase in cell replication with several agents administered at the maximum tolerated dose.

WILLIAMS: Yes. I'm not sure that I have really caught on to how this approach would be used to design better carcinogenesis studies. Personally, I believe that one of the objectives for realistic testing would be to test chemicals at nonhepatotoxic doses.

LOURY: If a non-DNA-reactive agent has produced neoplasia, this approach as well as other techniques will help determine if cytotoxicity may have played a role in the development of tumors. If the long-term study is in the planning stages, these techniques may be used to help determine the nontoxic dose range. Remember also that some agents produce hyperplasia without toxicity.

SWENBERG: We can test chemicals at doses that don't produce pathology and come away sensing that they are not carcinogenic. The reason for using a maximum tolerated dose is to have a benchmark for a top dose level that is somewhat toxic, but not life-shortening. The relevance of findings under those conditions to human exposures orders of magnitude away from that is a serious issue that, unfortunately, we don't have time to discuss now.

WILLIAMS: I question whether chemicals should be tested for carcinogenicity at doses that are overtly toxic.

SWENBERG: In fact, that is what we are trying to avoid. In reality, however, you come down to the definition of toxic. If you don't use the typical definitions such as not causing necrosis and severe pathology that shortens survival for factors other than tumors, what are you going to use to set your doses?

SCRIBNER: We do not like to test at doses that are overtly toxic. Unfortunately, often we don't find that out until after the fact; then we have the problem of having to explain the adverse effects.

Chemically Induced Cell Turnover in the Kidney and Its Possible Role in Carcinogenesis

ERNST D. WACHSMUTH
Research Department, Pharmaceuticals Division
CIBA-GEIGY Limited, CH 4002 Basel, Switzerland

OVERVIEW

The effects of chemicals on the kidney have been the object of various investigations (for references, see Bach et al. 1982; Bach and Lock 1985). One observation is especially striking, and its implication may not have been fully considered. This is the potential of renal tubular cells to proliferate and, in particular, to regenerate even after excessive tubular necrosis, which in some instances leads to renal hyperplasia. Toxicity studies with various chemicals in various species have revealed this fact, on which one may speculate with regard to carcinogenesis, since increased cell proliferation (but also abnormal nuclear morphology) is characteristic of various tumors. The percentage of proliferating cells, however, is even higher in tissues with stem cell compartments (e.g., bone marrow, lymphatic tissue, and intestinal crypts).

INTRODUCTION

To investigate the magnitude of the potential proliferative response, it is desirable to use an organ with only a minor percentage of proliferating cells (e.g., kidney) and a method by which the proliferating cells can easily be detected, and thus its frequency of occurrence determined. Counting mitotic figures is one approach; however, the short duration of mitosis makes it the most laborious, since the mitotic cells constitute the smallest fraction of the cells in the various cell cycle phases. A more sensible and workable approach is the determination of cells in the S phase of the cell cycle by tracing their DNA synthesis, e.g., by determining [^{3}H]thymidine incorporated in their nuclei. Autoradiographs of tissues obtained 1 hour after a single pulse of [^{3}H]thymidine almost always reveal those cells which, at the time of administration, had been in the S phase and can be visualized by a silver grain density above background levels. An increase in the percentage of labeled cells, the labeling index (LI), may thus be due to either a real increase in the number of proliferating cells or, within limits, to a prolonged duration of the S phase, or to both. The former explanation appears to be the most likely one in the kidney, after the administration of a nephrotoxin, in view of the manyfold increase of the LI and, on the basis of other morphological criteria, the repopulation with tubular cells after cell necrosis. For the magnitude of proliferation per organ, one must take into

Banbury Report 25: Nongenotoxic Mechanisms in Carcinogenesis
© Cold Spring Harbor Laboratory. 0-87969-225-1/87. $1.00 + .00

account that all values given in this paper are data from area measurements and thus should be corrected by calculating the third power of the square root of the respective value (e.g., a 10-fold increase of labeled nuclei per area is a 32-fold increase in the particular organ part).

Major problems in studying proliferative events and, in particular, regeneration by means of histology arise from the fact that only one time point, that of autopsy, can be evaluated and thus previous events may escape observation. These problems may be overcome in kidney studies after administration of a nephrotoxin. Enzymes of the cytosol (e.g., LDH and ALD) and of the mitochondria (e.g., MDH) correlate well with the histological lesions in the kidneys of rats and rabbits within 24–48 hours after administration of the nephrotoxin, and better than enzymes of the brush border membrane or of the lysosomes (Wachsmuth 1982a). Thus, means are available to estimate acute nephrotoxic lesions without histology and to gain insight into toxic and regenerative events in individuals.

The results of studies with five chemicals of nephrotoxic potential presented in this paper suggest that the initially increased cell proliferation is not related to tumor induction.

RESULTS AND DISCUSSION

Labeling Index (LI) in Normal Rat Kidney

Only a few cells of the adult rat kidney can be labeled with [^{3}II]thymidine (e.g., after a 1-hour pulse, 20 ± 5 labeled cells/mm^2 cortex, and after continuous administration for 72 hours with a minipump, 154 ± 14 cells/mm^2 cortex). Mitotic figures are hardly ever observed. Thus, the number of proliferating cells in the kidney at one time is extremely small, i.e., approximately 0.1%.

Acute and Subacute Toxicity of Cephaloridine

A single intravenous dose of 0.8–1.2 g/kg cephaloridine in rats causes cell necrosis within 24–48 hours and a correspondingly large increase in urinary enzymes (Atkinson et al. 1966a; Wachsmuth 1982a). The kidney recovers within days with or without further administration of the compound and then tolerates even larger doses of cephaloridine (Cuppage and Tate 1968; Wachsmuth 1982b). Determination of tubular cell proliferation by [^{3}H]thymidine reveals a fourfold increase and a ninefold increase of the LI in the cortical tubules 24 hours and 48 hours, respectively, after a single dose of cephaloridine (Fig. 1). The LI in other parts of the kidney increases to a lesser extent, consistent with the interpretation of a regenerative process, since these parts show also less tubular necrosis. Following several injections of cephaloridine, a similar response is observed, with a maximal

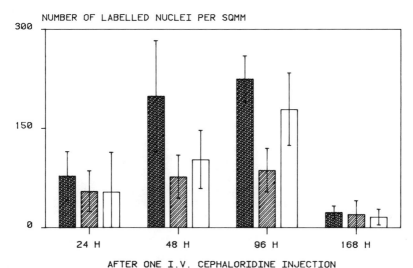

Figure 1

Acute toxicity: change of proliferation in rat kidney with time after a single intravenous injection of 0.8 g/kg cephaloridine. Male rats (230 g body weight, 3–4 per group, kept at 30°C in metabolic cages) received an intraperitoneal pulse of 2 μCi/g [^{3}H]thymidine 1 hr prior to autopsy; sections stained with PAS-haemalum were autoradiographed. Results are shown for the cortex (dark bar), outer stripe (medium bar), and inner stripe (open bar) of the outer medulla; mean and standard deviation are indicated.

eightfold increase of the LI in the cortex 24 hours after the second injection (Fig. 2). It should be noted that the LI becomes smaller with subsequent injections. Moreover, in the recovery period after multiple injections, the LI is low (3-fold above control on day 2 and 0.3-fold on day 9). Indeed, evaluation of the extent of necrosis in the same animals reveals that the extent of the lesions decreases with time after single or multiple doses. Taken together, the data indicate that young, regenerated tubular cells are more resistant than the original, established cells to the nephrotoxic action of cephaloridine.

The extent to which proliferation in rat kidney occurs becomes rapidly demonstrable when, instead of the 1-hour [^{3}H]thymidine pulse method, a technique is used in which [^{3}H]thymidine is administered for the major regeneration time of 3 days after injection of cephaloridine (Fig. 3) (Wachsmuth 1985). There were ten times more labeled nuclei in the cortex and five times more in the outer stripe (after cephaloridine injection) than in controls, indicating the tremendous proliferation. Evaluation of the sections by conventional means, however, revealed only minor evidence of lesions, and thus previous pathological changes may have escaped observation.

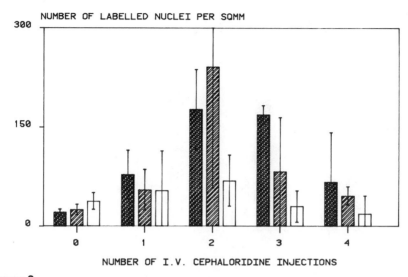

Figure 2

Subacute toxicity: proliferation in rat kidney 24 hr after various daily intravenous injections of 0.8 g/kg cephaloridine. Other experimental conditions and symbols are described in Fig. 1; mean and standard deviation are indicated.

Chronic Toxicity of Various Antibiotics

Investigation of proliferation in chronic toxicity studies must take into account the age of the animals, since proliferation rates in kidney decrease during maturation. Proliferation in 6-week-old healthy rats is approximately twice that of 10-week-old rats and is greater in the inner stripe of the outer medulla than in the outer stripe and the cortex (Fig. 4A). Here we compare the effects of three different antibiotics on proliferation in a chronic toxicity study in rats for 8 days and 25 days (Fig. 4).

As may be extrapolated from the acute toxicity studies described above, the LI at 8 days and 25 days after cephaloridine administration and the LI of controls are similar; however, the weight of the kidney is higher (Fig. 4B), which confirms previous findings (Atkinson et al. 1966b). The increased kidney weight may thus be taken as evidence of an earlier necrotizing event.

Although the nephrotoxic effect of gentamicin has been detected within hours of a single injection by means of electron microscopy (Faccini 1982), necrosis occurs slower and later than it does after cephaloridine. Both the LI and the kidney weight increase following continued gentamicin administration, and the extent of the rise of the LI is similar in all three renal segments (Fig. 4C). However, although the LI is larger than in controls, it is smaller after 25 days of administration than after 8 days. This finding is compatible with the observed development of increased renal

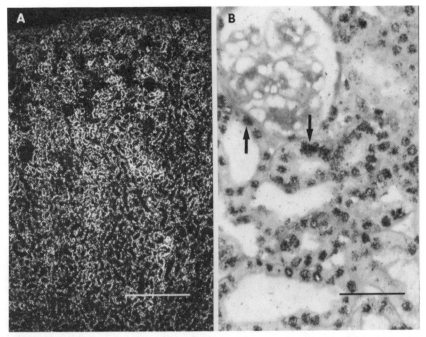

Figure 3

Regenerated renal tissue of the rat 96 hr after a single intravenous injection of 0.8 g/kg cephaloridine. [^{3}H]thymidine was continuously administered by a subcutaneous minipump (ALZET, osmet 2001) from 24 hr after cephaloridine injection for 3 days until autopsy. Autoradiographs of PAS-haemalum-stained paraplast sections: (A) dark-field illumination of cortex (top, 1500/mm^2) and outer medulla (800/mm^2), with numerous labeled cell nuclei visualized as white spots; (B) numerous heavily labeled nuclei in various tubules of the cortex (arrows). Bar, 50 μm.

tolerability to gentamicin (Cuppage et al. 1977; Luft et al. 1978) and in this respect is similar to the findings for cephaloridine.

Cefsulodin has been found to cause tubular necrosis virtually only in the outer stripe of the outer medulla (Wachsmuth and Thomann 1982), which is readily visualized by the LI after 8 days of continued administration, but less so after 25 days (Fig. 4D) and less than after gentamicin. However, the kidney weight after 25 days of administration is higher than it is in controls.

The results obtained with the three different antibiotics demonstrate that increased kidney weight may be caused by early necrotic events followed by regeneration; this cannot be readily demonstrated in the tissue at later times because the kidney develops increased resistance to the nephrotoxin. Increased incidence of renal tumors has not been reported with either of the three antibiotics, and, for instance, it does not occur in 6-month toxicity studies with cefsulodin (Takano 1979).

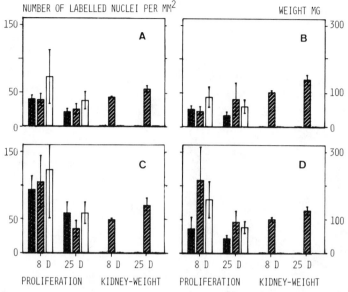

Figure 4

Chronic toxicity: proliferation in rat kidney at indicated day after daily subcutaneous injection of saline (A), 1.0 g/kg cephaloridine (B), 0.25 g/kg gentamicin (C), and 1.0 g/kg cefsulodin (D). Male rats (at start, ~150 g body weight, 5 weeks old) were kept at 21°C. Other experimental conditions and symbols are described in Fig. 1. Mean and standard deviation are indicated.

Acute Toxicity of *cis*-Platinum

The nephrotoxic effect of *cis*-platinum has been reported previously (Dobyan et al. 1980; Choie et al. 1981) and was also investigated by us in rats. A single intravenous dose of *cis*-platinum provokes no change for 24 hours in either urinary enzyme excretion or renal morphology, but changes become more frequent thereafter, with urinary enzyme levels peaking between day 3 and day 5 after injection. From day 2 onward, an increase in the sustained pattern of injury, with tubular atrophy, cystic changes, and interstitial nephritis, is obvious. The LI increased fivefold in the cortex and tenfold in the outer stripe (Fig. 5), the latter being also the major site of necrosis. Giant nuclei are also observed in tubules of the outer stripe, with an increase in frequency from day 4 to day 8 (Fig. 6). These giant nuclei are frequently labeled, and their grain counts per nucleus are approximately the same as in nuclei of normal morphological features. The occurrence of giant nuclei may be the first evidence of later tumor development, since *cis*-platinum has been shown to be carcinogenic (Leopold et al. 1979; Prestayko et al. 1980; Rosenberg 1985). The late occurrence of the nephrotoxic effect may be due to the protracted release of *cis*-platinum from the liver (Rosenberg 1985). Whether the

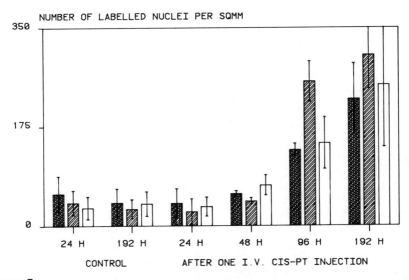

Figure 5

Acute toxicity: increase of proliferation in rat kidney after a single intravenous injection of 6 mg/kg *cis*-platinum in mannitol solution (platinol). Rats were kept at 21°C. Other experimental conditions and symbols are described in Fig. 1. Mean and standard deviation are indicated.

onset of proliferation is inhibited cannot be concluded from the data presented. The real differences between the antibiotics analyzed above and *cis*-platinum apparently can be recognized not on the basis of proliferation rates or disruption frequency of tubular basement membranes (though the latter is also observed with gentamicin), but on the basis of the occurrence of giant nuclei during the course of regeneration.

Acute Toxicity of Diethylnitrosamine

Diethylnitrosamine (DENA) is a well-known carcinogen, and its effect has been extensively studied in the livers of rats (Druckrey et al. 1963) and mice (Vesselinovitch et al. 1985). Bannasch et al. (1974, 1980), who investigated renal carcinogenesis with *N*-nitrosomorpholine (NNM), a similar carcinogen, in stop experiments, question tubular necrosis followed by hyperplasia as a pathogenic pathway. They detected tumorigenic cells only weeks and months after the start of administration of NNM. Supportive evidence is derived from proliferation studies with 3-hour [³H]thymidine pulse-labeling experiments in rats receiving 6–50 mg per 100 ml of drinking water (Braun 1976; Hagen 1977). By analysis of autoradiographs of liver sections (Braun 1976) and kidney sections (Hagen 1977), neither the percentage of labeled cells nor the percentage of labeled mitotic cells was found to change between day 1 and day 4. We have reexamined the problem by

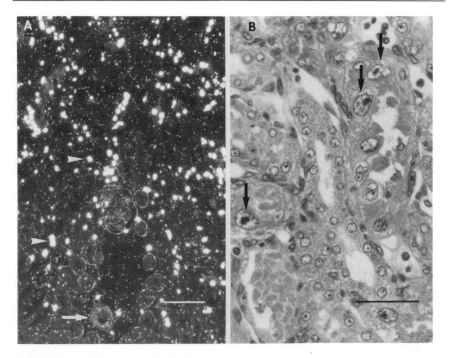

Figure 6

Juxtamedullary junction of rat kidney 192 hr after *cis*-platinum injection. Paraplast sections were stained with PAS-haemalum. Experimental conditions are described in Fig. 6. (*A*) Dark-field illumination of autoradiograph. The cortex is shown at the top. Arrow indicates art. arcuata, and arrowheads indicate labeled cell nuclei, visible as large white spots. (*B*) Giant nuclei in degenerating proximal tubules (arrow); signs of tubular regeneration are visible. Bar, 50 μm

investigating the LI at intervals from 6 hours to 96 hours after a single dose of DENA per gavage in mice, since it is conceivable that stimulated proliferation is an early event followed by a cell-cycle arrest. Six doses ranging from 0.25 μg to 10 mg per mouse were chosen; doses above 5 μg have been shown to be carcinogenic in mice (Vesselinovitch and Mihailovich 1983). The LI pattern (as a function of time after administration of DENA) in kidney (Fig. 7) and in liver (Fig. 8) were alike. No change in LI was seen with doses up to 2.5 μg per mouse. The LI decreases at doses above that level, and this is more marked at 6 hours than later. The incidence of cell necrosis or glycogen content were not affected within 96 hours after administration of up to 1 mg per mouse. Thus, these data indicate a dose-dependent cytostatic effect of DENA on both kidney and liver and do not provide evidence of an early stimulation of proliferation. Such a conclusion is in agreement with the ultrastructural findings in nephrotoxicity studies with DENA (Hard and Mackay 1985).

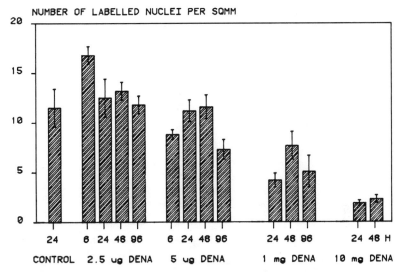

Figure 7

Acute toxicity: proliferation in mouse kidney after a single per oral dose of DENA. Female BALB/c mice (~25 g body weight) 3–4 months old were kept at 21°C; intraperitoneal pulse of 2 μCi/g [³H]thymidine was given 1 hr prior to autopsy. Sections were stained with PAS-haemalum and autoradiographed. The number of labeled nuclei in both cortex and outer stripe of outer medulla is indicated. Mean and standard deviation are also indicated.

CONCLUSION

Three chemicals (antibiotics) chosen for their known nephrotoxic potential were shown to induce tubular cell necrosis followed by extensive regeneration due to specific proliferation; regeneration continues to occur during further administration of the compounds. Shortly after a single administration, and during repeated administrations, the kidneys become less sensitive to the nephrotoxic agent. Similar development of tissue resistance to toxic agents has also been found in various other tissues (Balazs 1974) and appears to be due to properties of the renewed target-cell population. Evidence of a potential carcinogenic effect caused by either of the three antibiotics has not been obtained until now. In contrast, *cis*-platinum (Rosenberg 1985) and DENA apparently initially inhibit cell proliferation in the kidney. Both chemicals are known to be carcinogens. In addition, *cis*-platinum induces the appearance of giant tubular cells, which, in other cases, has been taken as early evidence of a carcinogenic event. Thus, the data presented on proliferation, although based on only a few chemicals, permit one to distinguish between two groups with respect to potential carcinogenesis. They do not provide evidence of a positive correlation between initially increased cell proliferation and carcinogenesis.

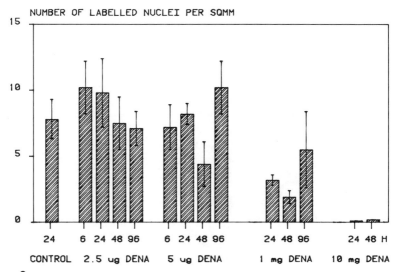

NUMBER OF LABELLED NUCLEI PER SQMM

Figure 8

Acute toxicity: proliferation in mouse liver after a single per oral dose of DENA. Sections were stained with Feulgen and autoradiographed. Livers of mice were prepared as described in Fig. 7. Mean and standard deviation are indicated.

REFERENCES

Atkinson, R.M., J.P. Currie, D.A.H. Pratt, H.M. Sharpe, and E.G. Tomich. 1966a. Acute toxicity of cephaloridine, an antibiotic derived from cephalosporin C. *Toxicol. Appl. Pharmacol.* **8:** 398.

Atkinson, R.M., J.D. Caisey, T.R. Middleton, D.A.H. Pratt, H.M. Sharpe, and E.G. Tomich. 1966b. Subacute toxicity of cephaloridine to various species. *Toxicol. Appl. Pharmacol.* **8:** 407.

Bach, P.H. and E.A. Lock, eds. 1985. *Renal heterogeneity and target cell toxicity.* John Wiley and Sons, Chichester, England.

Bach, P.H., F.W. Bonner, J.W. Bridges, and E.A. Lock, eds. 1982. *Nephrotoxicity, assessment and pathogenesis.* John Wiley and Sons, Chichester, England.

Balazs, T. 1974. Development of tissue resistance to toxic effects of chemicals. *Toxicology* **2:** 247.

Bannasch, P., U. Schacht, and E. Storch. 1974. Morphogenese und Mikromorphologie epithelialer Nierentumoren bei Nitrosomorpholin-vergifteten Ratten. II. Tubulaere Glykogenose und die Genese von klar- und acidophilzelligen Tumoren. *Z. Krebsforsch.* **92:** 63.

Bannasch, P., R. Krech, and H. Zerban. 1980. Morphogenese und Mikromorphologie epithelialer Nierentumoren bei Nitrosomorpholin-vergifteten Ratten. IV. Tubulaere Laesionen und basophile Tumoren. *J. Cancer Res. Clin. Oncol.* **98:** 243.

Braun, A. 1976. *Zur Zellproliferation der Rattenleber waehrend der Applikation von unterschiedlichen Konzentrationen von N-Nitroso-morpholin—Autoradiographische*

Untersuchungen mit 3H-Thymidin. Inaugural Dissertation, University of Wuerzburg, West Germany.

Choie, D.D., D.S. Longnecker, and A.A. Del Campo. 1981. Acute and chronic cisplatin nephropathy in rats. *Lab. Invest.* **44:** 397.

Cuppage, F.E. and A. Tate. 1968. Repair of the nephron in acute renal failure: Comparative eration following various forms of acute tubular injury. *Pathol. Microbiol.* **32:** 327.

Cuppage, F.E., K. Setter, L.P. Sullivan, E.J. Reitzes, and A.O. Melynkovych. 1977. Gentamycin nephrotoxicity. II. Physiological, biochemical and morphological effects of prolonged administration to rats. *Virchows Arch.* B **24:** 121.

Dobyan, D.C., J. Levi, C. Jacobs, J. Kosek, and M.W. Weiner. 1980. Mechanism of cis-platinum nephrotoxicity: II. Morphologic observations. *J. Pharmacol. Exp. Ther.* **213:** 551.

Druckrey, H., A. Schildbach, R. Schmaehl, R. Preussmann, and S. Ivankovic. 1963. Quantitative Analyse der carcinogenen Wirkung von Diaethylnitrosamin. *Arzneim. Forsch.* **13:** 841.

Faccini, J.M. 1982. A perspective on the pathology and cytochemistry of renal lesions. In *Nephrotoxicity, assessement and pathogenesis* (ed. P.H. Bach et al.), p. 82. John Wiley and Sons, Chichester, England.

Hagen, S. 1977. *Zur Zellproliferation der Rattenniere unter N-Nitroso-Morpholin in verschiedenen Konzentrationen—Autoradiographische Untersuchungen mit 3H-Thymidin.* Inaugural Dissertation, University of Wuerzburg, West Germany.

Hard, G.C. and R.L. Mackay. 1985. Dimethylnitrosamine nephrotoxicity: Ultrastructural evidence for a novel sequence of early target cell injury. In *Renal heterogeneity and target cell toxicity* (ed. P.H. Bach and E.A. Lock), p. 67. John Wiley and Sons, Chichester, England.

Leopold, W.R., E.C. Miller, and J.A. Miller. 1979. Carcinogenicity of antitumor cis-platinum (II) coordination complexes in the mouse and rat. *Cancer Res.* **39:** 913.

Luft, F.C., L.I. Rankin, R.S. Sloan, and M.N. Yumi. 1978. Recovery from aminoglycoside nephrotoxicity with continued drug administration. *Antimicrob. Agent Chemother.* **14:** 284.

Prestayko, A.W., S.T. Crooke, S.K. Carter, and N.A. Adler. 1980. *Cisplatin, current status and new developments.* Academic Press, New York.

Rosenberg, B. 1985. Fundamental studies with cisplatin. *Cancer* **55:** 2303.

Takano, K. 1979. Subacute and chronic toxicity studies on cefsulodin (SCE-129). *Chemotherapy* **2:** 113.

Vesselinovitch, S.T. and N. Mihailovich. 1983. Kinetics of diethylnitrosamine hepatocarcinogenesis in the infant mouse. *Cancer Res.* **43:** 4253.

Vesselinovitch, S.T., H.J. Hacker, and P. Bannasch. 1985. Histochemical characterization of focal hepatic lesions induced by single diethylnitrosamine treatment in infant mice. *Cancer Res.* **45:** 2774.

Wachsmuth, E.D. 1982a. Quantification of acute cephaloridine nephrotoxicity in rats: Correlation of serum and 24-hr urine analyses with proximal tubule injuries. *Toxicol. Appl. Pharmacol.* **63:** 429.

———. 1982b. Adaptation to nephrotoxic effects of cephaloridine in subacute rat toxicity studies. *Toxicol. Appl. Pharmacol.* **63:**446.

———. 1985. Renal cell heterogeneity at a light microscopic level. In *Renal heterogeneity and target cell toxicity* (ed. P.H. Bach and E.A. Lock), p. 13. John Wiley and Sons, Chichester, England.

Wachsmuth, E.D. and P. Thomann. 1982. Testing for renal tolerability: Cefsulodin in rats and rabbits. In *Nephrotoxicity, assessment and pathogenesis* (ed. P.H. Bach et al.), p. 498. John Wiley and Sons, Chichester, England.

COMMENTS

REITZ: Did you show us the control values for the minipump?

WACHSMUTH: The number of labeled cells per mm^2 was found to be approximately 10 times larger in the cortex and 5 times larger in the outer stripe than in controls.

NEWBERNE: How do you interpret that very large cell in the tubule of the *cis*-platinum?

WACHSMUTH: I don't know. It is a striking phenomenon that others may also have observed with *cis*-platinum. It consists of tubular cells with giant nuclei of abnormal appearance which have been taken as precancerous cells in some instances. They were found 4 days after a single injection of *cis*-platinum.

TRUMP: Those karyomegalic nuclei are found with a variety of known carcinogens, and even some compounds, I guess, that we really don't know. Following administration of some compounds they can occur very early, within a few weeks. They can incorporate thymidine, but I am not sure whether or not they can divide.

WACHSMUTH: Indeed, upon closer inspection of the histological specimens, many of these giant cells were labeled in a 1-hour pulse with [^{3}H]thymidine and thus are presumably in S phase.

TRUMP: Some of them certainly incorporate thymidine, but I'm not sure they can divide. However, many mutagenic carcinogens in the kidney give rise to them, and maybe some nonmutagenic carcinogens. It has been suggested as an early test.

WACHSMUTH: Searching for the occurrence of giant nuclei may be a more predictive approach than determining proliferative stages in order to gain evidence of the carcinogenic potential of a chemical.

TRUMP: On the cells with all of that labeling that you showed, were there any abnormal enzyme markers that you could find?

WACHSMUTH: No. Most kidneys had a perfectly normal appearance by means of conventional histology when rats were investigated 5 days or more following a single nephrotoxic dose of cephaloridine.

PITOT: Does the pattern of labeling and the kinetics that you see in these experiments differ significantly from compensatory hyperplasia or hypertrophy of the kidney after one kidney is removed?

WACHSMUTH: The effect of removal of one kidney in rats on the proliferation of the other has not been studied by us. However, it is known that under these circumstances the major site of increased proliferation is the outer stripe of the outer medulla, leading to renal hyperplasia.

SWENBERG: Have you looked with your minipump system at any old rats, where you have old-age nephropathy, to determine what is happening?

WACHSMUTH: Our studies were performed only with rats up to the age of approximately 3 months. The rate of proliferation in 10-week-old rats is certainly smaller than in 6-week-old rats, but the same as in 14-week-old rats.

SWENBERG: Could you reiterate to what extent carcinogenicity testing has been carried out on agents associated with an increase in proliferation? Have they been adequately tested or not? For instance, I am not aware of a 2-year bioassay on gentamicin.

WACHSMUTH: I am not aware of a carcinogenicity study with one of the chemicals studied here. If the incidence of renal tumors would be increased, one may have observed this in a 6-month or a 1-year study. But this has not been reported.

SWENBERG: I know that the National Toxicology Program is conducting a 2-year study of mercuric chloride, which is a pretty potent mitogen.

WACHSMUTH: Not only does mercuric chloride lead to tubular necrosis and regeneration, but lesions are often associated with rupture of the tubular basement membrane and interstitial nephritis. Moreover, HgCl also provokes changes of the immune system in some rat species. These and other differences in acute toxicity do not permit one to readily extrapolate to similar long-term effects, e.g., carcinogenesis. Moreover, antibiotics affect the microbial environment of the animal, certainly in the dose range used for toxicity testing.

MAGEE: In your experiments with diethylnitrosamine, what sort of dose induced tumors?

WACHSMUTH: The dose range used in our studies was approximately 0.01 mg/kg to 400 mg/kg as a single dose per gavage in mice. The lowest effective dose in reducing proliferation was 0.2 mg/kg, which was shown to be carcinogenic in mice by Vesselinovitch et al. (1985).

MAGEE: With 0.1 mg/kg, a single dose?

WACHSMUTH: Yes.

MAGEE: I would be surprised at that, wouldn't you, Henry?

PITOT: Yes, in the kidney.

SWENBERG: Usually, with diethyl- or dimethylnitrosamine, you need a large single dose to get kidney tumors.

MAGEE: That's why I am so surprised about diethylnitrosamine.

SARMA: Unless it's given in drinking water.

PITOT: That was the dose given continuously in the drinking water, though, not as a single dose.

WACHSMUTH: No, that was a single dose. We used a single dose of DENA administered orally by gavage in the mouse.

PITOT: Yes, in the mouse, which is very sensitive, but not in the rat.

TRUMP: In the mouse those aren't tubular tumors that are induced in the kidney, are they? They're nephroblastic lesions, or whatever they're called.

SWENBERG: That varies with the age of the animal. Young animals get nephroblastic tumors and old animals get cortical tumors.

Influence of Cytotoxicity on the Induction of Tumors

JAMES A. SWENBERG AND BRIAN G. SHORT
Department of Biochemical Toxicology and Pathobiology
Chemical Industry Institute of Toxicology
Research Triangle Park, North Carolina 27709

INTRODUCTION

Numerous chemicals that have been shown to lack genotoxic potential clearly can induce tumors in animals exposed to high doses in a carcinogenesis bioassay. A common feature of such studies is a corresponding induction of cytotoxicity and/or hyperplasia in the same tissue that developed neoplasia. Although there are several theories for carcinogenesis, including somatic mutation and chronic irritation, these theories do not have to be mutually exclusive. In fact, it is likely that multiple factors are involved in the chemical induction of most cancers. The proportionate role of mutational versus other factors can vary with the chemical and even the dose. For example, formaldehyde has a very nonlinear dose response for the induction of nasal squamous cell carcinomas in rats (Kerns et al. 1983; Swenberg et al. 1983). It is known that the amount of DNA-protein crosslinks/ppm formaldehyde increases by a factor of 4 between 2 ppm and 6 ppm and remains at that level at higher concentrations (Casanova-Schmitz et al. 1984). Thus, interaction with DNA alone does not explain the major nonlinearity in the tumor response that occurs between 6 ppm and 15 ppm. Rather, the major difference at these two concentrations appears to be related to the extent of cell proliferation (Swenberg et al. 1983, 1985, 1986a). The marked nonlinearity in the tumor dose-response most likely represents a combination of greater DNA binding and increased cell proliferation.

Control animals from strains of laboratory rodents commonly used in carcinogenesis bioassays develop many spontaneous tumors. It therefore follows that these animals have many spontaneously initiated cells. The incidence of spontaneous tumors varies greatly from tissue to tissue, strain to strain, sex to sex, and species to species. Certain tissues (i.e., mouse liver and lung; rat testis and pituitary) are very susceptible to developing spontaneous neoplasia. The mechanisms responsible for these spontaneous tumors remain unknown. One possibility is that cancer is an age-related disease, with the incidence of most tumor types increasing markedly with increasing age. Various hypotheses have been proposed for this, including the cumulative number of mutations from exogenous sources, free-radical damage to DNA and membranes, hormonal imbalance, and activation of protooncogenes. Since different factors may participate to different degrees in each tissue, strain, sex, and species, it would be unreasonable to insist that similar dose-response relationships exist for each tumor type. The objective of this paper is

Banbury Report 25: Nongenotoxic Mechanisms in Carcinogenesis
© Cold Spring Harbor Laboratory. 0-87969-225-1/87. $1.00 + .00

to explore several aspects of this issue, including the influence of age on spontaneous neoplasia and possible roles of increased cell proliferation on spontaneous and induced neoplasia, and to place data from such studies in perspective for regulatory decision-making.

INFLUENCE OF AGE ON SPONTANEOUS NEOPLASIA

The incidence of cancer is clearly age-related, with the greatest increases occurring late in life. This is true across the evolutionary tree, but it has been best studied in humans, rodents, and dogs. It is because of this strong association that data from epidemiologic studies and carcinogenesis bioassays are usually reported in an age-adjusted manner. This provides some assurance that incorrect comparisons have not been made. It is of considerable importance when data acquired under conditions of life-shortening toxicity are compared with those of controls. While such age adjustments work reasonably well for tumors that have consistent age-response relationships, they can be equally misleading for data on tumor types that exhibit variability in incidence. For example, astrocytomas of the brain occur in 0.4% of male Fischer 344 (F344) rats in conventional 2-year bioassays and in 2.7% of the animals carried for their life spans (Solleveld et al. 1984). However, when the same life span data were analyzed as five individual control groups, the

Table 1
Effect of Age on Spontaneous Tumor Incidence (%) in F344 Rats

Nonendocrine neoplasm	Males		Females	
	2-year	life span	2-year	life span
Brain				
astrocytoma	0.4	2.7	0.5	1.6
Kidney				
tubular cell adenoma	0.2	0.2	<0.1	0.4
tubular cell carcinoma	0.1	0.4	0.1	0.6
Liver				
neoplastic nodule	3.4	8.6	3.0	2.8
hepatocellular carcinoma	0.8	3.0	0.2	0.4
Mammary gland				
fibroadenoma	2.2	13.4	24.1	57.3
carcinoma	0.3	1.5	2.1	11.2
Pancreas				
acinar cell adenoma	0.3	7.0	<0.1	1.3
Skin				
squamous cell papilloma	1.2	2.1	0.3	1.3
basal cell tumor	0.9	3.6	0.3	0.9

Data from Solleveld et al. (1984).

Table 2
Effect of Age on Spontaneous Tumor Incidence (%) in F344 Rats

Endocrine neoplasm	Males		Females	
	2-year	life span	2-year	life span
Adrenal gland				
pheochromocytoma	17.9	30.1	3.9	15.0
Pancreatic islets				
adenoma	3.8	6.1	0.8	2.5
carcinoma	2.1	5.2	0.3	2.9
Parathyroid gland				
adenoma	0.1	3.1	0.1	0.6
Thyroid gland				
follicular cell adenoma	1.0	4.0	0.4	3.8
follicular cell carcinoma	0.8	4.4	0.4	3.8
C-cell adenoma	5.1	12.7	4.9	9.0
C-cell carcinoma	3.8	14.6	3.6	11.0

Data from Solleveld et al. (1984).

incidence of astrocytoma varied from 0% to 5.9%. In other studies, incidences of brain tumors in control rats ranged from 0% to 11% (Swenberg 1986b). Similar problems exist for other tumor types, such as pancreatic islet cell adenoma and mammary gland and thyroid C-cell adenomas (Solleveld et al. 1984).

The most comprehensive data set on age-response patterns of neoplasia currently available is from the National Toxicology Program (Solleveld et al. 1984). This study examined life span data from 529 F344 rats of both sexes and contrasted those data with historic control data on 2320 male and 2370 female F344 rats from 2-year bioassays conducted during the same time period. Several important observations were made. First, the same tumor types were formed in life span and 2-year studies. Second, the incidence of many tumor types increased 100–500% when data from 2-year studies (terminated at 110–116 weeks of age) were compared with those from rats on life span studies (terminated at 140–146 weeks). Since this represents only a 25% increase in age, it is clear that the age-response relationship for spontaneous neoplasia is highly nonlinear. Selected examples of data for nonendocrine neoplasms are shown in Table 1, and comparisons of endocrine tumors are listed in Table 2. The most extreme difference in incidence occurred for parathyroid gland adenomas, which increased 3100%! Solleveld et al. (1984) also provided data on age-specific prevalence rates for tumor types whose incidence exceeded 5% in aging F344 rats that demonstrated rapid increases in incidence between 85 and 123 weeks of age. The incidence of mononuclear cell leukemia went from 8% at 59–84 weeks to 21% at 85–97 weeks to approximately 40% at 98–140 weeks. The third feature demonstrated in the Solleveld et al. (1984) data was a tendency for progression from benign to malignant tumors of the same cell type with increasing age.

POTENTIAL INFLUENCE OF TOXICITY ON THE AGE-RESPONSE RELATIONSHIP OF CANCER

We have also examined data from carcinogenesis bioassays of nongenotoxic agents from the perspective of the potential influence of toxicity on the age-response relationships of neoplasms. One can pose the following questions. What is the "age" of a tissue chronically exposed for 2 years to cytotoxic doses of a chemical that increases organ- or tissue-specific cell proliferation? What incidence of neoplasia would be expected at this theoretical age? Does the untreated control rat from the same study provide the appropriate data base for comparison? At present, little hard data are available to answer these questions.

There are several features of the data from bioassays on nongenotoxic carcinogens that provide support for the role of toxicity-induced shifts in the age-response relationship of neoplasia. For example, several bioassays have been conducted by the National Cancer Institute/National Toxicology Program (NTP) to evaluate the carcinogenic potential of chlorinated hydrocarbons such as trichloroethylene, perchloroethylene, and pentachloroethane. A common finding was the induction of renal adenomas and renal carcinomas in male rats. Similar tumors have occurred in male rats exposed by inhalation to unleaded gasoline and by gavage to 1,4-dichlorobenzene. The incidence of renal tumors in treated male rats ranged from 2% to 14%, whereas the historical control incidence has been 0.3%. Increased renal tumors only occurred at doses that produced renal toxicity. B. G. Short (unpubl.) and T. L. Goldsworthy (unpubl.) have demonstrated a good correlation between the induction of protein droplets in the P_2 segment of the nephron, increased cell proliferation, and carcinogenicity for several chemicals (Table 3). Protein droplet nephropathy is a disease caused by a wide variety of chemicals that is specific for male rats. The major factor responsible for this appears to be the large amount of a low-molecular-weight protein, $\alpha_{2\mu}$ globulin, that is synthesized in the male rat's liver, passed through the glomerular filtrate, and reabsorbed primarily in the P_2 segment of the nephron (Roy and Raber 1972; Maack et al. 1985). When male rats are exposed to chemicals such as unleaded gasoline, decalin, 1,4-dichlorobenzene, perchloroethylene, or pentachlorethane, the normal handling of $\alpha_{2\mu}$ globulin is disturbed, leading to protein droplet nephropathy. As demonstrated with unleaded gasoline, this can result in a selective five- to sevenfold increase in the proliferation of cells in the P_2 segment of the nephron (Short et al. 1986).

Data comparing the dose response for cell proliferation following 3 weeks of inhalation exposure to unleaded gasoline and that for the induction of renal epithelial tumors in the API carcinogenicity bioassay (Kitchen 1984) are shown in Figure 1. Currently, studies are under way in our Institute to determine if a quantitative relationship exists between the increase in cell proliferation in the P_2 segment and the ability of unleaded gasoline to promote renal neoplasia in rats initiated with ethylhydroxyethylnitrosamine. This study should provide data to

Table 3
Comparison of Hyaline Droplets, Cell Proliferation, and Carcinogenicity in Kidneys of Male Rats Exposed to Chlorinated Hydrocarbons and Unleaded Gasoline

	Hyaline droplets	P_2 cell proliferation	Carcinogenicity
Controls	+	−	−
Trichloroethylene	+	−	+
Perchloroethylene	+ +	$2\times\uparrow$	+
Pentachloroethane	+ + +	$3\times\uparrow$	+
Unleaded gasoline	+ + + +	$5\times\uparrow$	+ +

Data from T.L. Goldsworthy et al. (in prep.) and B.G. Short et al. (in prep.).

better understand the mechanism by which unleaded gasoline causes kidney tumors in male rats, but not in female rats or in male or female mice.

Neoplasia of the thyroid follicular epithelium increases 400–900% in rats in life span studies, compared to the rate in animals from 2-year studies (Solleveld et al. 1984). It is well established that chemicals that cause thyroid toxicity, resulting in lower circulating T_3 and T_4 concentrations and chronically elevated levels of thyroid-stimulating hormone (TSH), also cause thyroid neoplasia. The follicular tumors only occur at doses that elevate TSH, causing chronic hyperplasia. It is also known that humans are less sensitive than rats.

A recent NTP bioassay on inhalation exposure of F344 rats and B6C3F$_1$ mice to perchloroethylene demonstrated increased numbers of liver tumors in mice, kidney tumors in male rats, and mononuclear leukemia in male and female rats (National Toxicology Program 1986). The mouse liver tumors and rat kidney tumors only occurred at doses causing considerable toxicity to these tissues. No data are available on the immunotoxicity of perchloroethylene. As mentioned earlier, however, mononuclear cell leukemia in F344 rats has a steep age-response relationship. It is entirely possible that perchloroethylene is toxic to the stem cells for mononuclear cell leukemia and that this causes a shift in the age-response relationship of this neoplasm. Thus, it is possible that a nongenotoxic chemical may cause toxicity in multiple organs, sexes, and species by altering the age-response relationship of neoplasia in the same tissues. Considerably more research will be required to fully establish a cause-and-effect relationship. Such information is much needed for developing scientifically based risk assessment for humans exposed to lower, nontoxic concentrations of chemicals.

ROLE OF ONCOGENES IN SPONTANEOUS AND INDUCED CANCER

Recent studies have reported the presence of an activated oncogene in spontaneous liver tumors of B6C3F$_1$ mice, a strain with a high spontaneous incidence of liver

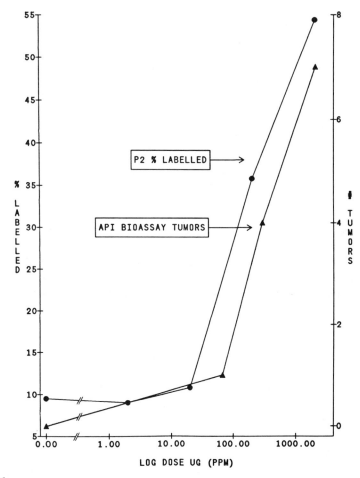

Figure 1
Effect of unleaded gasoline on P₂ cell proliferation at 3 weeks and renal tumors after 2 years in male rats.

cancer (Fox and Watanabe 1985; Reynolds et al. 1986). The 77% frequency of this genetic alteration in hepatocellular carcinomas of B6C3F₁ mice was the highest incidence ever observed in a spontaneous tumor of animal or human origin (Reynolds et al. 1986). These data strongly support the notion that B6C3F₁ mouse liver is predisposed to at least one of the events associated with carcinogenesis. One half of all the chemicals found to have carcinogenic potential in NTP bioassays have caused mouse liver tumors. Many of these chemicals are considered nongenotoxic on the basis of a battery of short-term tests. This raises a question regarding the mechanism by which such agents cause liver tumors in mice. These chemicals often cause hepatotoxicity, as defined by conventional histopathology. Few studies are available on the extent of cell proliferation and no data are available on the influence of chronic cell proliferation on oncogene activation. If an equal frequency of activated Ha-*ras* was present in treated and control liver tumors, such data would suggest that the chemical was enhancing or promoting spontaneously initiated cells. One could then examine whether or not the promoting activity was related to cell proliferation or some other factor. Conversely, if the chemical activated a different oncogene, such data would suggest that the chemical itself was the activating agent. Thus, molecular biology represents a promising frontier for determining mechanisms involved in carcinogenesis and the relevance of selected endpoints for human risk assessment.

SCIENTIFIC CONSIDERATIONS IN RISK ASSESSMENT

It is readily apparent that carcinogenesis is a complex multistage disease process. It is reasonable to invoke conservative regulatory policy in the absence of data. However, if risk assessment is to become scientifically based, it is equally important that mechanistic data be incorporated into the process when it is available. This includes taking into account cytotoxic phenomena, which only occur at relatively high doses. Such effects are likely to be responsible for many of the nonlinear responses of genotoxic agents as well as the carcinogenic effects of many, but certainly not all, nongenotoxic agents. Cytotoxicity is not likely to explain the promoting effects of chemicals working through specific receptors, such as dioxin. Although we still do not understand all of the mechanisms responsible for spontaneous tumor induction, it is clear that age plays a key role. What is the age of a tissue that has undergone a 500% increase in cell proliferation for 2 years? This scenario may not be atypical for tissue-specific toxicity at doses achieving a maximum tolerated dose based on conventional histopathology and body weight gain. Would it not be more appropriate to set the maximum tolerated dose using cell proliferation data? It is likely that a review of completed cancer bioassays would reveal data sets suitable for retrospective investigations of this issue. Future research must concentrate on developing techniques to both gather and apply relevant information to the risk assessment process if this process is expected to be accurate and scientifically defensible.

REFERENCES

Casanova-Schmitz, M., T.B. Starr, and H. d'A. Heck. 1984. Differentiation between metabolic incorporation and covalent binding in the labeling of macromolecules in the rat nasal mucosa and bone marrow by inhaled [^{14}C]- and [^{3}H]-formaldehyde. *Toxicol. Appl. Pharmacol.* **76**: 26.

Fox, T.R. and P.G. Watanabe. 1985. Detection of a cellular oncogene in spontaneous liver tumors of B6C3F1 mice. *Science* **228**: 596.

Kerns, W.D., K.L. Pavkov, D.J. Donofrio, E.J. Gralla, and J.A. Swenberg. 1983. Carcinogenicity of formaldehyde in rats and mice after long-term inhalation exposure. *Cancer Res.* **43:** 4382.

Kitchen, D.N. 1984. Neoplastic renal effects of unleaded gasoline in Fischer 344 rats. In *Renal effects of petroleum hydrocarbons* (ed. M.A. Mehlman et al.), p. 65. Princeton Scientific Publishers, Princeton, New Jersey.

Maack, T., C.H. Park, and M.J.F. Camargo. 1985. Renal filtration, transport, and metabolism of proteins. In *The kidney: Physiology and pathophysiology* (ed. D.W. Seldin and G. Giebisch), p. 1773. Raven Press, New York.

National Toxicology Program (NTP). 1986. *Toxicology and carcinogenesis studies of tetrachloroethylene in F344/N rats and B6C3F1 mice,* NTP technical report 311, NIH publ. no. 85-2567. U.S. Government Printing Office, Washington, D.C.

Reynolds, S.H., S.J. Stowers, R.R. Maronpot, M.A. Anderson, and S.A. Aaronson. 1986. Detection and identification of activated oncogenes in spontaneously occurring benign and malignant hepatocellular tumors of the B6C3F1 mouse. *Proc. Natl. Acad. Sci. U.S.A.* **83:** 33.

Roy, A.K. and D.L. Raber. 1972. Immunofluorescent localization of $\alpha_{2\mu}$-globulin in the hepatic and renal tissues of the rat. *J. Histochem. Cytochem.* **20:** 89.

Short, B.G., V.L. Burnett, and J.A. Swenberg. 1986. Histopathology and cell proliferation induced by 2,2,4-trimethylpentane in the male rat kidney. *Toxicol. Pathol.* **14:** 194.

Solleveld, H.A., J.K. Haseman, and E.E. McConnell. 1984. Natural history of body weight gain, survival and neoplasia in the F344 rat. *J. Natl. Cancer Inst.* **72:** 929.

Swenberg, J.A., E.A. Gross-Bermudez, and H.W. Randall. 1986a. Localization and quantitation of cell proliferation following exposure to nasal irritants. In *Toxicity of the nasal passages* (ed. C.S. Barrow), p. 291. Hemisphere Publishing, New York.

Swenberg, J.A. 1986b. Brain tumors—Problems and perspectives. *Food Cosmet. Toxicol.* **24:** 155.

Swenberg, J.A., H. d'A. Heck, K.T. Morgan, and T.B. Starr. 1985. A scientific approach to formaldehyde risk assessment. *Banbury Rep.* **19:** 255.

Swenberg, J.A., C.S. Barrow, C.J. Boreiko, H. d'A. Heck, R.J. Levine, K.T. Morgan, and T.B. Starr. 1983. Nonlinear biological responses to formaldehyde and their implications for carcinogenic risk assessment. *Carcinogenesis* **4:** 945.

COMMENTS

GHOSHAL: Dr. Ward reported 2 or 3 years ago that in the rat liver there are spontaneous tumors, but when he tried to promote it by phenobarbital, the number didn't increase. This shows that these tumors are just not promotable. They never developed into cancer, but just remained as foci.

SWENBERG: These are already tumors. I am not talking about foci. Ward's paper was on foci.

GHOSHAL: No, no. He showed that at old age, in a small percentage of rats, there were tumors. But also, when he tried to promote with phenobarbital, if there were some spontaneous foci, then naturally phenobarbital would promote more tumors.

TENNANT: You are equating just a temporal situation. That additional 25% or 30% of life span doesn't imply that there is likewise the same degree of proliferation in an animal.

SWENBERG: Absolutely not. I am saying that cancer in these rats is very definitely age-related. We know that cells undergo a certain number of replications in the life span of a control animal. One can at least hypothesize that, if you have five times that amount of proliferation going on for 2 years, that is very likely, for reasons we have heard earlier today, to result in an increase in tumors. The question then is, Is that a carcinogen? You could also take it further into the regulatory arena and ask, What are the risks of doses that don't cause such increases in proliferation?

TENNANT: Relating to the point on the phenobarbital, too, there is some implication that tumorigenicity is overtoxicity, and I don't think that is necessarily the case; I mean, there are toxic noncarcinogens. The impetus of compensatory proliferation may be important in allowing expression of some tumors, but it is not really a causative agent itself.

SWENBERG: I don't think we really know that for a fact. I guess my plea is that we start trying to think about how can we design experiments to try to get at this kind of an issue. We don't know what is responsible for the increase in tumors with a 25% increase in life span. It could be oxidative damage, since these older cells contain increased lipofuscin.

PITOT: Have you determined cell proliferation rates during the period of initiation? It seems to me that variations in rates of cell proliferation during this period would be important in the later outcome of the experiment.

SWENBERG: We haven't looked at it, but we are going to. It should have returned to control levels by the time the promoter is started, because we have a full month in between.

PITOT: But actually during the period of initiation, does this initiator act in a manner similar to that of DEN, that is, actually decrease the rate of all proliferation?

SWENBERG: Those studies are under way, but we don't have the data yet. We are also looking at the alkylation in those kidneys. It doesn't affect the interpretations of the promotion study, however, since animals were randomized after initiation.

CERUTTI: I would like to bring this discussion back to genotoxicity. It has been speculated that the number of replication cycles might be proportional to mutagenicity. This could explain the type of model you are proposing. On the other hand, recent data from experiments where plasmids were transfected into human cells and mutations were analyzed in the rescued plasmid showed that the deletion of the replication origin (totally inhibiting replication of the plasmid) had no effect on the mutation rates. The present data, disappointingly, argues against a simple relationship between mutagenicity and numbers of replication cycles.

REITZ: Yes, but that still leaves the possibility that DNA repair is less effective.

SWENBERG: I think that any time you have a genotoxic agent replication is very important.

SLAGA: We have to be very careful when we say a toxic noncarcinogenic compound, because in a lot of cases it's related to our ignorance. We just really have not adequately looked at them in a large dose-response study.

SWENBERG: That was why I asked my question about the antibiotics and the extent of testing. You call them noncarcinogenic if they haven't been tested, but it's really a state of ignorance.

TRUMP: Getting back to the aging kidney, there is a lot going on there in terms of tubular lesions and inflammation. A lot of the so-called basophilic atrophic areas may reflect cell turnover. Have you done the minipump studies in the old animals?

SWENBERG: No, but I can assure you we will.

TRUMP: Because almost anything in the bioassay program that is nephro-carcinogenic seems to also intensify what would be called the old rat nephropathy; and conversely, aging itself may be a promoter in the male rat. There is nothing new on that.

ROE: In relation to your last slide, surely more than one mechanism must be implicated. Insofar as we know that a wide variety of mechanisms is involved in carcinogenesis, I cannot believe that it is sensible to make general statements about the role of one factor in the causation of cancers of quite different sites and kinds. Pituitary and mammary tumors arise because animals are seriously abnormal, from a hormonal viewpoint, as a consequence of overfeeding. These problems increase with age, but they do not necessarily have anything to do with an aging process per se.

SWENBERG: Those data were obtained in control animals; they do not involve a chemical.

ROE: I know that. Overfeeding renders untreated control animals endocrinologically abnormal, as well as animals in the treated groups.

MAGEE: Some years ago, we showed that trichloroethylene in the liver does bind to DNA, but it does it to a very, very small extent. We regard it as being so low as to be nongenotoxic, but this may not be the case.

SWENBERG: We were actually quite surprised when it didn't cause more cell proliferation, but not necessarily surprised that it didn't induce hyaline droplets.

STEVENSON: Since food reduction or the use of a semisynthetic diet reduces tumors so dramatically and increases life span so much, do you have any information as to whether that affects the rate of cell turnover?

SWENBERG: No, I don't.

ROE: Ames is presently investigating this and is looking for DNA breakdown products in urine.

TRUMP: But protein deprivation in the case of the kidney really can modify downward the old rat nephropathy. That's the one thing we know that can control it—protein in the diet.

ROE: It doesn't have to be protein. You can just do it with food (i.e., total calories not just protein).

ANDERSON: Masoro did that with the 40% reduction of diet intake, where he eliminated the kidney lesion of aged rats.

ROE: You don't have to submit animals to such severe restrictions. Nephropathy can be largely eliminated with just 20% restriction.

ANDERSON: He happened to use 40%, but he increased the life span something like 40% and the end-stage kidney was not an issue in those animals; whereas, with the full-fed animals, 80% were diagnosed with end-stage kidneys at death.

Session 3:
Rodent Bioassays

Nongenotoxic Mouse Liver Carcinogens

PAUL M. NEWBERNE, VORA SUPHAKARN, PHAIBUL PUNYARIT,
AND JOAO DE CAMARGO
Department of Pathology
Boston University School of Medicine
Boston, Massachusetts 02118

OVERVIEW

There has been growing concern in recent years in the scientific community and the lay public regarding the validity of using rodent studies to evaluate the risk of drugs and other chemicals to human populations. A number of prominent substances, some of which have been used by humans for long periods without apparent harm, have recently been declared carcinogenic on the basis of the appearance of liver neoplasms in rodents exposed to them (The Nutrition Foundation 1983). In some instances (Table 1), it has been only the mouse liver that has been affected, and often there was no further evidence that the substance in question possessed other characteristics typical of carcinogens. These chemicals, more often than not, do not exhibit evidence of mutagenicity and must therefore be considered nongenotoxic. Despite this, however, they may induce tumors in mouse and rat liver. Such observations, in many instances, have raised questions about the interpretation of the data and point toward the need for a better understanding of mechanisms in carcinogenesis by nongenotoxic agents.

INTRODUCTION

A large number of chemicals are associated with liver tumors in rodents (Butler and Newberne 1975; Newberne and Butler 1978), many of which produce neoplasms in mice only (The Nutrition Foundation 1983). Some of these substances are widely distributed in the environment (e.g., pesticides) and others are drugs ingested by humans for a variety of therapeutic purposes. Such chemicals are often enzyme inducers and promoters of liver neoplasms that may be initiated by other agents (Kunz et al. 1983; Williams and Numoto 1984; Glauert et al. 1986). Moreover, many of the chemicals that induce liver nodules and tumors in mice are generally negative in a variety of short-term tests for DNA effects. This is in contrast to human chemical carcinogens, most of which are DNA-reactive genotoxic agents (IARC 1982). These differences create problems in the interpretation of animal data and its meaning relative to human risk.

We have conducted investigations in rodents in which we examined the effects of hepatotoxic agents on the liver of mice, as well as a dietary deficiency that induces liver neoplasia. None of these are DNA-reactive agents and should

Banbury Report 25: Nongenotoxic Mechanisms in Carcinogenesis
© Cold Spring Harbor Laboratory. 0-87969-225-1/87. $1.00 + .00
165

Table 1
Chemicals That Induced Liver Tumors in Mice Only: NCI Bioassay

Aldrin	1,1,2,2,-Tetrachloroethane
Captan	Tetrachloroethylene
Chloramben	Tetrachlorvinphos
Chlordane	Toxaphene
Chlordecone	1,1,2-Trichloroethane
Chlorobenzilate	Trichloroethylene
Chloroform	Trifluralin
Chlorothalonil	3'-Nitro-p-acetophenetide
p,p'-DDE	5-Nitro-o-anisidine
Dibromochloropropane	6-Nitro-benzimidazole
1,2-Dibromoethane	Nitrofen
1,2-Dichloroethane	2-Nitro-p-phenylenediamine
Dicofol	3-Nitropropionic acid
1,4-Dioxane	N-Nitrosodiphenylamine
Heptachlor	p-Nitrosodiphenylamine
Hexachloroethane	5-Nitro-o-Toluidine
Nitrofen	Phenazopyridine HCl
Sulfallate	Piperonyl sulfoxide

therefore be considered nongenotoxic, acting through mechanisms other than damage to genetic material. The substances or conditions reported on here are (1) the pesticide DCB (3,5-dichloro [N-1,1-dimethyl-2-propynyl] benzamide), (2) phenobarbital, and (3) choline deficiency. Some pertinent results are described for each of the studies. Generally, we have given DCB and phenobarbital in the diet, or we have provided rigidly controlled, semipurified diets low in, or devoid of, choline and other lipotropic factors (Newberne et al. 1983). Male hybrid mice (B6C3F$_1$) were used in studies reported here.

RESULTS

Pesticide Toxicity/Carcinogenicity

Groups of mice were either untreated or were fed the pesticide DCB at varying levels for 12, 18, or 24 months (Essigmann and Newberne 1981); DCB was incorporated into NIH-07 open formula natural product diet. A few mice from each group were sacrificed at 12, 18, and 24 months to evaluate potential tumorigenicity characteristics and to assess the enzyme alterations associated with nodule and tumor formation. A short-exposure study was also conducted to determine if the preponderance of tumors in the median lobe and, to a lesser extent, the right lobe were associated with early and continuous hepatonecrosis. Each mouse was given [^{3}H]thymidine (1 μCi/g body weight); after 1.5–2 hours they were sacrificed. Sections of left, median, and right lobes were prepared for routine hematoxylin and eosin staining, and additional slides of the same areas were prepared for autoradiography. Counts were

Table 2
Proliferative Liver Lesions in Mice Treated with DCB

	Dietary DCB (PPM; % tumor-bearing animals)				
Lesions	none(294)[a]	20(147)	100(147)	500(147)	2500(146)
Nonneoplastic (hyperplastic nodule)	15.0	21.0	23.8	35.3	34.9
Neoplastic (adenoma/carcinoma)	7.1	15.6	20.4	26.5	39.7
Total nonneoplastic and neoplastic	22.0	36.7	44.2	61.9	74.6

Abridged data from Essigmann and Newberne (1981).
[a]Number in parentheses is total in group.

made in ten high-power fields in the periportal and centrilobular zones of each mouse liver and combined to arrive at a mean $\pm$ s.d. number.

There was a clear dose response, in terms of neoplasms (Table 2), with a preference for the median and right lobes of the liver. This correlated well with necrosis and hepatocyte [^{3}H]thymidine labeling (Table 3) in a short-term study. Hypertrophy and necrosis were most prominent in the centrilobular zone. This strain of mouse exhibits a variable but significant incidence of liver tumors in untreated controls; about 22% of the untreated animals in this study had liver nodules (Table 2). However, in the short-term study, evidence for necrosis in this group was not detected, implying that one population of cells developed tumors without significant evidence for necrosis.

Serum glutamic pyruvic transaminase (SGPT) concentrations clearly indicated

Table 3
DCB, Serum Enzyme Levels, Liver Necrosis, and [^{3}H]Thymidine Labeling of Hepatocytes in Median Lobes of Male B6C3F$_1$ Mice

Pesticide level (ppm)	SGPT (IU/liter)	Necrotic index[a]		[^{3}H]Thymidine[b] labeled nuclei (%)	
		periportal	centrilobular	periportal	centrilobular
0	n.d.	0.0	0.0	0.1±0.1	0.1±0.1
100	62±30	0.1±0.1	0.2±0.1	0.2±0.1	0.3±0.1
200	88±18	0.3±0.2	0.9±0.2	0.4±0.1	1.0±0.1
500	98±21	0.6±0.2	1.4±0.4	0.8±0.2	1.1±0.3
1000	140±20	1.1±0.2	3.0±0.8	2.1±0.5	6.9±1.2
1500	243±25	1.9±0.3	3.6±1.0	2.5±0.9	7.2±1.8
2000	334±31	1.7±0.2	3.4±0.9	3.1±0.7	10.1±1.6
2500	420±34	1.6±0.4	2.8±0.7	3.0±0.6	8.3±1.1

Ten weanling male mice per group were fed DCB 6 weeks prior to sacrifice. n.d. = none detected.
[a]Mean $\pm$ s.d. necrotic hepatocytes, ten high-power fields/mouse in ten mice (100 total).
[b]Mean $\pm$ s.d. hepatocytes with nuclei labeled with 6 or more grains in ten high-power fields per mouse in ten mice (100 total).

increasing hepatocellular injury with increasing dose of chemical. Liver cell injury correlated closely with the chronic effects. Thus, liver injury, necrosis, nuclear labeling with [^{3}H]thymidine (higher in the centrilobular zone), and the chronic results all point to a correlation between liver necrosis and the induction of liver tumors.

Phenobarbital Tumorigenesis

Phenobarbital is used widely in human and veterinary medicine, and the many effects it exerts on the morphology and metabolism of hepatocytes have been described by a number of investigators (Jones and Fawcett 1966; Peraino et al. 1966, 1971; Conney 1967; Kuntzman 1969; Smuckler and Arcasoy 1969; Thorpe and Walker 1973; Ponomarkov et al. 1976). It causes proliferation of smooth endoplasmic reticulum, increased synthesis of RNA and drug metabolizing enzymes, and increased mitotic activity of hepatocytes (Conney and Gilman 1963; Burger and Herdson 1966; Japundzic et al. 1967; Peraino et al. 1971). These observations and other considerations led to testing of phenobarbital for carcinogenic activity (Peraino et al. 1973; Thorpe and Walker 1973; Ponomarkov et al. 1976). It has thus been established that phenobarbital is a carcinogen for the mouse liver.

More recently, phenobarbital has been used to promote carcinogenesis initiated by other chemicals (Peraino et al. 1971; Weisburger et al. 1975; Glauert et al. 1986). Our interest in phenobarbital stemmed from observations made during studies comparing phenobarbital with pesticides that induce hypertrophy, necrosis, and liver tumors in mice (Essigmann and Newberne 1981). The hypertrophy and necrosis appeared to be similar to that induced by chronic exposure to phenobarbital (Burger and Herdson 1966; Smuckler and Arcasoy 1969; Newberne and Rogers 1986). Some of our observations are reported below.

Most studies with phenobarbital have used 500 ppm, administered either in the drinking water or mixed into the diet. If a chemical is an enzyme inducer, we usually do a 3–4-week preliminary exposure study in groups of animals as a guide to setting doses for chronic studies. This was done with phenobarbital to groups of nine mice each, with the various groups exposed to dietary concentrations ranging from 200 ppm to 1000 ppm, as shown in Figure 1. On the basis of these 30-day exposures, enzyme induction (paranitroanisole), and relative liver weight, we established two dietary exposure levels (500 and 800 ppm) and maintained them for 80 weeks. Some mice from each group were examined for morphologic changes, serum enzyme (SGPT) concentrations, [^{3}H]thymidine labeling, and hepatocyte necrotic index. Table 4 lists results of some of the short-term studies, and Table 5 shows survival rate, tumor incidence, and liver/body weight ratios in the control and two treated groups. The SGPT levels correlated with levels of phenobarbital at both 1 and 3 months, as did the labeling index and necrosis of hepatocytes. In the 500-ppm group, the mice appeared to adjust to the injury and the indices declined after 3 months. This was not the case, however, in the 800-ppm group, where all

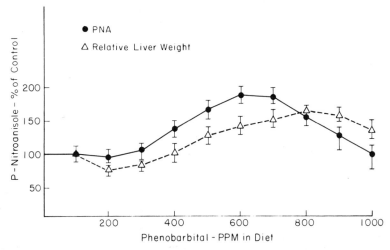

Figure 1

Nine male $B6C3F_1$ hybrid mice in each group were fed a semipurified diet containing sodium phenobarbital at the various concentrations indicated. After 30 days, the mice were sacrificed, the livers were weighed, and samples were taken for paranitroanisole assay. The resulting data were used to construct this plot. We chose 500 ppm as a lower dose that the mice could metabolize without evidence of compromising liver function; 800 ppm exceeds the capability of normal enzyme induction and detoxification, as shown by a plateau in relative liver weight and by a decrease in enzyme induction. This level, over a long period (80 weeks) of exposure, could be expected to exceed the maximum tolerated dose, which proved to be the case.

Table 4

Liver Injury and Repair in Liver of Mice Exposed to Phenobarbital at Two Dietary Concentrations

	Control	500 ppm	800 ppm
SGPT			
IU/liter			
1 month	n.d.	62±21	485±35
3 months	n.d.	40±8	740±54
[³H] Thymidine labeling index[a]			
1 month	0.7±0.07	0.8±0.2	4.7±0.4
3 months	0.4±0.09	0.3±0.07	6.3±0.6
Necrotic index[b]			
1 month	n.d.	1.2±0.4	4.6±1.2
3 months	n.d.	0.5±0.1	5.2±1.1

Ten mice per group per time point. n.d. indicates not determined.
[a]Percentage of hepatocyte nuclei labeled.
[b]Mean ± s.e. number of necrotic hepatocytes, ten high-power fields.

Table 5
Survival Rate, Liver and Body Weights, and Tumor Incidence in Mice Fed Phenobarbital

	Control	500 ppm	800 ppm
Survival (%)			
52 weeks	98	100	89
80 weeks	90	85	75
Body weight	42±3.8	44±6.5	36±4.8
Liver weight (g)[a]	1.40±0.16	2.40±0.21	2.41±0.43
Ratio (liver/body weight)	3.32	5.45	6.70
Tumor incidence			
52 weeks	5	9	35
80 weeks	21	52	82

100 male B6C3F$_1$ mice each group.
[a]Nontumorous livers only (mean ± s.e.).

parameters increased (compared to the 500-ppm group) and were higher after 3-month exposure than after 1-month exposure.

Choline Deficiency and Liver Carcinogenesis

Choline deficiency as a promoter for hepatocellular tumors has been used by many investigators in recent years (Rogers and Newberne 1980; Abanobi et al. 1982; Newberne et al. 1982; Ghosal and Farber 1983; Mikol et al. 1983). Almost all of these studies have used rats, which accounts for a preponderance of data associated with this species. Most strains of mice have been resistant to choline deficiency, but the discovery that the hybrid B6C3F$_1$ is susceptible not only to choline deficiency (Newberne et al. 1982), but also to aflatoxin B$_1$ (AFB$_1$) gave us an interesting additional model to investigate mechanisms for carcinogenesis. Table 6 lists the effects of a single dose of AFB$_1$ combined with choline deficiency. Under these conditions, the normal, supplemented control mice were not sensitive to AFB$_1$. However, when the mice were fed a choline-deficient diet, there was a significant incidence of liver tumors (80%). Furthermore, this relatively high incidence could be reduced to near control levels by feeding the antioxidant butylated hydroxyanisole (BHA). Tissue peroxidation has been associated with lipid peroxidation (Newberne et al. 1969, 1986; Wilson et al. 1973; Ghoshal et al. 1984). This suggested acute, short-term studies, designed and conducted to evaluate this possibility and factors that might account for the susceptibility to AFB$_1$. Table 7 lists some of the results of the short-term studies.

Earlier studies had shown that choline deficiency has little, if any, effect on the concentration of glutathione (GSH) in the liver. However, as noted in table 7, when AFB$_1$ was superimposed on the choline-deficient mouse, liver GSH levels were depressed. This decrease was, in part, moderated by BHA. Since a major route for detoxification of AFB$_1$ is by conjugation with GSH, we examined the livers of some

Table 6
Influence of Choline Deficiency and BHA on AFB$_1$-Induced Liver Tumors in Mice

	Incidence of liver tumors	
Group treatment	no.	%
None - controls	3/25	12.0
Control + AFB$_1$	5/25	20.0
Choline-deficient	7/25	28.0
Choline-deficient + AFB$_1$	20/25	80.0
Choline-deficient + AFB$_1$ + BHA	6/24	24.0

Male mice, B6C3F$_1$ 9 weeks of age, given 6 mg/kg body weight in DMSO, by gavage. BHA was included in semisynthetic diet at 1% level. Mice were sacrificed at 60 weeks. Abridged data from Newberne et al. (1986).

of the mice in this study for GSH-AFB$_1$ conjugates. There appeared to be less conjugation in the choline-deficient liver. In the choline-deficient liver exposed to AFB$_1$, supplementation with BHA increased GSH-AFB$_1$ conjugation significantly.

Necrosis of hepatocytes was increased in groups given AFB$_1$, whether deficient or supplemented with choline, but the choline-deficient group given AFB$_1$ had the most severe necrosis, measured either by SGPT determinations or by counting necrotic cells. The thiobarbituric acid (TBA) reactants were highest in this group as well, suggesting that GSH metabolism, peroxidation, and necrosis were interacting

Table 7
Effects of AFB$_1$ on Lipid Peroxidation, Liver Necrosis, GSH, and AFB$_1$-GSH Conjugates in B6C3F$_1$ Male Mice

				Choline-deficient	
	Control	Control + AFB$_1$	Choline-deficient	+ AFB$_1$	+ AFB$_1$ + BHA
GSH					
(μmole/g liver)	8.11±0.6	5.23±1.4	8.30±0.8	4.1±0.5	6.0±0.7
GSH-AFB$_1$ conjugate					
(nmole/g/hr)	0	0.11 (0.07–0.14)	0	0.06 (0.04–0.08)	0.15 (0.11–0.19)
SGPT					
(IU/liter)	93±21	360±36	342±29	466±42	206±26
Necrotic index					
(mean no./10 fields)	0	6.3	2.4±0.4	9.6±1.1	2.6±0.6
TBA reactants					
(μg MDA equiv./g dry fat-free liver)	8.3±2.1	14.2±3.1	210±8.2	301±14.1	29.6±3.4

Mice sacrificed 24 hr after exposure to intragastric dose AFB$_1$, 6 mg/kg, when acute injury has peaked. Data abridged from Newberne et al. (1986).

in some manner that might contribute to enhancement of AFB$_1$ carcinogenesis observed in the chronic study.

DISCUSSION

The three examples of carcinogenesis described here, in mice exposed to non-genotoxic carcinogens or to a dietary deficiency that results in increased liver tumors, provide a basis for arguing that hepatocellular necrosis contributes to and is significantly involved in mice fed increasing levels of the pesticide. The tumor incidences in the various groups correlated well with continued chronic liver injury and regeneration.

Injury of the mouse liver by pesticides of many different chemical structural configurations is a well-known phenomena. Many such compounds are potent enzyme inducers and, where given at maximum tolerated doses, result in marked hepatocellular hypertrophy and in liver cell necrosis. The study with the pesticide DCB is a good example of a substance that causes the development of liver tumors in mice through a nongenotoxic mechanism. DCB is not mutagenic; it has been tested in a variety of systems and is negative. Thus, the tumorigenic effect occurs by way of some other mechanism. We prefer to consider that its necrogenic effect is an important factor.

Similar to many pesticides, DCB results in enzyme induction, and after a period of time, in the centrilobular zone, parenchymal cell hypertrophy, necrosis, and compensatory hyperplasia takes place. This occurs in a dose-response relationship. Focal hepatocellular hyperplasia is observed in the same area as necrosis, and it is in this area that nodules and tumors are first observed.

Phenobarbital at two different dietary concentrations resulted in significant hepatocellular injury, particularly at the 800-ppm level. All of the parameters measured suggested that the 800-ppm level exceeded the capacity of the hepatocytes to detoxify the chemical. The hepatocytes, perhaps through exhaustion and death, set the stage for uncontrolled compensatory hyperplasia terminating in neoplasia. The similarity between the effects of a tumorigenic pesticide and phenobarbital are striking and suggest that similar mechanisms are extant.

The choline-deficient mouse model is an important tool for elucidating mechanisms for hepatocellular carcinogenesis. Table 6 shows the effects of choline deficiency combined with AFB$_1$ on tumor induction. Under the conditions of this study, only the deficient liver exposed to AFB$_1$ had a significant increase in tumors, and this was inhibited by the antioxidant BHA. This strongly suggests that peroxidation was in some way involved with the development of tumors, a hypothesis supported further by the presence of TBA-reactive materials in high concentrations in those two groups with the increased tumor incidence (choline-deficient and choline-deficient plus AFB$_1$). It is not surprising, then, that tumors occurred in the choline-deficient mice; we have observed that previously (Newberne et al. 1982). Evidence for necrosis (SGPT and necrotic index) and for peroxidation generally agree with tumor appearance.

The roles of glutathione and other thiols in cellular toxicity have been demonstrated by many investigators (Jallou et al. 1974; Stacey and Klassen 1981; Jewell et al. 1982; Orrenius et al. 1983; Casini et al. 1985; Helliwell et al. 1985). There is little doubt that GSH, lipid peroxidation, and necrosis are important aspects of tissue injury, regeneration and, in some cases, tumor formation. However, the significance of these factors, their interactions, and the relative importance of each await further studies. It is our belief that many factors, including liver lipid, cell injury, enzyme induction beyond the capacity of the cell to sustain itself, and the availability of glutathione or other biological antioxidants, can all play variable but significant roles in hepatocellular necrosis and subsequent hyperplasia and neoplasia.

Although these data are circumstantial, it would be difficult to deny an important correlation between hepatocellular necrosis, hyperplasia, and tumor induction. A similar pattern is seen in mice fed phenobarbital for long periods of time, and the tumors that develop under these conditions probably have much in common with DCB and other enzyme-inducing, necrogenic agents that are not DNA-reactive. The data of Ying et al. (1981) appear to support our hypothesis.

CONCLUSION

The data provided here in three animal models for mouse liver tumorigenesis point to a multicausal mechanism for the induction of tumors by non-DNA-reactive chemicals or conditions. It is our hypothesis that chronic cell death, regeneration, and loss of regulatory control over liver cell proliferation result in neoplasia. The concomitants of tissue peroxidation, aberrations of detoxifying enzyme systems, or aberrant methylation of nucleic acid bases (Becker et al. 1981; Newberne et al. 1986; Wainfan 1986), all acting in concert, contribute to neoplasia.

ACKNOWLEDGMENTS

The work described in this paper was supported by grants from Rohm and Haas, Eli Lilly, Hoffmann LaRoche, and the National Institutes of Health (CA-32520, CA-26731 and AM-32959).

REFERENCES

Abanobi, S.E., B. Lombardi, and H. Shinozuka. 1982. Stimulation of DNA synthesis and cell proliferation in the liver of rats fed a choline-devoid diet and their suppression by phenobarbital. *Cancer Res.* **42:** 412.

Becker, R.A., L.R. Barrows, and R.C. Shank. 1981. Methylation of DNA guanine in hydrazine hepatotoxicity: Dose response and kinetic characteristics of 7-methyl-guanine and O^6-methyl guanine formation and persistance in rats. *Carcinogenesis* **2:** 1181.

Burger, P.C. and P.B. Herdson. 1966. Phenobarbital induced fine structural changes in rat liver. *Am. J. Pathol.* **48:** 793.

Butler, W.H. and P.M. Newberne, eds. 1975. *Mouse liver neoplasia*. Elsevier, New York.

Casini, A.F., A. Pompella, and M. Comporti. 1985. Liver glutathione depletion induced by bromobenzene, iodobenzene, and diethylmaleate poisoning and its relation to lipid peroxidation and necrosis. *Am. J. Pathol.* **118:** 225.

Conney, A.H. 1967. Pharmacological implications of microsomal enzyme induction. *Pharmacol. Rev.* **19:** 317.

Conney, A.H. and A.G. Gilman. 1963. Puromycin inhibition of enzyme induction by 3-methylcholanthrene and phenobarbital. *J. Biol. Chem.* **238:** 3682.

Essigmann, E.M. and P.M. Newberne. 1981. Enzymatic alterations in mouse hepatic nodules induced by a chlorinated hydrogen pesticide. *Cancer Res.* **41:** 2823.

Ghoshal, A.K. and E. Farber. 1983. Induction of liver cancer by a diet deficient in choline and methionine. *Proc. Am. Assoc. Cancer Res.* **24:** 98.

Ghoshal, A.K., T. Rushmore, Y. Lim, and E. Farber. 1984. Early detection of lipid peroxidation in the hepatic nuclei of rats fed a diet deficient in choline and methionine. *Cancer Res.* **25:** 94.

Glauert, H.P., M. Schwarz, and H. Pitot. 1986. The phenotypic stability of altered hepatic foci: Effect of the short-term withdrawal of phenobarbital and of the long-term feeding of purified diets after the withdrawal of phenobarbital. *Carcinogenesis* **7:** 117.

Helliwell, T.R., J.H.K. Yeung, and B.K. Park. 1985. Hepatic necrosis and glutathione depletion in captopril-treated mice. *Br. J. Exp. Pathol.* **66:** 67.

International Agency for Research on Cancer (IARC) 1982. *Monographs on the evaluation of the carcinogenic risk of chemicals to humans: Chemicals, industrial processes and industries associated with cancer in humans,* suppl. 4. Lyon, France.

Jallou, D.J., J.R. Mitchell, N. Zampaglione, and J.R. Gillette. 1974. Bromobenzene-induced liver necrosis. Protective role of glutathione and evidence for 3,4-bromobenzene oxide as the hepatic metabolite. *Pharmacology* **11:** 151.

Japundzic, M., B. Knezenic, V. Djordjemic-Camba, and I. Japundzic. 1967. The influence of phenobarbital sodium on the mitotic activity of parenchymal cells during rat liver regeneration. *Exp. Cell Res.* **48:** 163.

Jewell, S.A., G. Bellows, H. Thor, S. Orrenius, and M.T. Smith. 1982. Bleb formation in hepatocytes during drug metabolism is caused by disturbances in thiol and calcium ion homeostasis. *Science* **217:** 1257.

Jones, A.L. and D.W. Fawcett. 1966. Hypertrophy of the agranular endoplasmic reticulum in hamster liver induced by phenobarbital. *J. Histochem. Cytochem.* **14:** 215.

Kuntzman, R. 1969. Drugs and enzyme induction. *Annu. Rev. Pharmacol.* **9:** 21.

Kunz, H.C., H.A. Tennekes, R.E. Port, M. Schwarz, D. Lorke, and G. Schaude. 1983. Quantitative aspects of chemical carcinogenesis and tumor promotion in liver. *Environ. Health Perspect.* **50:** 113.

Mikol, Y.B., K.L. Hoover, D. Creasia, and L.A. Poirier. 1983. Hepatocarcinogenesis in rats fed methyl-deficient, amino acid defined diets. *Carcinogenesis* **4:** 1619.

Newberne, P.M. and W.H. Butler, eds. 1978. *Rat liver neoplasia*. MIT Press, Cambridge, Massachusetts.

Newberne, P.M. and A.E. Rogers. 1986. Labile methyl group and the promotion of cancer. *Annu. Rev. Nutr.* **6**: 407.

Newberne, P.M., M.R. Bresnahan, and N. Kula. 1969. Effects of two synthetic antioxidants, vitamin E and ascorbic acid on the choline deficient rat. *J. Nutr.* **97**: 219.

Newberne, P.M., J.L.V. deCamargo, and A.J. Clark. 1982. Choline deficiency, partial hepatectomy and liver tumors in rats and mice. *Toxicol. Pathol.* **10**: 95.

Newberne, P.M., A.E. Rogers, and K. Nauss. 1983. Choline, methionine and related factors in oncogenesis. In *Nutritional factors in the induction and maintenance of malignancy* (ed. C.E. Butterworth and M. Hutchinson), p. 247. Academic Press, New York.

Newberne, P.M., P. Punyarit, J.L.V. deCamargo, and V. Suphakarn. 1986. The role of necrosis in hepatocellular proliferation and liver tumors. Proceedings of conference on mouse liver tumors: Relevance to human cancer risk. *Arch. Pathol.* **10**: 54.

The Nutrition Foundation. 1983. *The relevance of mouse liver hepatoma to human carcinogen risk. A report of the International Expert Advisory Committee to the Nutrition Foundation.* The Nutrition Foundation, Washington, D.C.

Orrenius, S., K. Armstad, H. Thor, and S.A. Jewell. 1983. Turnover and functions of glutathione studied in isolated hepatic and renal cells. *Fed. Proc.* **42**: 3177.

Peraino, C., R.J.M. Fry, and E. Staffeldt. 1971. Reduction and enhancement by phenobarbital of hepatocarcinogenesis induced in the rat by 2-acetylaminofluorene. *Cancer Res.* **31**: 1506.

———. 1973. Enhancement of spontaneous hepatic tumorigenesis in C3H mice by dietary phenobarbital. *J. Natl. Cancer Inst.* **51**: 1349.

Peraino, C., C. Lamar, Jr., and H.C. Pitot. 1966. Studies on the induction and repression of enzymes in rat liver. IV. Effects of cortisone and phenobarbital. *J. Biol. Chem.* **241**: 2944.

Ponomarkov, V., L. Tomatis, and V. Turusov. 1976. The effect of long-term administration of phenobarbitone in CF-1 mice. *Cancer Lett.* **1**: 165.

Rogers, A.E. and P.M. Newberne. 1980. Lipotrope deficiency in experimental carcinogenesis. *Nutr. Cancer* **2**: 104.

Smuckler, E.A. and M. Arcasoy. 1969. Structural and functional changes of the endoplasmic reticulum of hepatic parenchymal cells. *Int. Rev. Exp. Pathol.* **7**: 305.

Stacey, N.H. and C.D. Klassen. 1981. Inhibition of lipid peroxidation without prevention of cellular injury in isolated rat hepatocytes. *Toxicol. Appl. Pharmacol.* **58**: 8.

Thorpe, E. and A.I.T. Walker. 1973. The toxicology of dieldrin (HEOD). II. Comparative long-term oral toxicity studies in mice with dieldrin, DDT, phenobarbitone, B-BHC and Y-BHC. *Food Cosmet. Toxicol.* **11**: 433.

Wainfan, E., M. Dizik, M. Hluboky, and M.E. Balis. 1986. Altered tRNA methylation in rats and mice fed lipotrope-deficient diets. *Carcinogenesis* **7**: 473.

Weisburger, J.H., R.M. Madison, J.M. Ward, C. Viguera, and E.K. Weisburger. 1975. Modification of diethylnitrosamine liver carcinogenesis with phenobarbital but not with immunosuppression. *J. Natl. Cancer Inst.* **54**: 1185.

Williams, G.M. and S. Numoto. 1984. Promotion of mouse liver neoplasms by the organochlorine pesticides chlordane and heptachlor in comparison to dichlorodiphenyltrichloroethane. *Carcinogenesis* **5**: 1689.

Wilson, R.B., N.S. Kula, P.M. Newberne, and M.W. Conner. 1973. Vascular damage and lipid peroxidation in choline-deficient rats. *Exp. Mol. Pathol.* **18**: 357.

Ying, T.S., D.S.R. Sarma, and E. Farber. 1981. The role of acute hepatic necrosis in the induction of early steps in liver carcinogenesis by diethylnitrosamine. *Cancer Res.* **41:** 2096.

COMMENTS

SLAGA: What compound doesn't work with choline deficiency?

NEWBERNE: The liver carcinogen that doesn't work in our hands with lipatrope-deficient diets is dimethylnitrosamine (DMN). Virtually every other one works about the same.

SLAGA: Did you use a dose at which the tumor response could increase?

NEWBERNE: I don't know. We have done straight DMN carcinogenesis in the noncholine-deficient liver. The deficient liver didn't seem to affect it any; that is, we obtained the same incidence and frequencies, deficient or not. With all the others, though, it really does elevate the frequency and incidence. The tumors develop sooner, and all of the bits and pieces you see that are indicative of the induction begin much earlier. You can see the focal areas of cellular alteration and hyperplasia at the end of treatment with the carcinogen; this usually takes 3 or 4 months in a control animal.

GHOSHAL: You said that fat accumulation due to choline deficiency is centrilobular. Your diet is not only deficient in choline, but also deficient in methionine, B_{12}, and folic acid. Our diet is like that of Lombardi's diet, only deficient in choline and marginally deficient in methionine, but not deficient in B_{12} and folic acid. When we give this diet to rats, we found that fat accumulation starts from zone 1 on the first day, then zone 2, and then after 5 days, all over. We also found that out of 45 rats, only 2 or 3 had liver cirrhosis. We did not get any cirrhosis of liver, most probably due to added B_{12}.

NEWBERNE: I know that the four lipatropes—B_{12}, choline, folate, and methionine—all interact and ratios influence the effects, overall. B_{12} can have an enhancing effect in addition to the other members, particularly when dietary protein is low. It is an interesting model because you do not have to add a carcinogen to it. You take important dietary constituents out and you get tumors.

REITZ: When you looked at the thymidine-labeling index, did you notice any time dependency? I presume that the numbers you showed us were at the time that the animals were sacrificed, or right before.

NEWBERNE: No. We have done sequential studies with labeling to follow development of the nodules. They label from the beginning of the period after exposure to the carcinogen. At 48 hours and 72 hours after administration of the last dose of a carcinogenic regimen of chlorinated hydrocarbon, aflatoxin, AAF, or diethylnitrosamine, there is marked labeling, more frequent in the periportal area, but afterward scattered throughout the lobule. It is unlike the labeling you see with a partial hepatectomy, which is uniform throughout the lobules. Labeling in this case is typical of what you see with other carcinogens, patchy and focal.

DI GIOVANNI: What does choline deficiency do to the liver in other strains of mice, for example, C57BL/6 mice?

NEWBERNE: It results in a fatty liver, but I have never been able to produce cirrhosis with it in other strains. That was the difference in the $B6C3F_1$ hybrid. This mouse develops cirrhosis as well as fatty liver, and in that respect it is similar to the rat. Most strains of mice are not sensitive to aflatoxin, as the $B6C3F_1$ mouse is; it takes an extremely high dose in other mouse strains to produce an effect. They metabolize it and detoxify and excrete the metabolites very efficiently.

DI GIOVANNI: But would choline deficiency, take a strain like C57BL/6 which has virtually no spontaneous or very, very low spontaneous tumor incidence in the liver, and increase that to any extent?

NEWBERNE: It hasn't in our hands.

GHOSHAL: We tried strain A mouse; we couldn't even produce fatty liver due to choline deficiency.

NEWBERNE: The mouse certainly is different.

TENNANT: The liver tumors that you observed with phenobarbital occurred after 1 year?

NEWBERNE: The tumors started to appear at about 1 year into the study. At about 50 weeks, we had a few; between 50 and 80 weeks, the incidence increased progressively.

TENNANT: Do you interpret that as a property of phenobarbital or as a consequence of the conditions under which the animals were exposed, that is, both the genotype of the B6 and dietary combination? Do you think you are looking at a property of phenobarbital? Is phenobarbital tumorigenic?

NEWBERNE: I think phenobarbital is tumorigenic. We are pushing beyond its usual effect with this type of diet, i.e., a semipurified high-protein diet, which in my view is a type of promotion. I think we have some interaction, but, nevertheless, you would get tumors in the phenobarbital-treated animal anyway. The parenchymal cell injury and death, with compensatory hyperplasia, is in my view the basis for enhanced tumor induction. Hypomethylation in choline deficiency is crucial to the end result, as Shank and I have shown in other systems.

TENNANT: I would like to push just slightly further for a semantic clarification then, because we clearly have a substance that under the right conditions of observation creates neoplastic lesions that do have the capacity to regress, which Dr. Pitot showed yesterday.

NEWBERNE: In the rat.

TENNANT: Yes. But, if under one circumstance we can see evidence of independent neoplastic induction, and where phenobarbital did demonstrate capacity to mutagenize *Salmonella,* then it seems that we have nothing but a conditional description for the actions of phenobarbital. It is conditionally a promoter, it is conditionally a mutagen, conditionally a carcinogen. It seems to me that this is at the heart of our problem. It is partially semantic, but what do we call phenobarbital?

STEVENSON: Was it positive in the Ames test with or without activation?

TENNANT: I can't recall.

STEVENSON: We couldn't show any microsomal metabolism of phenobarbital at all; so I would really question the Ames system.

TENNANT: It was tested under code in the standard protocol. It did produce a reproducible positive response. That is the extent that I can recall those data, but it was a tangible result.

ROSENKRANZ: It was tested in five different laboratories in the International Study and they all found it positive in the absence of metabolic activation.

NEWBERNE: If it is a mutagen, it certainly is not like MNNG. Therein is where we need a lot more study. Perhaps under certain conditions, it would be.

BUTTERWORTH: Let's assume that in the whole animal phenobarbital is not a mutagen. In your opinion, if you had gone to very low doses of phenobarbital where you saw no increase in S phase and no necrosis, do you think you would have eliminated the stimulus for the tumors?

NEWBERNE: That would be pure conjecture, but I suspect there is a level at which you would not get tumors.

Induction of Cancer by Dietary Deficiency without Added Carcinogens

AMIYA GHOSHAL, THOMAS RUSHMORE, AND EMMANUEL FARBER
Departments of Pathology and of Biochemistry
University of Toronto
Toronto, Ontario M5S 1A8, Canada

OVERVIEW

Of all the deaths due to cancer, 30–40% have been related to important effects of diet. One goal of the National Cancer Institute is to irradicate cancer caused by dietary imbalance by the end of this century. Imbalance of fat, protein, and many microconstituents, either singly or in combination, seems to be involved in the carcinogenic process. The main role of diet has so far been thought to be only as a modifier of carcinogenesis initiated by a carcinogen. The realization that an imbalance in the diet by itself might act as a carcinogen is now slowly emerging. Recently, it has been observed that a diet deficient in choline and methionine is carcinogenic to rat liver, with a 50% incidence of liver cell cancer and a 100% incidence of hepatic nodules within 2 years. Attempts to understand the mechanism by which a diet alone, in the absence of any added chemical carcinogen, induces hepatocellular carcinoma revealed that such a diet induces DNA alterations, perhaps mediated by nuclear lipid peroxidation. Since this diet also induces persistent liver cell proliferation, it appears that the mechanism by which the choline-methionine diet induces liver cell cancer is similar to that proposed for liver cell cancer induced by chemical carcinogens. The significance of these observations lies in the prospect that the interplay between diet, nutrition, and cancer can now be examined at a mechanistic level.

INTRODUCTION

The interplay between diet, nutrition, and cancer, even though recognized for a long time, has not been clarified at a mechanistic level in any depth, largely because of the lack of experimental models. Recently, three laboratories, including ours, have shown with purified and analyzed diets that dietary deficiency of choline and methionine (CD diet), without any added carcinogen, can induce hepatocellular carcinoma in the rat (Ghoshal and Farber 1983, 1984; Mikol et al. 1983; Yokoyama et al. 1985). This finding has a profound significance from the mechanistic point of view because of the knowledge already accumulated on experimental liver carcinogenesis models. To gain insight into the possible mechanism(s) by which a diet with no added chemical carcinogen causes liver carcinogenesis, we have

Banbury Report 25: Nongenotoxic Mechanisms in Carcinogenesis
© Cold Spring Harbor Laboratory. 0-87969-225-1/87. $1.00 + .00

undertaken this study to determine whether the CD diet induces changes in the liver similar to those induced by chemical carcinogens.

RESULTS

It is generally believed that chemical carcinogens interact with DNA either directly (covalent) or indirectly (e.g., free radicals including reactive oxygen species) to cause DNA damage (Slaga et al. 1981; Emerit and Cerutti 1982; Rajalakshmi et al. 1982; Ames 1983). Cell proliferation prior to the repair of critical lesions appears to be an important component in the initiation process. Amplification of initiated cells, with or without associated alterations in gene expression, is believed to result in promotion of the initiated cells to form nodules, papillomas, or polyps which as a population are precancerous. It thus became important to determine whether the CD diet would induce any alterations in liver DNA. Interestingly, the results obtained clearly indicated that the CD diet does indeed induce certain alterations in the liver DNA monitored either by alkaline sucrose density gradient (Fig. 1) or by alkaline elution techniques (Fig. 2). This DNA alteration is repaired when the CD diet is replaced by a choline-supplemented (CS) diet after 5 days for 2 weeks (see Figs. 1B and 2B).

Since the CD diet does not have any obvious exogenously added chemical carcinogen, it was reasoned that such DNA alterations could have arisen by some free radicals generated by the CD diet. Attention was directed toward the induction of lipid peroxides, especially in the nucleus, mainly because of the close proximity of the DNA. Indeed, within a period of 1 day, the CD diet induced nuclear lipid peroxidation (Rushmore et al. 1984).

In addition to the DNA damage, the second prerequisite to achieve initiation is liver cell proliferation prior to the repair of critical lesions. Interestingly, the CD diet does induce liver cell proliferation (Rogers and Newberne 1969). Thus, the CD diet, like chemical carcinogens, induces changes in the liver that have been postulated as necessary to achieve initiation (Fig. 3).

From the mechanistic viewpoint, it became important to determine the nature of free radicals induced by choline deficiency. This question was approached initially by determining whether a radicophile can inhibit the early effects induced by the CD diet. Recently, a group of compounds consisting of acylated enamide, which are potentially useful for free-radical trapping, have been synthesized and tested by Viehe and Roberfroid (Louvain University, Belgium) for their potential as antipromoters in chemically induced experimental cancers. The acylated enamide compound preferred for its peroxidation preventive action is designated as AD_5; its structural formula is shown in Figure 4. Oral administration of AD_5 to rats exposed to the CD diet prevents nuclear lipid peroxidation (Table 1).

The results are consistent with the hypothesis that the CD diet induces free

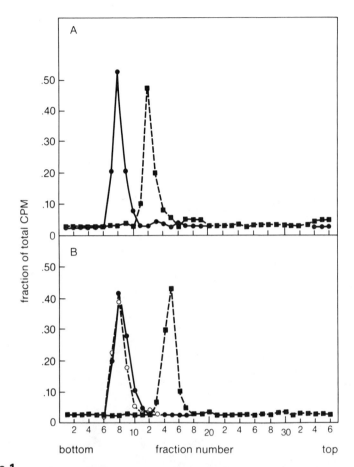

Figure 1

Alkaline–sucrose gradient profiles of DNAs from the livers of rats exposed to (■) CD or CS diet. (*A*) Control (CS) diet for 3 days (○), and CD diet for 3 days (■). (*B*) Control (CS) diet for 5 days (○), CD diet for 5 days (■), and CD diet for 5 days followed by CS diet for 14 days (●). Sedimentation is from right to left.

radicals. In the next series of experiments, attempts were made to characterize the free radicals by determining whether certain more specific antioxidants would inhibit the early effects induced by choline deficiency. Unfortunately, several antioxidants, BHA, BHT, DPPD, and Trolox-C, could not inhibit the nuclear lipid peroxidation induced by choline deficiency. This is not too surprising in view of the fact that these antioxidants are only marginally effective in preventing the liver injury induced by CCl_4 and other hepatotoxins, whose mechanism of action is known to be due, at least in part, to lipid peroxidation.

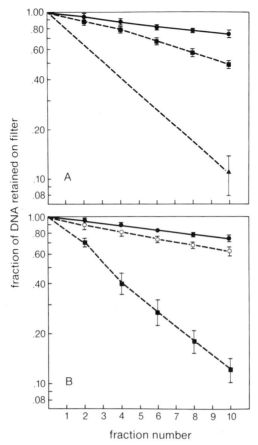

Figure 2

Alkaline elution profiles of rat liver DNA after exposure to a CS or CD diet. (*A*) Control (CS) diet for 3 days (○) CD diet for 3 days (■), and DMN 10 mg/kg (●). (*B*) Control (CS) diet for 5 days (○), CD diet for 5 days (■), and CD diet for 5 days followed by CS diet for 7 days (●). Each profile represents the mean of 8–16 values. Vertical bars represent the standard error.

Recently, in in vitro experiments, it was shown that lipid peroxidation could be detected in liver cells suspended in a Ca^{++}-free medium. Addition of Ca^{++} prevented lipid peroxidation in those cells (Fariss et al. 1984). Also, addition of excess calcium to the diet decreased cellular damage in the colon induced by carcinogen (Newmark et al. 1984). These observations prompted us to study the effect of Ca^{++} on the nuclear lipid peroxidation induced by the CD diet. The results indicated that Ca^{++} could inhibit the nuclear lipid peroxidation (Fig. 5). It also was found that extra dietary calcium could inhibit several other early changes, such as cell death and cell proliferation induced by the CD diet (Ghoshal et al. 1985a), but

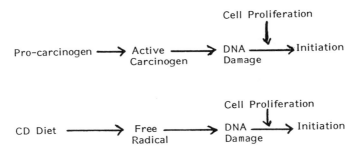

Figure 3
CD diet and chemical carcinogens induce changes in the liver postulated as necessary to achieve initiation.

not the accumulation of triglyceride ("fatty liver"). It is not yet established whether the nuclear lipid peroxidation induced by the CD diet is due to the increased generation of the free radicals, the decreased availability of competing free-radical scavengers, an increased susceptibility of the membranes, or combinations of these. Also of interest is whether the alterations observed in DNA are secondary to nuclear lipid peroxides or whether both DNA and nuclear lipid are the targets for some free radicals generated by choline deficiency (Fig. 6).

The results obtained thus far clearly indicate that the CD diet can induce changes that are relevant for initiation of liver carcinogenesis. The pertinent question now is, Does CD diet induce initiation? The relevance of this question stems from the argument that perhaps the induction of liver cell cancer by choline deficiency occurs because of its promoting effect on the preexisting initiated hepatocytes rather than on the independent initiation/promotion potential of the CD diet. The results clearly suggest that choline deficiency has the potential to induce initiated hepatocytes (Ghoshal et al. 1985b). The reason it takes 10 weeks of exposure to the CD diet to achieve initiation in spite of the fact that this diet can induce alterations in DNA and liver cell proliferation within the first few days of exposure is not clear and needs further study.

$$AD_5$$

$$CH_2{=}C\Big\langle\genfrac{}{}{0pt}{}{\text{COOH}}{\text{NH}{-}\overset{\overset{\text{O}}{\|}}{\text{C}}{-}\overset{\overset{\text{H}}{|}}{\text{CH}}}\!\!-\!\!\bigcirc\!\!-\text{OCH}_3$$

Figure 4
Structural formula of AD_5.

Table 1

Modification of Early Aberrations due to Choline Deficiency by AD_5 (7-day Exposure)

Treatment	Body weight (g)	Liver weight (g/100 g b.w.)	SDH (units/liter)	Diene conjugates $\left(\Delta E \; ^{1\%}_{1 \; cm} \right)$
CS diet	213±12.3 (12)	4.0	4.4±0.1	0.00
CD diet	210±12.8 (12)	5.1	27.21±2.8	0.89
CD diet + AD_5	208±11.8 (8)	4.2	5.0±0.5	0.00

Dose of AD_5: 40 mg/100 g in propylene glycol every day from day −1 to day 6 of exposure to a CD diet. (Data from Recknagel and Ghosal 1966.)

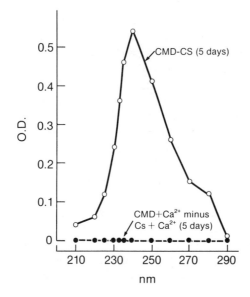

Figure 5

Diene conjugate absorption spectra of liver nuclear lipid. Rats were fed a CD diet or a CD diet + Ca^{++} for 5 days. Control rats were exposed to a CS diet or a CS diet + Ca^{++}.

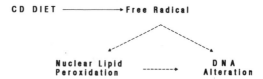

Figure 6

DNA and nuclear lipid as targets for free radicals generated by choline deficiency.

DISCUSSION

The discovery that rats develop liver cancer when exposed to the CD diet is not new. Copeland and Salmon (1946), and Buckley and Hartroft (1955) between 1946 and 1955, reported the occurrence of hepatocellular carcinoma in rats, mice, and chickens fed lipotrope-deficient diets. With the discovery of aflatoxin in 1958 and of its carcinogenic effects shortly thereafter, the significance of the CD diet was thrown in total disarray when it was observed that the peanut meal used in the lipotrope deficiency studies might have been contaminated with aflatoxin B_1 (Salmon and Newberne 1963; Newberne 1965). These observations concerning possible contamination with aflatoxin completely changed the direction of the studies on diet and liver disease, including liver cancer, with an ever-increasing focus on the diets as modulators (promoters, cocarcinogens, etc.) of carcinogenesis rather than as prime movers.

The discovery that dietary deficiency alone can cause cancer indicates that certain internal imbalances in metabolism might precipitate a condition leading to cancer. Whether the imbalance caused by dietary deficiency of choline is similar to the imbalance caused by chemical carcinogen has yet to be shown, but our demonstration of DNA damage and cell proliferation due to choline deficiency suggests that the initiation process due to dietary deficiency might follow a pattern similar to that with chemical carcinogens.

To our knowledge, the choline deficiency model to study liver carcinogenesis is one of very few systems available today that has the potential for mechanistic understanding. For example, the system is less complicated than those using xenobiotics. With the slower initiation process, early changes such as fat accumulation, free-radical generation, membrane alterations, DNA damage, cell death, and cell proliferation can be detected in a stepwise fashion. This allows for a step-by-step mechanistic analysis of the initiation process. Also, the choline deficiency model offers an unusually interesting opportunity to study the possible roles of free radicals in acute cell injury and in cancer.

CONCLUSION

So far, this is the only dietary model known and partly characterized to study carcinogenesis without a carcinogen. This study points directly to the importance of maintaining the internal metabolic balance in the body by proper dietary manipulation and the possible neoplastic consequences of some imbalances.

ACKNOWLEDGMENTS

We would like to express our sincere thanks to Lori Cutler for her excellent secretarial help. This work was supported in part by grants from the U.S. Public

Health Service (CA-41537 and CA-21157) and from the National Cancer Institute, the National Cancer Institute of Canada, and the Medical Research Council of Canada.

REFERENCES

Ames, B.N. 1983. Dietary carcinogens and anticarcinogens. *Science* **221:** 1256.

Buckley, G.F. and W.S. Hartroft. 1955. Pathology of choline deficiency in the mouse. *Arch. Pathol.* **59:** 185.

Copeland, D.H. and W.D. Salmon. 1946. The occurrence of neoplasms in the liver, lungs and other tissues of rats as a result of prolonged choline deficiency. *Am. J. Pathol.* **22:** 1059.

Emerit, I. and P.A. Cerutti. 1982. Tumor promoters phorbol 12-myristate 13-acetate induces a clastogenic factor in human lymphocytes. *Proc. Natl. Acad. Sci. U.S.A.* **79:** 7509.

Fariss, M.W., K. Olztsdottier, and D.J. Reed. 1984. Extracellular calcium protects isolated hepatocytes from injury. *Biochem. Biophys. Res. Commun.* **121:** 102.

Ghoshal, A.K. and E. Farber. 1983. Induction of liver cancer by a diet deficient in choline and methionine (CMD). *Proc. Am. Assoc. Cancer Res.* **24:** 98.

———. 1984. The induction of liver cancer by dietary deficiency of choline and methionine without added carcinogens. *Carcinogenesis* **5:** 1367.

Ghoshal, A., T. Rushmore, and E. Farber. 1985b. Cancer induction with a choline-methionine deficient diet: A working hypothesis. *Proc. Can. Fed. Biol. Soc.* **28:** 217.

Ghoshal, A., F. Willemsen, R. Chown, T. Rushmore, H. Newmark, and E. Farber. 1985a. Amelioration of nuclear lipid peroxidation and cell death by Ca^{2+} in a choline-methionine deficient (CMD) diet fed rat. *Fed. Proc.* **44:** 521.

Mikol, Y.B., K. Hoover, D. Creasia, and L.A. Poirier. 1983. Hepatocarcinogenesis in rats fed methyl-deficient, amino acid defined diets. *Carcinogenesis* **4:** 1619.

Newberne, P.M. 1965. Carcinogenicity of aflatoxin-contaminated peanut meals. In *Mycotoxins in foodstuffs* (ed. G.N. Wogan), p. 187. M.I.T. Press, Cambridge, Massachusettes.

Newmark, H.L., M.J. Wargovich, and W.R. Bruce. 1984. Colon cancer and dietary fat, phosphate and calcium: A hypothesis. *J. Natl. Cancer Inst.* **72:** 1323.

Rajalakshmi, S., P.M. Rao, and D.S.R. Sarma. 1982. Chemical carcinogenesis: Interactions of carcinogens with nucleic acids. In *Cancer: A comprehensive treatise* (ed. F.F. Becker), vol. 1, p. 335. Plenum Publishing, New York.

Recknagel, R.O. and A.K. Ghoshal. 1966. Quantitative estimation of peroxidative degeneration of rat liver and mitochondrial lipids after carbontetrachloride poisoning. *Exp. Mol. Pathol.* **5:** 413.

Rogers, A. and P. Newberne. 1969. Aflatoxin B_1 carcinogenesis in lipotrope deficient rats. *Cancer Res.* **29:** 1965.

Rushmore, T.H., Y.P. Lim, E. Farber, and A.K. Ghoshal. 1984. Rapid lipid peroxidation in the nuclear fraction of rat liver induced by a diet deficient in choline and methionine. *Cancer Lett.* **24:** 251.

Salmon, W.D. and P.M. Newberne. 1963. Occurrence of hepatomas in rats fed diets containing peanut meal as a major source of protein. *Cancer Res.* **23:** 571.

Slaga, T.J., A.J.P. Klein-Szanto, L.L. Triplett, L.P. Yotti, and J.E. Trosko. 1981. Skin tumor promoting activity of benzoyl peroxide, a widely used free radical generating compound. *Science* **213:** 1023.

Yokoyama, S., M.A. Sells, T.V. Reddy, and B. Lombardi. 1985. Hepatocarcinogenic and promoting action of a choline-devoid diet in the rat. *Cancer Res.* **45:** 2834.

COMMENTS

MAGEE: Are you suggesting that the mechanism is very similar for carbon tetrachloride and the choline deficiency?

GHOSHAL: The mechanism for carcinogenesis is similar with respect to choline deficiency and chemically induced initiation. The carbon-tetrachloride-induced lipid peroxidation mechanism is different because carbon tetrachloride causes lipid peroxidation only in the microsomes and later in mitochrondria, but it doesn't touch the nuclei. Choline deficiency, on the contrary, causes lipid peroxidation in the nuclei and mitochondria later, but it doesn't touch the microsomes. So, it is different.

PITOT: I believe the data you showed exemplify a very important advantage of three-dimensional analysis of focal lesions in the liver as contrasted with two-dimensional analysis. Your data demonstrated that the number of foci in animals on the choline-deficient diet alone was approximately half those on the choline-deficient diet followed by the selection regimen, while at the same time the average diameter of the foci enlarged from 0.2 to 0.4. These measurements were made from a two-dimensional analysis of focal area.

GHOSHAL: Yes. This was measured by computerized program and corrected for variation in size.

WACHSMUTH: Dr. Pitot's remark is reasonable, in particular when large nodules occur rarely and only these sections were evaluated. One would have to look at the histogram, which should be skewed, and then apply a method like that of Weibel and Gomez (1962) for determining the mean nodule size.

PITOT: The standard deviation of the smaller foci is always larger than that parameter of larger foci, since the rate of growth of the former varies in a more uniform manner. Even if one assumed a 25% or 50% increase in the standard deviation of the larger foci, the conclusions stated above would not be altered.

CERUTTI: I have a comment to your paradox, that upon replenishing calcium, lipid peroxidation actually went down, but the effect on necrosis stayed the same.

GHOSHAL: Lipid peroxidation was totally inhibited; cell death stopped; cell proliferation stopped. But it had minimal effect on lipid accumulation.

CERUTTI: I see. I just wondered, because you were measuring total lipid peroxidation. It might be more revealing to determine the stimulation of the formation of particular products in the prostaglandin and the leukotriene pathways, which may be secondarily stimulated by lipid peroxides.

GHOSHAL: What we are measuring is diene conjugates in the membrane.

CERUTTI: It's not just a matter of toxicity. Whether you damage or not, very small amounts of general lipid peroxidation stimulate cyclooxygenase and lipoxygenase, changing the paracrine milieu of the liver.

GHOSHAL: That is a possibility, but in our system aspirin did not exhibit any effect.

SWENBERG: Have you looked at any of the peroxisomal proliferators for diene conjugates?

GHOSHAL: No, we did not.

SLAGA: Shinizuka showed that chemical promoters, like phenobarbital, do not lead to an increase in lipid peroxidation, whereas dietary manipulations like this do. Do you have any comments on that?

GHOSHAL: CD diet is unique in the sense that it induces lipid peroxidation in the nucleus, so close to DNA. All promoters need not induce lipid peroxidation.

The Problem of Pseudocarcinogenicity in Rodent Bioassays

FRANCIS J.C. ROE
Independent Consultant in Toxicology
Wimbledon Common, London SW19 5BB, England

OVERVIEW

Pseudocarcinogenicity is defined as the enhancement of tumor risk by a nongenotoxic mechanism in physiologically abnormal animals. In the case of rats, severe endocrine disturbance secondary to overfeeding is the commonest cause of physiological abnormality. Pseudoanticarcinogenicity is the counterpart of pseudocarcinogenicity. The literature abounds with, and is seriously confused by, examples of these phenomena, which could be largely avoided by sensible choice of animal strain and intelligent animal husbandry. The fact that pseudocarcinogenic effects are reported alongside true carcinogenic effects while pseudoanticarcinogenic effects are usually ignored not only adds to the confusion, but also introduces serious bias into the overall picture.

INTRODUCTION

It is now reasonable to subdivide carcinogens into two categories: genotoxic and nongenotoxic. However, we need a term to describe apparent effects on tumor incidence that are neither examples of genotoxic carcinogenicity nor examples of nongenotoxic carcinogenicity but which are, in effect, laboratory artifacts. To fill this need, I have proposed the term pseudocarcinogenicity (Roe 1983), which applies to the enhancement of tumor risk by a nongenotoxic mechanism in physiologically abnormal animals but not in physiologically normal animals.

It is not intended that pseudocarcinogenicity should apply to apparent effects which, in reality, are due to the statistical mismanagement of data, e.g., failure to age-standardize data or failure to allow for the fact that the expectation of encountering statistically significant differences apparently attributable to treatment increases with the number of comparisons made. Nor is it intended that the term should apply to a situation in which animals are inadvertently exposed to carcinogens.

The commonest source of both pseudocarcinogenic and pseudoanticarcinogenic phenomena is overfeeding. In rats, overfeeding profoundly influences hormonal status and increases the incidence of hormonally mediated neoplasia. Effects of overfeeding on other forms of neoplasia are less evident in the rat. In mice, overfeeding increases the incidences of lung, liver, and lymphoreticular neoplasia by mechanisms about which we can at present only speculate.

Banbury Report 25: Nongenotoxic Mechanisms in Carcinogenesis
© Cold Spring Harbor Laboratory. 0-87969-225-1/87. $1.00 + .00

ANIMAL MODEL

A rat, or mouse, is a highly complex, intricate, and integrated living system that has taken millions of years to evolve. It is not simply a list of protocol tissues to be checked by a Quality Assurance officer. Animals are subject to a myriad of variables, both genetic and environmental. The experimentalist must strive to avoid interference by these variables and must not imagine that good experimental design is proof against possible bias from such interference. This is particularly true if animals are obtained from a breeder according to requirements specified only in terms of strain, sex, and weight. Littermates vary in birth weight and in growth rate before weaning, and birth weight and growth before weaning vary with litter size. Thus, a batch of young animals of similar body weight may be of different ages and have different expectations of maximum achievable weight. It is normal for an experienced breeder to cull runts and to discard young animals with obvious abnormalities, such as hydrocephalus or other birth defects, that have not already been rejected by the dam. However, animals with inobvious abnormalities find their way into long-term studies. Bias from undetected variation between animals can be largely obviated by a proper system of randomization of animals between groups. But let no one imagine that there is no inhomogeneity between animals of the same sex and weight even if they are derived from the same inbred strain.

EFFECTS OF OVERFEEDING IN RATS

Historically, the current practice of supplying animals with overnutritious food ad libitum for 24 hours each day has several roots. First, nutritionists have led experimentalists to believe that maximum growth is a hallmark of optimal nutrition. Arguably, this may be true for those responsible for fattening turkeys for Thanksgiving Day, but as pointed out by Berg and Simms (1960), it certainly is not true for rats and mice in untreated control groups in long-term toxicity/carcinogenicity tests. Second, in the bad old days when animal houses were left unattended on weekends and public holidays, it was obviously convenient to supply animals with an excess of food. Third, in the eyes of animal lovers, to deprive animals of food savors of cruelty and is therefore something to be avoided. Today, no animal house is left unattended for as long as 24 hours, so there is no need to supply excessive amounts of food. Furthermore, it is now clear that it is more inhumane to allow animals to become obscenely obese, and to predispose them to renal disease, endocrine disturbances, cancer, and an early grave, than to control what, when, and how much they eat. Three aspects of the effects of overfeeding merit separate attention: (1) effects on survival, progressive nephropathy, and other nonneoplastic diseases in rats, (2) effects on risk of tumor development, and (3) effects on hormonal status.

OVERFEEDING AS A CAUSE OF NEPHROPATHY AND OTHER NONNEOPLASTIC DISEASES IN THE RAT

Berg (1960) and Berg and Simms (1960) were among the first to demonstrate the role of caloric intake in the etiology of three particular nonneoplastic life-shortening diseases in the rat: chronic progressive glomerulonephritis, polyarteritis, and myocardial degeneration. They found that diet restriction from the time of weaning to 67% or 54% of the food intake of rats fed ad libitum greatly reduced the age-standardized incidence of these three increasingly debilitating and fatal diseases (see Table 1). A quarter of a century later, in the course of a routine carcinogenicity study involving Sprague-Dawley rats fed ad libitum on a standard laboratory chow, I observed in the male control group a 67% incidence of severe glomerulonephritis and an 83% incidence of chronic degenerative myocarditis. The animals had simply been fed ad libitum on a standard diet. Parathyroid hyperplasia secondary to nephropathy was evident in two thirds of the animals and, in half of these, metastatic calcification of the aorta and other tissues had occurred.

Bras and Ross (1964) concluded the following from a study involving 1000 male Sprague-Dawley rats: "A remarkable reduction in the prevalence of progressive glomerulonephrosis (PGN) was found in those experimental groups which were restricted in their intakes of protein, of carbohydrates, or of calories. The most beneficial effects were obtained in those groups whose carbohydrate intake and concomitant calorie intake was reduced regardless of the level of protein intake. The

Table 1
Effect of Food Intake on Survival and Incidence of Glomerulonephritis, Polyarteritis, and Myocardial Degeneration

	Days	Ad libitum %	67% of Ad libitum	54% of Ad libitum
Males				
deaths	0–800	52	13	19
G	0–800	97	0	7
	800+	100	36	0
P	0–800	83	0	0
	800+	63	17	3
MD	0–800	69	17	0
	800+	96	29	3
Females				
deaths	0–800	6	4	5
G	0–800	69	0	0
	800+	57	0	0

Data from Berg and Simms (1960).
Abbreviations: (G) glomerulonephritis; (P) polyarteritis; (MD) myocardial degeneration.

Table 2
Effect of Overnutrition on Survival and Renal Disease in Rats

	Sex	24 hr access/day	6.5 hr access/day
Survival to 2 years	male	8/20	18/20
	female	14/20	16/20
Incidence of moderate	male	13/20	1/20
or severe nephropathy	female	12/20	0/20

Data from Harleman et al. (1984).

greatest prevalence as well as the earliest appearance of PGN was found in those rats fed a commercial diet (Purina Chow) ad libitum.''

In the literature there are many examples of treatment-related and dose-related reductions in incidence/severity of chronic progressive nephropathy in rats. Indeed, one should expect to see such reductions wherever reduced body weight gain is a feature of response. It is somewhat ironic that by poisoning animals with high doses of test substances, we end up rendering them healthier than untreated controls!

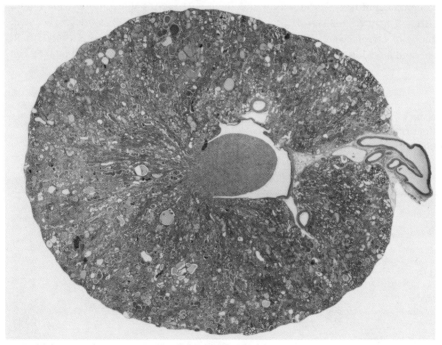

Figure 1
Kidney of a 25-month-old male Wistar rat given free access to a standard laboratory diet for 24 hr/day. There is gross enlargement because of advanced chronic glomerulonephritis.

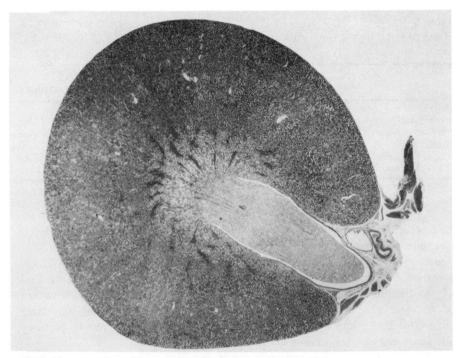

Figure 2
Kidney of a 25-month-old male Wistar rat given free access to the same standard diet (see Fig. 1) but for only 6.5 hr/day. It is histologically normal.

Recently, we (Harleman et al. 1984) reported that the survival of rats can be improved and the incidence of chronic renal disease dramatically reduced by the simple stratagem of reducing the number of hours per day during which they have free access to food from 24 to 6.5 (see Table 2). Figures 1 and 2 illustrate the appearance of the kidneys from rats fed 24 hours/day and 6.5 hour/day, respectively. In the same small study, we witnessed a significantly lower incidence of testicular arteriolitis in the 6.5 hour/day group.

OVERFEEDING IN RELATION TO NEOPLASIA

Many investigators have reported a direct association between food intake and tumor risk in laboratory rodents. In the rat study of Berg and Simms (1960) referred to above, there was a marked reduction in the incidence of benign tumors, particularly in females, but no effect on the incidence of malignant tumors (see Table 3). Tucker (1979) reported an even more striking effect of 20% diet restriction on tumor incidence in rats despite improved survival (see Table 4). In a survey of

Table 3

Effect of Food Intake on Tumor Incidence in Rats Surviving for 25 Months or More

	Ad libitum (%)	67% of Ad libitum	54% of Ad libitum	Trend
Males				
benign/malignant tumor	58	36	26	$p < 0.01$
malignant tumor	0	2	5	n.s.
Females				
benign/malignant tumor	43	14	12	$p < 0.1$
malignant tumor	2	5	0	n.s.

Data from Berg and Simms (1960). n.s. indicates not significant.

25 2-year cancer bioassay studies in F344 rats, Haseman (1983) found that reduced weight gain during the studies was associated with reduced incidences not only of pituitary and mammary tumors, but also of adrenal medullary, thyroid C-cell, and pancreatic islet-cell tumors (see Table 5). Ross and Bras (1971) found that a period of restriction in food intake early in life permanently influenced the growth pattern of rats and was associated with a decreased risk of development of benign connective tissue tumors and tumors of epithelial tissue, particularly pituitary adenomas and islet-cell tumors of the pancreas.

Clearly, the predominant pattern in rats is that overfeeding predisposes them to

Table 4

Effect of 20% Food Restriction on Percentage of Survival to 2 Years and Percentage of Tumor Incidence in Rats

	Ad libitum (%)	20% Restricted
Males		
survival to 2 years	72	88
one or more tumors	66	24[a]
>1 tumor	22	2[b]
pituitary	32	0[a]
dermis	12	2[c]
Females		
survival to 2 years	68	90
one or more tumors	82	57[b]
>1 tumor	26	10[c]
pituitary	66	39[b]
mammary benign or malignant	34	6[a]
malignant	12	2[c]

Data from Tucker (1979).
[a] $p < 0.001$.
[b] $p < 0.01$.
[c] $p < 0.05$.

Table 5
Relation between Low Weight Gain and Tumor Incidence in 25
Carcinogenicity Tests on F344 Rats

Site	Incidence
Males	
pituitary	down
thyroid (C-cell)	down
adrenal medulla	down
pancreas (islet-cell)	down
monocytic leukemia	up
Females	
pituitary	down
mammary (fibroadenoma)	down
monocytic leukemia	up

Data from Haseman (1983).

endocrine and mammary tumors. In contrast, overfeeding predisposes mice toincreased incidence of a wide variety of tumors, but mainly of a nonendocrine origin. Both Conybeare (1980) and Tucker (1979) found the biggest effects to be on tumors of the lung, liver, and lymphoreticular system (Table 6). An important feature of Conybeare's study was the significant difference he saw between ad-libitum-fed and diet-restricted mice of both sexes in the overall incidence of malignant tumors.

Table 6
Effect of Overfeeding on Percentage of Tumor Incidence in a Mouse Study of
18 Months Duration

Tumor site	Ad libitum	75% of Ad libitum
Males (160 per group)		
any tumor at any site	44	22.5[a]
any malignant tumor	11	4[b]
lung	19	12[c]
liver	29	7.5[a]
lymphoreticular	2.5	0.6
other	5	2.5
Females (160 per group)		
any tumor at any site	31	11[c]
any malignant tumor	14	4[c]
lung	15	5[c]
liver	4	0.6[b]
lymphoreticular	7	2.5[b]
other	7.5	2.5[b]

Data from Conybeare (1980).
[a] $p < 0.001$.
[b] $p < 0.05$.
[c] $p < 0.01$.

EFFECT OF OVERNUTRITION ON HORMONAL STATUS

The pattern of enhancement of endocrine and mammary tumor incidence in overfed rats is clearly associated with disturbance of hormonal status. Most of the pituitary tumors that arise in rats fed ad libitum are prolactinomas, and the high circulating levels of prolactin to which these tumors give rise increases the risk of development of mammary tumors in rats of both sexes.

A recent study by G. Conybeare (pers. comm.) has provided important information about the influence of overfeeding on the sex hormone status of female rats. He found that female rats given free access to food for 24 hours each day reached sexual maturity a week or so earlier than females given free access to food for only 6 hours each day. However, by 1 year of age, most of the animals fed ad libitum were cycling irregularly and subfertile while most of the restricted animals were still normal in these respects (see Table 7). In the normally cycling young female rat, serum prolactin levels range from 20 to 80 ng/ml, according to the stage of the cycle. In the irregularly cycling 1-year-old ad-libitum-fed females, Conybeare found higher serum prolactin levels ranging over 310 ng/ml. But even this latter level is modest compared to the levels of over 1000 ng/ml that may occur in older ad-libitum-fed females with hyperplasia or neoplasia of prolactin-producing cells in the pituitary.

The influence of food intake on other hormones awaits further study. Disturbances of growth hormone, insulin, calcitonin, and the hormones produced by the adrenal medulla almost certainly occur in association with the increased incidences of tumors at sites where these hormones are produced in overfed rats. However, published data are generally lacking.

Table 7
Effects of Overfeeding on Onset of Sexual Maturity, Regularity of Estrus Cycling, and Reproductive Performance in Female Wistar Rats (Ten per Group)

	Ad libitum	80% of Ad libitum
Opening of vagina		4 days later than in ad libitum
Success of mating at 8 weeks of age (no. of litters)	10	7
Success of mating at 10 weeks of age (no. of litters)	—	10
Cycling irregularly at 12 months of age (no. of litters)	8	2
Success of mating at 12 months of age (no. of litters)	2	6
Mean litter size of successfully mated females	2	5
Total offspring from mating at 1 year	4	30

Data from G. Conybeare (pers. comm.)

DO HIGH LEVELS OF CIRCULATING PROLACTIN PREDISPOSE TO NEPHROPATHY IN RATS?

The results of a 2-year feeding study on bromocriptine, which blocks prolactin release, revealed a number of dose-related beneficial effects not only on the incidences of prolactin-associated pituitary and mammary tumors, but also on the incidences of nephropathy and polyarteritis nodosa (see Table 8) (Richardson et al. 1983). It was suggested (Richardson and Luginbuehl 1976) that excessively high levels of circulating prolactin adversely affect the rat kidney directly. It was also suggested that the reduction in prolactin levels caused by bromocriptine permit estrogen dominance and that this explains the treatment-related increase in inflammatory, hyperplastic, metaplastic, and neoplastic uterine changes that they saw. Richardson et al. (1983) further suggested that the reduction in adrenocortical tumors in males is a consequence of prolactin suppression. In support of this, they point out that prolactin has been found to support the growth of experimentally induced tumors of this kind (Thomson et al. 1973).

INCREASED CALCIUM ABSORPTION AS A RISK FACTOR FOR PHEOCHROMOCYTOMA IN THE RAT

In a recent review of this topic, we (Roe and Bär 1985) sought to bring together scattered data relating increased calcium absorption with increased incidence of

Table 8
Effects of Bromocriptine in Rats (50/sex/group)

	% Incidence per dose (mg/kg/day)			
	0	1.8	9.9	44.5
Males				
survival to 2 years	28	44	58[a]	62[a]
moderate/severe nephropathy	84	62[b]	62[b]	44[c]
polyarteritis nodosa	50	16[c]	32[b]	24[a]
tumor-bearing rats	56	60	56	38
adrenal cortical tumors	38	24	28	6[a]
Females				
survival to 2 years	36	50	54	36
moderate/severe nephropathy	16	8	0[a]	0[a]
polyarteritis nodosa	18	4[b]	6	0[a]
tumor-bearing rats	88	58[a]	52[a]	40[a]
mammary tumors	80	30[a]	20[a]	16[a]
estrogen-associated				
endometrial changes	10	70[c]	82[c]	84[c]
uterine tumors	0	4	8[a]	9[a]

Data from Richardson et al. (1983).
[a]$p < 0.01$.
[b]$p < 0.05$.
[c]$p < 0.001$.

adrenal medullary hyperplasia and neoplasia in the rat. This association is seen when rats, but not mice, are fed on diets containing high levels (e.g., 10% or more) of lactose or various polyols, including sorbitol, mannitol, lactitol, and xylitol. With these substances, there is evidence of both increased calcium absorption from the gut and increased urinary output of calcium. Secondary to the latter, one observes pelvic, and sometimes other forms of, nephrocalcinosis. Brion and Dupuis (1980) reported that the adrenal medullary hypofunctioning secondary to hypocalcemia associated with vitamin D deficiency can be corrected by the administration of lactose in the diet. Even in rats deficient in vitamin D, dietary lactose can increase calcium absorption sufficiently to bring serum calcium levels into the physiological range, which is necessary for the normal functioning of the adrenal medulla. We suggest that excessive calcium absorption can give rise in the rat to hypercalcemia and that this predisposes them to adrenal medullary hyperfunctioning as evidenced histologically by hyperplasia and neoplasia.

An important cause of hypercalcemia in the rat is parathyroid hyperplasia secondary to severe nephropathy. Thus, we were not surprised to find (see Fig. 3) a highly significant ($p < 0.01$) correlation between metastatic calcification (secondary to hypercalcemia) and adrenal medullary hyperplasia/neoplasia in the carcinogenicity study referred to earlier.

Gilbert et al. (1958) dramatically brought down the incidence of adrenal medullary tumors in ad-libitum-fed rats of both sexes by reducing the level of carbohydrate in the diet (Table 9). This effect was probably mediated by reduced calcium absorption, since calcium is absorbed from the gut lumen along with monosaccharides.

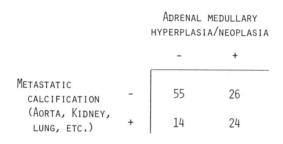

ADRENAL MEDULLARY
HYPERPLASIA/NEOPLASIA

		−	+
METASTATIC CALCIFICATION (AORTA, KIDNEY, LUNG, ETC.)	−	55	26
	+	14	24

SIGNIFICANCE OF POSITIVE ASSOCIATION

P = 0.01

Figure 3

Correlation between hypercalcemia, as indicated by histologically evident metastatic calcification, and incidence of adrenal medullary hyperplasia and/or neoplasia among 119 male Wistar rats that survived for 64 weeks or longer in a routine oral carcinogenicity test on a nongenotoxic agent.

Table 9
Effect on Dietary Composition on Incidence of Pheochromocytoma in Rats
Fed Ad Libitum

Diet (%)			Lifetime incidence of pheochromocytomas	
carbohydrate	protein	fat	male	female
64.4	15.2	11.3	63	47
3.6	81.6	10.2	13	15

Data from Gilbert et al. (1958).

In a survey of 25 cancer bioassay feeding studies in F344 rats, Haseman (1983) found that the incidence of tumors of the adrenal medulla in males was lower in animals that put on less weight than in those that put on more weight. Also, Berg and Simms (1960) reported that diet restriction reduced the incidence of pheochromocytomas in rats. It is not at present clear whether overfeeding predisposes directly to adrenal medullary proliferation disease in rats or whether the effect is mediated by high calcium absorption under conditions of overfeeding. I suspect that both factors are implicated.

In my opinion, most laboratory rat diets contain too much phosphate and too much calcium. In addition, some are deficient in magnesium. These faults render the laboratory rat prone to develop corticomedullary and pelvic nephrocalcinosis. They also stretch to the limit the ability of rats to maintain mineral homeostasis. For this reason, these rats are easily pushed into states of pathological nephrocalcinosis and adrenal proliferative disease by agents that increase calcium absorption.

CONCLUSIONS

At present, the literature is full of examples of what are almost certainly pseudocarcinogenic and pseudoanticarcinogenic phenomena that have been observed in studies in which control animals exhibit evidence of markedly abnormal physiological status. However, proof that these are not examples of true nongenotoxic carcinogenicity is usually lacking, since there are no parallel data derived from tests involving physiologically normal animals. Pending such proof, some may feel that pseudocarcinogenicity is simply a concept and not an actuality. If so, then the sooner we upgrade it from the status of concept to accepted fact the better.

ACKNOWLEDGMENTS

I am very grateful to Mr. Peter Lee, Dr. A.J. Cohen, and Mr. Geoffrey Conybeare for their critical and constructive comments during the preparation of this paper.

REFERENCES

Berg, B.N. 1960. Nutrition and longevity in the rat. I. Food intake in relation to size, health and fertility. *J. Nutr.* **71:** 242.

Berg, B.N. and H.S. Simms. 1960. Nutrition and longevity in the rat. II. Longevity and onset of disease with different levels of food intake. *J. Nutr.* **71:** 255.

Bras, G. and M.H. Ross. 1964. Kidney disease and nutrition in the rat. *Toxicol. Appl. Pharmacol.* **6:** 247.

Brion, F. and Y. Dupuis. 1980. Calcium and monoamine regulation: Role of vitamin D nutrition. *Can. J. Physiol. Pharmacol.* **58:** 1431.

Conybeare, G. 1980. Effect of quality and quantity of diet on survival and tumor incidence in outbred Swiss mice. *Food Cosmet. Toxicol.* **18:** 65.

Gilbert, G., J. Gillman, P. Loustalot, and W. Lutz. 1958. The modifying influence of diet and the physical environment on spontaneous tumor frequency in rats. *Br. J. Cancer* **12:** 565.

Harleman, J.H., F.J.C. Roe, and G.K. Salmon. 1984. Life span and spontaneous lesions in rats. The effects of ad libitum versus controlled feeding. In *Proceedings Joint Meeting of European Society of Veterinary Pathology, American College of Veterinary Pathologists and World Association of Veterinary Pathologists,* Utrecht, Netherlands. Sept. 4–7, 1984. Abstract No. 49.

Haseman, J.K. 1983. Patterns of tumor incidence in two-year cancer bioassay feeding studies in Fischer 344 rats. *Fundam. Appl. Toxicol.* **3:** 1.

Richardson, B.P. and H-R. Luginbuehl. 1976. The role of prolactin in the development of chronic progressive nephropathy in the rat. *Virchows Arch.* **370:** 13.

Richardson, B.P., I. Turkalj, and E. Fluckiger. 1983. *Bromocriptine.* Sandoz Ltd., Basel, Switzerland.

Roe, F.J.C. 1983. Carcinogenesis. Testing for carcinogenicity and the problem of pseudocarcinogenicity. *Nature* **303:** 657.

Roe, F.J.C. and A. Bär. 1985. Enzootic and epizootic adrenal medullary proliferative disease of rats: Influence of dietary factors which affect calcium absorption. *Hum. Toxicol.* **4:** 27.

Ross, M.H. and G. Bras. 1971. Lasting influence of early caloric restriction on prevalence of neoplasms in the rat. *J. Natl. Cancer Inst.* **47:** 1095.

Thomson, M.J., M.R. Garland, and J.F. Archards. 1973. Hormonal effects on thymidine kinase and thymidylate kinase activity of oestrogen dependent tumors in the rat. *Cancer Res.* **33:** 220.

Tucker, M.J. 1979. The effect of long-term food restriction on tumors in rodents. *Int. J. Cancer* **23:** 803.

COMMENTS

TENNANT: In terms of the implication of the observations, would it not tend to mitigate against the classification of the substance X or Y as a carcinogen where the background frequency is increased? Just on a statistical basis the higher the spontaneous frequency of tumors in the control population, the lower the probability that the chemical would be identified as a carcinogen simply because of the magnitude of effect that one has to see in order to statistically resolve between those. So, overall, one group of people would argue that in using the current dietary regimen we would be underidentifying substances as carcinogens because of the background statistical problem associated with it.

ROE: I expect you are right, but we haven't got enough data to support or refute that argument. However, that isn't really what I am worried about. Irrespective of the effect of background tumor incidence on the sensitivity of animal tests, surely it is just plain stupid to use as a model animals that are endocrinologically completely messed up. Methods are becoming available whereby it is possible to measure hormone levels repeatedly in individual living rats. Using such a technique for prolactin, we know that, from the age of 6 months onward, prolactin levels begin to rise far above the normal range. The main difficulty at present is that there are not enough comparative data for known carcinogens tested in diet-restricted and nonrestricted animals. The few data we have suggest that true carcinogenic effects are not missed if diet restriction is practiced. Diet restriction may reduce the age-standardized risk of tumor development, but the significance of the difference between the responses of treated and control animals may nevertheless have been increased because of the lower intensity of background noise.

TENNANT: I agree. What I was really speaking to was in terms of the overall issue of hazard identification. Of the last 75 substances that have been tested under the aegis of the National Toxicology Program, there has been, I believe, only one that has been classified as carcinogenic on the basis of endocrine tumors alone. I agree with you. On an individual chemical basis, you are absolutely right, in particular if you want to study the effects of that chemical. But, in terms of the overall use of these animals in their current state. . . .

ROE: The regulatory viewpoint is a very narrow one. Our main concern should be with the impact pseudocarcinogenic data have when they find their way to scientific data bases such as the data base provided by the IARC monographs. The consequences of this are not only serious with respect to the substance tested but also because chemically analogous substances fall under the same cloud.

TENNANT: That is the point I was speaking to. I can't answer for the IARC data base. The summary of the National Toxicology Program results released (related to a spontaneous high level of endocrine tumors in the rodent) have, with one exception, not contaminated the literature by identifying substances as carcinogenic.

ROE: Oh, yes they have. They have done it for a different reason.

NEWBERNE: Perhaps it is fortuitous that the National Toxicology Program uses the Fischer rat, which doesn't really get very fat. If you look at other strains, they all get obese if you hold them for 2 years.

ROE: I understand they get a very high incidence of renal disease, though.

NEWBERNE: Yes, they do, but I'm not sure we can correlate that directly with overfeeding in the Fischer rat. That doesn't eliminate the other causes.

ANDERSON: Masoro showed that very clearly. He restricted diet in male F344 rats and went from 80% end-stage kidney to zero, plus a great lengthening of life span.

HECK: Could you clarify one thing for me? In your slides you show the percentage ad libitum for a number of studies, but it is not clear to me what amount of food intake that represented. Does that represent any decrease in food intake?

ROE: In the studies which showed percentage of ad libitum food intake, the animals were rationed. The amount of food which the controls ate was measured. On each day during the following week, restricted animals were offered only 75% or 80% of the food consumed by the ad-libitum-fed animals during the previous week. Rats given access to food for only 6.5 hours per day ate only about 80% of the food consumed by rats fed 24 hours per day.

Session 4:
Solid State Carcinogenesis

Solid State Carcinogenesis

K. GERHARD BRAND
University of Minnesota Medical School
Department of Microbiology
Minneapolis, Minnesota 55455

OVERVIEW

Methodological approaches to the study of foreign body (FB) or "solid state" carcinogenesis are described at the beginning of this paper. Experimental results, interpretations, and conclusions are then presented that give evidence for the nongenotoxic nature of this carcinogenic process. (References are listed in reviews by Bischoff and Bryson 1964; Brand et al. 1976; Brand 1982.) Initiation appears to be due to a spontaneous genome error in a rapidly proliferating cell population. Progression does not involve further mutational steps. Rather, it depends on physiological effects mediated by the fibrotic state of chronic FB reaction. Furthermore, it requires the preneoplastic cells to attach onto the FB surface whereby structural and/or physiological effects are exerted on the cell membrane.

INTRODUCTION

We started our research on FB tumorigenesis in the mid-60s with several questions in mind. The most intriguing one happens to be the topic of this volume. At the time, it was particularly startling to us that a large, inert, biologically nondegradable FB, one that was definitely not cell-invasive by either physical or chemical mechanisms, would induce cancer. We thought that an experimental cancer induction model of this kind would be closest to what was regarded as "spontaneous carcinogenesis," and that it might also serve as a useful model for human FB cancers associated with asbestosis, schistosomiasis, and other similar conditions.

During the 1950s, several laboratories, especially the Oppenheimer group, showed that sarcomas are easily produced in rats and mice by implantation at various body sites of solid materials such as inert plastics, metals, and glass. My co-workers and I routinely employed plates of rigid unplasticized polyvinyl chloride acetate (PVCA), 0.2 mm thick. Other materials (plastics of different kinds, sizes, and shapes, as well as Millipore filters, glass, and metals) were used as controls or for special purposes.

The tumors that resulted were studied histologically, histochemically, karyologically, immunologically, and virologically. The main target of our research was, however, the preneoplastic period, i.e., the time span between FB implantation and tumor emergence. First, we studied the histological and histochemical developments at the FB surface and in the surrounding FB-reactive tissue. The most revealing data, however, were obtained through experiments of the following kind:

Banbury Report 25: Nongenotoxic Mechanisms in Carcinogenesis
© Cold Spring Harbor Laboratory. 0-87969-225-1/87. $1.00 + .00

Segments were cut from implants and from surrounding FB-reactive tissue at various time points during preneoplasia; the segments were transplanted to histocompatible yet karyologically distinguishable mice (e.g., from CBA/H to CBA/H-T6, or vice versa); specific characteristics of resulting tumors permitted retrospective conclusions as to the presence and state of preneoplastic cells. Experiments were extended and the results were refined when we succeeded in culturing and cloning the cancer precursor cells in vitro at chosen time points of preneoplasia. Such cells were tested for degree of preneoplastic maturation by reimplantation into recipient mice. Thus, it was possible to simulate certain phases of progression and to search for essential promotion factors.

RESULTS

Induction and Characteristics of FB Tumors

Implantation in mice (subcutaneously or at other sites) of nonbiodegradable solid materials with smooth surfaces evokes sarcomas after latencies of 6 months to over 30 months. Histopathologically, we recorded fibro-, myxo-, hemangio-, leiomyo-, and osteogenic sarcomas and, infrequently, still other types. This variety suggests different cell types of origin or a uniform cell type with pluripotentiality. If the material is implanted as a powder, no tumors emerge. This and several other experimental findings exclude chemical components as carcinogenic factors. Tumor incidence correlates with implant size and surface continuity. Reduction in overall size or perforation of the implant lowers tumor yield. Surface roughness or porosity delays tumor appearance.

Tumor-specific neoantigens were not detected, not even in tumors produced in immunosuppressed animals. On the contrary, transplantation antigens are frequently lost. When produced in a hybrid mouse strain, 80% of the tumors and 60% of preneoplastic cell specimens prove transplantable to one of the parent strains. These findings invalidated the concept of immunosurveillance as a general defense mechanism against cancer. Virological investigations failed to establish an etiological role of oncoviruses in FB tumorigenesis.

Preneoplastic Events

Within 1–2 weeks postimplantation, the FB surface is covered by firmly attached mono- and multinuclear macrophages. Very little change is seen during later months, except that giant cells may become more numerous and occasional fibroblasts or other cell types may appear among the macrophages. The surrounding tissue is characterized by a typical FB reaction. At first the reaction is acutely inflammatory, dominated by an influx by masses of macrophages and few granulocytes and lymphocytes. From 2 to 3 weeks, fibroblasts can be seen lining up opposite the FB surface. Blood capillaries begin to sprout into the FB-reactive tissue. Within 2–3 months, the fibroblasts take over in number, produce collagen, and develop a firm fibrotic capsule around the FB. Gradually, the capsule becomes more collagenous and less cellular; many of the capillaries begin to obliterate.

The data presented below were obtained by in vivo preneoplastic transplantation experiments and by in vitro culture of preneoplastic cells and reimplantation in recipient mice. The resulting tumors were analyzed by criteria and parameters indicated below.

FB sarcomas were found to be of monoclonal origin. Homologous tumors (i.e., those derived from cells of the same preneoplastic clone) are identical or closely related with respect to duration of tumor latency, numerical and morphological chromosome aberrations as well as banding alterations, histopathological tumor characteristics, degree of anaplasticity and invasiveness, and growth behavior in vivo and in vitro. It was established that these tumor properties are predetermined and already fixed in the earliest demonstrable clonal cells. The determinants remain virtually unchanged through many preneoplastic cell generations. Two conclusions can be drawn from these results: (1) Tumor determinants originate early in conjunction with an initiating carcinogenic key event in a primary "parent" cell and (2) no consecutive mutational steps occur that would alter the determinants or create additional ones.

In our attempts to find the cell type of tumor origin, we suspected at first the predominating macrophages or fibroblasts; however, both cell types were excluded from consideration in our laboratory and others. Instead, we identified the pluripotential stem cells of the microvasculature, the pericytes, that generate new blood capillaries sprouting into the FB-reactive tissue.

The number of initiated parent cells and clones to be expected in an FB reaction correlates with the size of the implant. Direct clone-counts were carried out by transplanting to recipient mice minimum-size segments of implants and capsule tissue. Statistical calculations were done applying the Poisson distribution. By either method, it was found that upon subcutaneous implantation of a $0.2 \times 15 \times 22$ mm^3 PVCA plate in CBA/H mice, the most probable number (MPN) is 3. If the size of the plate is cut to $0.2 \times 7 \times 15$ mm^3, the MPN is 1. Obviously, the size of an implant determines the extent of the FB reaction. It thus appears that preneoplastic parent cells emerge with higher probability as the number of FB-reactive proliferating cells increases. (The MPN differs between mouse strains and is also influenced by implant properties; e.g., glass evokes a weaker FB reaction and fewer preneoplastic parent cells than PVCA does.)

Carcinogenic Initiation

The initiating key event takes place within 4–8 weeks following FB implantation, at the time when the pluripotential mesenchymal stem cells proliferate at a high rate to supply the FB-reactive tissue with a network of new blood vessels. The parent cells in which the initiating key event occurs and their immediate clonal progeny are never found in contact with the FB, but at a distance in the acutely FB-reactive tissue. Hence, the FB does not induce the key event in a direct way. Rather, it appears to be an intrinsic, spontaneous event whose probability increases with forced cell proliferation.

A possible clue as to the nature of the initiating key event is the regular observation of chromosomal aberrations with regard to number, morphology, and banding patterns. These occur in the primary parent cell and persist without major changes through clonal generations of preneoplastic and tumor cells. This is also true for the determinants of specific tumor characteristics. Marked differences exist, however, between clones with regard to both specific chromosomal aberrations and tumor characteristics. It is therefore concluded that different patterns of genetic disorder or imbalance can constitute a basic defect causing initiation of the tumorigenic process. This hypothesis is supported by experiments that provide evidence for nonuniformity of initiation events in FB tumorigenesis. These observations are not incompatible with the proto-oncogene hypothesis of carcinogenesis. Our data would support the notion that oncogenes could result from spontaneous defects or mutations of normal genes involved in cellular growth regulation.

Progression and Promotional Factors

During the preneoplastic period, which may last for months or even years, the cells pass through distinct stages of progression, whereas the determinants of later tumor characteristics remain mostly unchanged. An essential factor that promotes preneoplastic cell maturation in vivo is bound to the chronic stage of FB reaction. This stage is characterized by macrophage dormancy and fibrosis as a result of fibroblast activity. The macrophages have lost most of their organelles, such as mitochondria and lysosomes; they show no signs of phagocytic activity. In this state, they give off substances known to stimulate fibroblast activity and collagen production. Experimental interference with the development of the fibrotic stage of FB reaction affects the tumorigenic process significantly. Tumor latency is prolonged by several months, in case of persistent acute inflammation, when phagocytizable substances are applied, when the implant surfaces are mechanically roughened, or when corticosteroids are given. Under such circumstances, the acute stage of FB reaction is protracted as indicated by minimal fibrosis and dense vascularization in the presence of active macrophages, particularly giant cells, and perhaps granulocytes.

While residing in the fibrotic capsule tissue, separate from the implant, the preneoplastic cells reach a certain degree of maturation. The final step to neoplastic autonomy, however, is accomplished only when the cells attach to the FB surface. Firm scars, calcium deposits, or osseous metaplasia can exert the same surface effect. The structural and physiological alterations of the cell membrane remain to be studied at the ultrastructural and molecular level. Nevertheless, it must basically be assumed that the affected cell membrane sends a signal to the hereditary apparatus ordering the expression of the neoplastic properties as they were predetermined by the initiation event.

Data from combined in vivo and in vitro experiments make it possible to describe phases of cellular progression more distinctly. Four phases are described below.

Phase T: The initiation event usually occurs (i.e., in 80% of animals) within 4–8 weeks following FB implantation. The presence of clonal preneoplastic cells can be demonstrated by transplantation experiments, but until the fourth month after implantation, they cannot be cultured in vitro by standard methods.

Phase tS: During the following 3–8 months, the cells normally stay in the FB-reactive tissue. However, now they can be cultured with increasingly greater ease. It appears that proliferative barriers are gradually removed. If early in phase tS the preneoplastic cells are transferred to in vitro culture on a plastic or glass surface, they often speed up preneoplastic progression by some weeks or even months. (Upon reimplantation of such cultured cells into recipient mice, they produce tumors sooner than their clonal sister cells, which were left in vivo continuously.) The pace of progression in vitro during phase tS can be accelerated even more if the preneoplastic cells are cocultured with normal fibroblasts. This effect is abolished if fibroblasts and phase-tS cells are cultured on either side of, and thus separated by, a 0.45-μm Millipore filter disk. Apparently, direct cell-to-cell contact is required to make this mode of promotion work. Coculture with a pure macrophage population is ineffective. Also interesting is the finding that by placing phase-tS cells on collagen-coated surfaces in vitro, the pace of progression is not accelerated but remains as slow as the pace recorded for clonal sister cells in vivo.

Phase S: It has consistently been observed that FB-surface attachment of preneoplastic cells is an indispensable condition before neoplastic autonomy can be attained. This condition can be fulfilled equally well in vivo and in vitro. Various kinds of surfaces, including roughened plastic and collagen-coated glass plates, were found equally effective. Thus, it is plausible that if the FB implant is removed from the animal, the preneoplastic cells residing in the FB-reactive tissue at that time will not develop into a tumor (unless the fibrotic capsule contains calcium deposits, osseous metaplasia, or hardened scar tissue that may substitute for an FB surface). If, on the other hand, we let preneoplastic cells pass through phase S and then remove them from the implant surface and reimplant them as a suspension without an FB, a tumor will develop.

Phase St: During this final phase, the cells stay normally on the implant surface. They reach full neoplastic autonomy within 1–2 months and then detach from the implant and start to grow as a tumor. If we remove the cells from the implant surface at the beginning of phase St and then reimplant them as a suspension without an FB, phase ST will last much longer and tumor appearance will be delayed by 4 months or more.

DISCUSSION

The experiments, results, and conclusions described above give evidence that in murine FB tumorigenesis neither the carcinogenic initiation event nor the stages of promotion are brought about by genotoxic mechanisms. Undoubtedly, the initiation event is due to an alteration at the genome level, but it appears to be a spontaneous chance event in a susceptible cell population in a state of forced proliferation. Accordingly, the probability of an initiation event occurring correlates with the size of the FB implant and the extent of the FB reaction.

The results of experimental FB tumorigenesis permit some comments on issues raised in other papers in this volume.

Sivak alluded to the possible role of genome or chromosome imbalance. This is entirely in line with our observations. Genetic imbalance is invariably seen in connection with the initiation event in FB carcinogenesis.

Both Cerutti and Trump related carcinogenic initiation to inflammation and inflammatory products secreted by granulocytes, macrophages, or other cells involved. The fact that initiation in FB tumorigenesis occurs during early FB reaction may be seen as generally supportive of this concept. However, a number of observations are more or less inconsistent with it: (1) Granulocytes and lymphocytes do not usually participate in carcinogenic FB reaction. (2) Initiation seems to occur at the time of capillary sprouting and early fibrosis rather than during the exudative-inflammatory stage when macrophage activity is at its peak. (3) The initiation event is delayed in experiments that protract or enhance the exudative-inflammatory phase. (4) Regarding L. Diamond's (Wistar Institute) comment about the possibly contributing role of viruses and viral infections in carcinogenesis, Brinton-Darnell and my wife (Brinton-Darnell and Brand 1977) found that FB tumor latency is significantly lengthened in mice that had been infected with lactate dehydrogenase elevating virus (LDV). This virus affects the macrophage population and stimulates these cells to greater activity. If inflammatory cell activity were indeed causally related to the initiation event, one should expect shorter latencies and a higher incidence of FB tumors in LDV-infected mice.

Trump emphasized involvement of the cell membrane in tumor promotion. Our results provide complete support for his thesis. Marked acceleration of promotion is seen when preneoplastic cells are attached onto solid surfaces, and in fact temporary attachment is an indispensable requirement for the completion of the promotional process. It might be worthwhile to study structural and molecular changes in the surface-attached parts of cell membranes in relation to promotion of FB tumorigenesis.

Boreiko and Yamasaki discussed the role of intercellular communication in promotion. Our results confirm the importance of direct intercellular contact. As pointed out, the promotional pace during the tS phase of FB tumorigenesis is markedly accelerated when preneoplastic cells are grown in mixed coculture with normal fibroblasts, but not when preneoplastic cells and fibroblasts are separated by a 0.45-μm Millipore filter disk. Acceleration is also seen when (instead of living fibroblasts) homogenized FB-reactive capsule tissue or normal liver tissue is added to the culture medium. The latter observation is in line with Pitot's statement that liver tissue is rich in cancer-promoting factors.

Several authors alluded to cell differentiation in context with carcinogenesis. The results of experimental FB tumorigenesis confirm this relationship in two ways: (1) The histopathological variety of sarcoma types arising from a common stem-cell type can only be explained as a result of differentiation along divergent pathways. (2) The preneoplastic cells appear initially in early cultures as spindly pericyte-like cells arranged in the form of a spongy network. Later, in single-cell-derived clonal subcultures, these cells differentiate into flat "endothelial" cells arranged as coherent pavement-like monolayers.

FB carcinogenesis is easily induced in mice and rats. In humans, FB cancers commonly result from asbestosis, schistosomiasis, and similar diseases after latencies of several decades. Implant-associated cancers, in contrast, have been reported infrequently so far. Until recently, it was thought that this might just be a matter of latency. Considering that methods of artificial implantation (pacemakers, endoprostheses, etc.) came into widespread use not before the late 1950s, it was feared that an epidemic of implant-associated cancers may erupt by the early nineties. This fear was dispelled on grounds of two studies, one statistical and the other experimental. First, we screened cases of human implant-associated cancers reported in the literature and found that 25% had developed within 15 years and 50% had developed within about 25 years. Since hundreds of thousands of implantations were done during the 1960s, a substantial number of cancers should have been recorded by now if human susceptibility were as high as that of experimental mice. Second, we studied tissue and implant-specimens from over 50 patients with chronic FB reactions against a variety of implant materials. The implants had been in place for up to 25 years. Methods developed on our mouse model were employed in a search for preneoplastic cells. In none of the specimens did we detect cells that resembled murine preneoplastic cells morphologically or karyologically. No clonal cells with chromosomal aberrations were discovered. Thus, it was concluded that human, in contrast to murine, pericytes are rarely the site of carcinogenic genome errors and chromosomal defects.

Among the human FB cancers reported in the literature, most were carcinomas. This indicates that human FB cancers usually arise from an ectodermal cell type, whereas the mouse produces invariably sarcomas of mesodermal origin. It appears that murine pericytes (the stem cells of the microvasculature that are the originator cells of FB sarcomas) possess an unusually labile genome. This would explain their proneness to spontaneous genome errors, especially when in a state of forced proliferation. Accordingly, the rarity of human FB sarcomas would reflect a high degree of genome stability in human pericytes.

Although carcinogenic initiation in murine FB tumorigenesis is likely to be due to a spontaneous nongenotoxic genome error, the mechanism of initiation in human asbestos or schistosomiasis cancers may well be genotoxic. To be considered as initiating carcinogens are chemical inhalants, e.g., cigarette smoking in asbestos-related bronchial carcinoma, or X-rays in mesothelioma, or chemical ingestants such as nitrosamines in bladder cancer associated with schistosomiasis. On the other hand, the factors of promotion may be the same in these human and murine cancers. Fibrosis, being one of the main promotional elements of murine FB tumorigenesis, is also the most conspicuous pathological feature of asbestosis and schistosomiasis. And by the very nature of this group of cancers, interaction between cell membranes and FB surfaces is likewise a common occurrence.

As a research tool, the murine FB tumorigenesis model is far from being exhausted. In fact, we feel that our investigations have barely scratched the surface. Still unanswered questions include the nature, location, and functional consequences of carcinogenic genome errors, the molecular nature and the structural and physiological effects of promotion factors connected with fibrosis and cellular surface attachment, and the communication between cell membrane and genetic apparatus.

CONCLUSION

I have presented a summary of our research on murine FB tumorigenesis as it relates to the question of nongenotoxic mechanisms of carcinogenesis. In this model, initiation of the carcinogenic process appears to be due to a spontaneous genome error in genome-labile mesenchymal stem cells during forced proliferation. No further events at the genome level or mutational steps are demonstrable during progression. Instead, preneoplastic progression is dependent on structural and/or physiological effects exerted by two specific promotional situations in sequence: (1) fibroblast activity and the state of fibrosis and (2) cell attachment onto a solid surface.

ACKNOWLEDGMENTS

This research was supported by the U.S. Public Health Service (CA-10712 and ES-02101) and the American Cancer Society (IN-13-Q-34).

REFERENCES

Bischoff, F. and G. Bryson. 1964. Carcinogenesis through solid state surfaces. *Prog. Exp. Tumor Res.* **5**: 85.

Brand, K.G. 1982. Cancer associated with asbestosis, schistosomiasis, foreign bodies, and scars. In *Cancer: A comprehensive treatise* (ed. F.F. Becker), 2nd ed. vol. I, p. 661. Plenum Publishing, New York.

Brand, K.G., K.H. Johnson, and L.C. Buoen. 1976. Foreign body tumorigenesis. *CRC Crit. Rev. Toxicol.* **4**: 353.

Brinton-Darnell, M. and I. Brand. 1977. Delayed foreign body-tumorigenesis in mice infected with lactate dehydrogenase-elevating virus. *J. Natl. Cancer Inst.* **59**: 1027.

COMMENTS

BARRETT: When do you see the earliest chromosomal changes? Is it at the tS stage in your model?

BRAND: That's right. As soon as we can culture the first preneoplastic cells (and that is about 3 months after implantation at the very earliest), then we already see these chromosomal aberrations.

BARRETT: There is a very nice analogy, I think, between what you see in vivo and what is seen during spontaneous transformation of cells in culture, in that the earliest change is a growth alteration, i.e., what is termed immortalization; whereas normal cells senesce and die off, partially altered cells continue to grow indefinitely. This is associated with chromosomal changes. These immortal cells (for instance, mouse 3T3 cells) are not tumorigenic in vivo unless they are attached to some anchor, either glass beads or plastic disks, as shown originally by Boone. That is very analogous to the second phase of your model, which requires attachment of the cells to the foreign body.

BRAND: In my opinion, 3T3 cells are derivatives of microvascular stem cells. They are at what I have called the tS phase. They only need a surface to attach to and then they go on to neoplasia.

BARRETT: Yes. It has actually been speculated that they are indeed of pericyte origin.

BUTTERWORTH: Please comment on what you think this means for the human situation.

BRAND: FB tumors in humans are rare, although they do occur. It is interesting that when they occur they are usually carcinomas, which immediately shows that these are tumors of ectodermal origin, and certainly not of the same origin as in our model. I propose that the mouse pericyte has a very labile genome prone to error under forced proliferation, in contrast to pericytes in man. The fact that we see carcinomas in the human FB situation, as well as in asbestosis, schistosomiasis, etc., suggests that we are dealing not only with a different cell type of origin, but also with a different kind of initiation event. It might very well be a genotoxic initiation process (e.g., smoking in the case of asbestosis, nitrosamines in schistosomiasis, and possibly X-rays in mesothelioma). However, I think what is identical here is the promotional situation, the fibrosis, and maybe also the membrane effects that come about by interaction with whatever FB is involved.

Biogenic Silica Fibers and Skin Tumor Promotion

TARLOCHAN BHATT, MAURICE COOMBS, AND CHARLES O'NEILL
Imperial Cancer Research Fund Laboratories
Lincoln's Inn Fields
London WC2A 3PX, England

OVERVIEW

In an area of the world where the incidence of esophageal cancer is high, the grain is commonly contaminated with seeds of various grasses of the genus *Phalaris*. These seeds are covered with microsopic sharp silica fibers that can be detected in the bread made locally. In experiments designed to explore the biological properties of these fibers, mice fed on a diet of the seeds suffered no apparent ill effects, but when they were first initiated by injection of a polycyclic aromatic carcinogen, numerous small skin tumors developed around their mouths. Whether these tumors were caused by the silica fibers was investigated by repeatedly rubbing the pure isolated fibers on the backs of mice after topical initiation. Both papillomas and carcinomas were induced, apparently similar to those found by conventional promotion with croton oil. It seems likely that it is the shape and size of these fibers, rather than their chemical composition, that is the cause of their interesting and unexpected tumor promoter activity. Fibers of this length act as powerful stimuli for division of cells in culture.

INTRODUCTION

Silica is one of the most common elements of the earth's crust, but a relatively rare and inconspicuous part of any living organism (Simpson and Volcani 1981; Parry et al. 1984). The only inorganic silica minerals known to cause cancer are the various forms of asbestos. We have found that biogenic silica can mimic some of the shapes of asbestos fibers and cause cancer just as effectively. Minute, sharply pointed silica hairs are borne by the seeds of several different species of grass of the genus *Phalaris*. These species contaminate the grain grown in northeast Iran, where esophageal cancer reaches extremely high incidences (O'Neill et al. 1980). Among these species, *Phalaris canariensis* has commercial importance as a fodder crop that is resistant to drought (Fig. 1). Seed merchants clean it before sale to remove the hairs, which are very irritating to human skin. The dust collected in this way is one of the richest forms of biogenic silica. Physical studies have shown it to have an opaline (disordered) structure (Mann et al. 1983; Newman and MacKay 1983). It develops initially as a deposit in the walls of the hairs on the influorescence bracts, and it eventually completely fills the lumen so as to form a solid fiber (Sangster et al. 1983a,b; Hodson et al. 1985).

Banbury Report 25: Nongenotoxic Mechanisms in Carcinogenesis
© Cold Spring Harbor Laboratory. 0-87969-225-1/87. $1.00 + .00

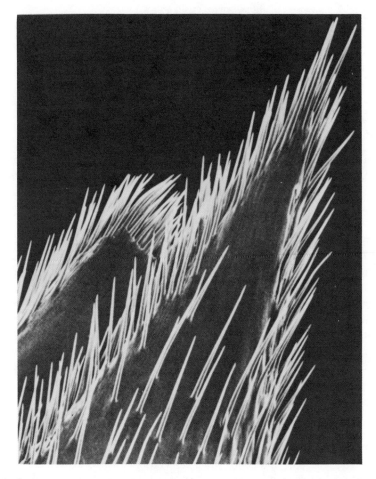

Figure 1

Grain of *P. canariensis*. Apex of two grains. The sharp silica hairs are about 200 μm long. Magnification, 50×. (Reprinted, with permission, from Bhatt et al. 1984.)

We have found that these fibers can be isolated in quantity by digestion with hot nitric acid. They form a soft flocculent white powder, have a mean length of 0.25 mm, and are 15 μm in diameter. We have set out to investigate the biological properties of these fibers and, in particular, whether they can cause cancer in rodents (Bhatt et al. 1984). The animals we used were Theiler's Original strain (T.O.), outbred within a closed colony at the Imperial Cancer Research Fund for many years and with which we have had much experience (Coombs and Croft 1969; Coombs et al. 1973, 1979).

RESULTS

Animal Experiments

In our first experiment, we added whole, unpolished seeds to the diet of T.O. mice by grinding the seed into a coarse meal and mixing this with an equal weight of egg white, allowing the mixture to dry, and then breaking the cake into small fragments. We did this because we observed that when the mice were given the whole seeds, they carefully stripped off the unpalatable husks and consumed only the kernels. The mice were given this seed cake for 4 days and then standard laboratory pellets for the remaining 3 days of each week. They seemed to suffer in no way from this treatment and after 1 year were 15% heavier than the controls fed entirely on laboratory pellets. Silica hairs were recoverable from the gut throughout its length in these mice, but no tumors or other evidence of toxicity was found. Other groups of mice first received an initiating dose of a polycyclic aromatic carcinogen. We used 15,16-dihydro-11-methylcyclopenta[a]phenanthren-17-one (Fig. 2) because we were very familiar with this carcinogen (Coombs 1966; Coombs et al. 1973, 1979), but more especially because, unlike many polycyclic aromatic hydrocarbon carcinogens, this polycylic aromatic ketone when injected at a moderate dose fails to induce local sarcomas, although it efficiently initiates skin remote from the injection site (Coombs et al. 1979). As we had previously found, after intramuscular injection of 3 mg of this carcinogen in oil, many of the animals on a normal diet (group 3 in Table 1) later spontaneously developed ventral skin tumors and a few tumors elsewhere on the skin. When another similar group initiated with the carcinogen (group 4) received twice-weekly applications of croton oil to their shaved backs, skin tumors developed at that site in addition. Treatment of uninitiated mice on a normal diet with croton oil in this way was ineffective in producing dorsal skin tumors (group 5). Of the two groups fed the *Phalaris* diet, the uninitiated animals (group 2) suffered no skin tumors, as already mentioned. In contrast, however, the initiated mice (group 1) showed a remarkable incidence of tumors on the face, in addition to those that occurred as expected on ventral skin. These facial tumors appeared mostly around the mouth and nose; the tumor shown in Figure 3 is typical. They grew to about 2–3 mm in diameter, and all were classi-

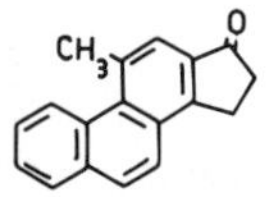

15,16-Dihydro-11-methylcyclopenta[a]phen-
-anthren-17-one

Figure 2

Structure of the carcinogen used to initiate the mice. The compound is numbered like a steroid.

Table 1
Skin Tumor Induction with 15,16–Dihydro–11–methylcyclopenta[a]phenanthren–17–one in Theiler's Original Mice

Group	Treatment	Initiation[a]	No. of mice	head and face	dorsal trunk	ventral trunk	other sites	all sites
				Total number of skin tumors observed on				
1	Seed diet	+	30	35	1	30	9	75
2	Seed diet	−	20	0	0	0	0	0
3	Normal diet	+	20	2	0	15	4	21
4	Normal diet + croton oil	+	20	0	10	12	7	29
5	Normal diet + croton oil	−	20	0	2	0	0	2

[a]Carcinogen (3 mg) in olive oil (0.2 ml) injected into the right shoulder once.

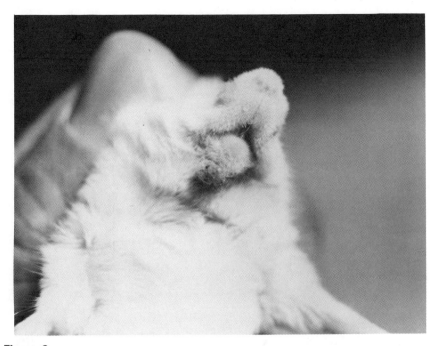

Figure 3

Typical skin tumor near the mouth of a mouse injected with the cyclopenta[a]phenanthrene carcinogen and fed a *Phalaris* seed diet.

fied as squamous papillomas on histology. Of the initiated mice kept on the normal diet (groups 3 and 4), only two suffered facial skin tumors, and both of these were on the eyelids. This quite unexpected incidence of facial tumors therefore seemed to indicate that the silica hair diet was in some way causing promotion of initiated skin around the mouth, an effect we had set out to observe in the esophagus. However, as before, no tumors at this site, or indeed of any part of the alimentary tract, were detected among the 30 initiated mice fed the *Phalaris* seed diet.

To study this apparent promotion by silica hairs further, we went back to a well-tried system (Coombs et al. 1979). The dorsal skin of three groups of 20 mice was shaved and then initiated by painting on the same carcinogen (400 mg in 40 μl of toluene per mouse). One group was promoted by painting the same area with croton oil twice weekly, and another initiated group was left untreated. The initiated dorsal skin of mice in the third group was gently rubbed twice weekly with the pure isolated silica fiber; we used ten strokes, running forward toward the head each time. Mice of a fourth group were rubbed in this way with the fiber but were not initiated with the carcinogen. The results of this experiment are shown diagrammatically in Figure 4. Croton oil produced the expected effect, with a skin tumor

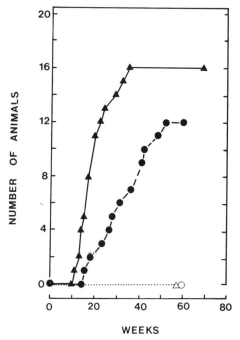

Figure 4

Times of first appearance of dorsal skin tumors (first tumor per animal) in groups of 20 T.O. mice. (●) Initiated mice rubbed with silica fiber; (▲) initiated mice painted with croton oil; (○) uninitiated mice rubbed with silica fiber; (△) initiated mice left untreated. (Reprinted, with permission, from Bhatt et al. 1984.)

incidence of 80% and mean latent period of 20 weeks. Dorsal skin tumors also occurred on initiated mice rubbed with *Phalaris* fiber, but they made their appearance somewhat later (the mean latent period was 33 weeks). Nevertheless, the tumor incidence was finally 60%, and the total number of skin tumors produced in this way was, in fact, larger—23 with fiber versus 16 with croton oil, both from groups of 20 mice. On average, the diameter of the tumors produced with fiber were smaller (1–8 mm) than those observed after application of croton oil (1–18 mm). A typical example is shown in Figure 5. Histologically, the tumors from both treatments were mostly papillomas and noninvasive tumors of the hair follicles and sebaceous glands; however, a few squamous carcinomas occurred also in both groups. No skin tumors were observed among the initiated mice left unpromoted or among the uninitiated mice rubbed repeatedly with *Phalaris* fibers. Thus, this experiment seems to prove conclusively that these silica fibers can act as a tumor promoter, at least on mouse skin. Since the fibers were prepared by exposure to hot, concentrated nitric acid, it seems unlikely that their promoting activity can be due

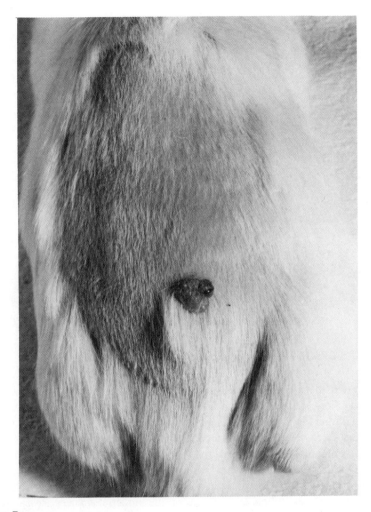

Figure 5

A typical dorsal skin tumor on a T.O. mouse initiated by topical application of the cyclopenta[a]phenanthrene carcinogen, followed by repeated rubbing with *Phalaris* silica fiber.

to any chemical contaminant. The only relevant factors are their size, shape, and chemical stability.

Cell Biology: The Anchorage Hypothesis

The appearance of the *Phalaris* silica fibers prepared as described above is shown in Figure 6, and Figure 7 illustrates their size distribution. The mean width is

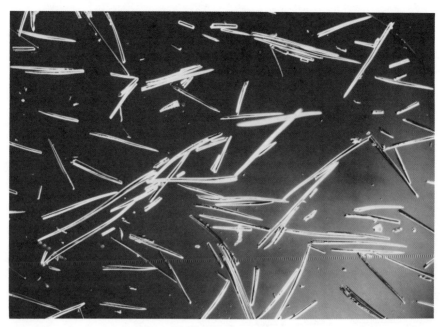

Figure 6
Biogenic silica fibers isolated from *P. canariensis* by nitric acid treatment.

14.6 μm and mean length is 150 μm, although as can be seen, there are many individual fibers between 150 μm and 250 μm long, i.e., the same length as the undamaged fibers found on the *Phalaris* seed (see Fig. 1). They consist exclusively of hydrated silica of composition $[Si(OSi)_n (OH)_{4-n}]$ (Mann et al. 1983), and there are approximately 1×10^7 fibers/g. Their surface area (in two dimensions) is therefore in the region of 3000 μm^2.

A clue to the possible significance of this surface area came from another line of research in progress at the laboratories of the Imperial Cancer Research fund, namely, investigations into anchorage dependence and growth control in cultured cells. It is well known that normal cells in culture soon cease to proliferate unless they become attached to a solid surface. One reason for this may be that unattached cells are unable to spread adequately to expose the surface area necessary for interchange with the medium. Recently, this has been investigated quantitatively by experiments of the following type (O'Neill et al. 1986). Cell-culture dishes are coated with HEMA (polyhydroxyethyl methacrylate) to which cells are unable to adhere. Circular palladium islands of defined position and surface area (Fig. 8) are then placed on the HEMA layer by a vacuum deposition technique. Cells introduced into these dishes attach only to these islands, and conditions can be arranged so that,

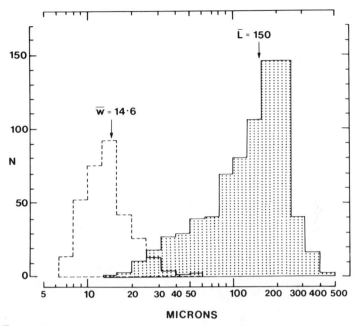

Figure 7

Size distribution of the isolated *Phalaris* fibers (L = mean length and W = mean width). (Reprinted, with permission, from Bhatt et al. 1984.)

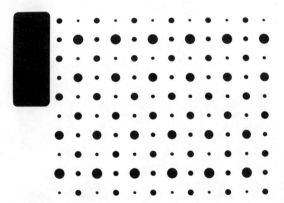

Figure 8

Pattern of palladium islands on a nonadhesive HEMA-coated dish. At the left are two large adhesive and nonadhesive areas; the size of the islands in the left-hand row are, reading from the top, 1625, 1230, 2155, 930, 2855, 700, 3770, 530, 5000, and 400 μm^2. This sequence is reversed alternately. The real size of this unit is 1.5 × 2.1 mm, and over one hundred of these units occupy each dish. (Reprinted, with permission, from O'Neill et al. 1986.)

on average, only one cell attaches to each island. The appearance of cells attached to islands is shown in Figure 9; on the smallest islands (400 μm^2), the cell remains small and spherical, whereas on the largest islands (5000 μm^2), the cell spreads out to cover more than 3000 μm^2. By incubating these cells in media containing [^{3}H]thymidine, those which have undergone DNA synthesis can subsequently be detected by autoradiography. As shown in Figure 10, it is found that the amount of

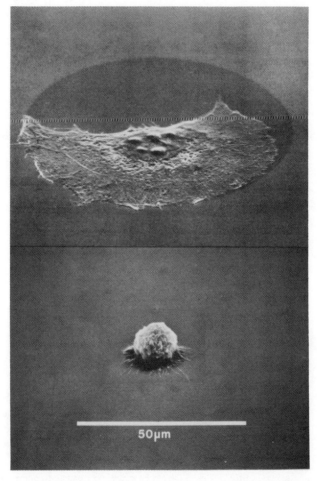

Figure 9
Appearance of cells attached to palladium islands of the largest (*top*) and smallest (*bottom*) size. (Reprinted, with permission, from O'Neill et al. 1986.)

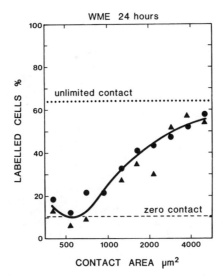

Figure 10

Effect of area of cell attachment on DNA synthesis in whole mouse embryo fibroblasts. Indicated is the percentage of cells found to have incorporated [^{3}H]thymidine after 24 hr in culture. Circles and triangles represent the results from two separate dishes. Zero contact refers to cells in suspension. (Reprinted, with permission, from O'Neill et al. 1986.)

cell division is strongly dependent on the cell surface area exposed to the medium, which is itself dependent on the area of attachment. On the smallest islands, no more cells undergo division than is seen in suspension, whereas on the largest, it is scarcely less than that observed for nonconfluent cells growing on a continuous surface. These findings give rise to the anchorage hypothesis that mineral fibers cause cancer by allowing cells to spread.

The significance of the surface area of the *Phalaris* silica fibers ($\sim$3000 μm^2) thus becomes apparent; they should act as a powerful stimulus to cell division. Indeed, this can readily be demonstrated in cell culture, for once a cell adheres to a fiber as shown in Figure 11, it soon undergoes repeated divisions to form a colony. Since these fibers are strong and sharply pointed, it seems probable that when they are rubbed on the skin, some will penetrate and become lodged in the epidermis, where they will stimulate local cell division. If the skin contains initiated cells, these too will form colonies, and the process of tumor promotion will have begun. We are now beginning to accumulate evidence for an association between the presence of silica fragments and microscopic papillomas detected in histological sections prepared from skin treated in this way. This is, of course, required by this model of tumor promotion, but until recently, we have had difficulty in obtaining this evidence. We think this may be due to the fact that silica fibers are extremely hard

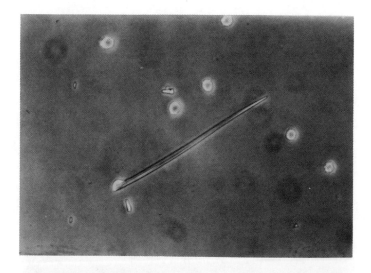

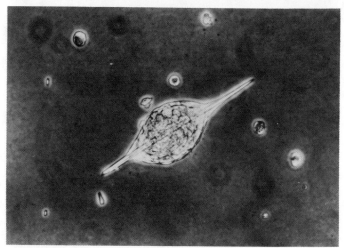

Figure 11

Cell division stimulation by *Phalaris* silica fiber. (*Top*) Cell has just attached to one end of the fiber; (*bottom*) the same field 21 days later. The fiber has stimulated this cell to divide to form a colony of more than 200 cells.

and are not cut by the microtome knife. When conventional wax-embedded sections are used, it instead tends to displace the fiber from its original site in the tissue. Embedding in epoxy resin may solve this problem but, of course, limits the size of the section we can cut.

DISCUSSION

P. canariensis silica fibers are very much more massive than typical biologically active mineral fibers such as those of asbestos. In fact, mineral fibers occur in a very wide range of lengths and diameters, but their cancer-inducing activity seems to be confined to those over 10 μm long and less than 0.2 μm wide (Stanton et al. 1977, 1981; Selikoff and Lee 1980; Wagner and Berry 1980). Typically, there are about 1×10^{11} fibers in one gram of asbestos (Wagner et al. 1982) compared with 1×10^7 for *Phalaris* fibers prepared by the method described; the absolute number of 200-μm fibers in each sample may therefore not be dissimilar. This is of particular interest because it has been established for some time that contact with a solid surface, such as a very thin (~0.5 μm) fiber of glass, acts as a stimulus to growth of cultured fibroblasts and reaches maximum efficiency at about this length (Maroudas et al. 1973). The reason for this appears to be that, under these conditions, the cell attached to the fiber grows in an ellipsoid form, which gives it a surface area of about 3000 μm^2, similar to one growing on an unrestricted solid surface. Moreover, this stimulation is exerted as effectively by *Phalaris* silica fibers as by glass (O'Neill et al. 1980). This leads us to expect that if the silica fiber length were to be considerably reduced, its promoting effects would disappear. This is obviously open to experimental confirmation or refutation. Industrial exposure to asbestos fibers is, of course, associated with the induction of lung cancer and, less frequently, with mesotheliomas of the pleura and peritoneum (Wagner 1984). Tumors of the latter type can be produced by implantation of asbestos or other fibers of similar dimensions within the pleural and peritoneal cavities of rats, and it was interesting to determine whether *Phalaris* fibers would also be effective despite their much greater diameter. In a small pilot experiment, two thus far uncharacterized pleural tumors have been obtained, and the experiment is now being repeated on a much larger scale.

It has recently been reported (Mirvish et al. 1985) that a plant found in the diet of a high-incidence region of South Africa has a small promoting effect on the incidence of esophageal carcinoma in rats induced by methyl *n*-amylnitrosamine. Since this plant (*Bidens pilosa*) is rich in silica fibers (Parry et al. 1986), it has brought us back to our original interest in the possible connection between *Phalaris* fibers and esophageal cancer in Iran. On the assumption that our failure to observe esophageal tumors in the mice kept on the *Phalaris* diet was due to lack of initiation of this tissue by the polycyclic carcinogen used, we have begun another large experiment with rats treated with benzylmethylnitrosamine, which is known to induce esophageal tumors in this species. Our aim is to determine whether the fibers, added to the diet, will have any effect on the incidence or latent period of these tumors.

Finally, returning to the mouse skin tumors described in this paper, it will clearly be necessary to establish dose-response curves and relationships with other carcinogens. It is noticeable that the mouse tumors are, on average, smaller than similar tumors formed with croton oil promotion. This leads us to speculate whether the fiber acts mainly on the first stage of promotion (Boutwell 1964). This idea is also open to test, for a short treatment with fiber followed by repeated application of a second-stage promoter such as mezerein (Slaga et al. 1980) should be more effective than either treatment alone. At present, we are investigating Sencar mice, which we hope will facilitate this and other projected experiments with *P. canariensis* silica fibers.

CONCLUSION

We have shown here that the biogenic silica fiber from *Phalaris* acts as a new tumor promoter with interesting properties. In shape the fibers share some similarities with asbestos, but unlike the latter, they are robust enough to behave as a classical tumor promoter in mouse skin-painting experiments. The mechanism of action is not yet clear, although the promoting effect may result simply from anchorage stimulation of cell growth. Obviously, it will be much easier to study promotion with these biogenic fibers than with mineral fibers such as asbestos because of their much greater uniformity in size and shape. The biogenic fibers may be important in human cancer. Moreover, they can be expected to throw new light on the mechanism of mineral fiber and foreign body carcinogenesis.

REFERENCES

Bhatt, T., M. Coombs, and C. O'Neill. 1984. Biogenic silica fibre promotes carcinogenesis in mouse skin. *Int. J. Cancer* **34**: 519.

Boutwell, R.K. 1964. The function and mechanism of promoters of carcinogenesis. *Crit. Rev. Toxicol.* **2**: 419.

Coombs, M.M. 1966. Potentially carcinogenic cyclopenta[a]phenanthrenes (1,2-cyclopentenophenanthrenes). Part I. A new synthesis of 15,16-dihydro-17-oxocyclopenta [a]phenanthrene and the phenanthrene analogue of oestrone methyl ether. *J. Chem. Soc. C.* p. 955.

Coombs, M.M. and C.J. Croft. 1969. Carcinogenic cyclopenta[a]phenanthrenes. *Prog. Exp. Tumor Res.* **11**: 69.

Coombs, M.M., T.S. Bhatt, and C.J. Croft. 1973. Correlation between carcinogenicity and chemical structure in cyclopenta[a]phenanthrenes. *Cancer Res.* **33**: 832.

Coombs, M.M., T.S. Bhatt, and S. Young. 1979. The carcinogenicity of 15,16-dihydro-11-methylcyclopenta[a]phenanthren-17-one. *Br. J. Cancer* **40**: 914.

Hodson, M.J., A.G. Sangster, and D.W. Parry. 1985. An ultrastructural study on the developmental phases and silicification of the glumes of *Phalaris canariensis* L. *Ann. Bot.* **55**: 649.

Mann, S., C.C. Perry, R.J.P. Williams, C.A. Fyfe, G.C. Gobbi, and G.S. Kennedy. 1983. The characterisation of the nature of silica in biological systems. *J. Chem. Soc. Chem. Commun.* p. 168.

Maroudas, N.G., C.H. O'Neill, and M. Stanton. 1973. Fibroblasts anchorage in carcinogenesis by fibre. *Lancet* **i**: 807.

Mirvish, S.S., S. Salamasi, T.A. Lawson, P. Poser, and D. Sutherland. 1985. Test of catechol, tannic acid, *Bidens pilosa,* croton oil, and phorbol for co-carcinogenesis of oesophageal tumors induced in rats by methyl *n*-amylnitrosamine. *J. Natl. Cancer Inst.* **74**: 1283.

Newman, R.H. and A.L. MacKay. 1983. Silica spicules in canary grass. *Ann. Bot.* **52**: 927.

O'Neill, C., P. Jordan, and G. Ireland. 1986. Evidence for two distinct mechanisms of anchorage stimulation in freshly explanted and 3T3 Swiss mouse fibroblasts. *Cell* **44**: 489.

O'Neill, C.H., G.M. Hodges, P.N. Riddle, P.W. Jordan, R.H. Newman, and R.J. Flood. 1980. A fine fibrous silica contaminant of flour in the high oesophageal cancer area of North East Iran. *Int. J. Cancer* **26**: 617.

Parry, D.W., M.J. Hodson, and A.G. Sangster. 1984. Some recent advances in studies of silica in higher plants. *Philos. Trans. R. Soc. Lond. B Biol. Sci.* **304**: 537.

Parry, D.W., C.H. O'Neill, and M.J. Hodson. 1986. Opaline silica deposits in the leaves of *Bidens pilosa* L. and their possible significance in cancer. *Ann. Bot.* **58**: 641.

Sangster, H.G., M.J. Hodson, D.W. Parry, and J.A. Rees. 1983a. A developmental study of silification in the trichomes and associated epidermal structures of the inflorescence bracts of the grass *Phalaris canariensis. Ann. Bot.* **52**: 171.

Sangster, A.G., M.J. Hodson, and D.W. Parry. 1983b. Silica deposition and anatomical studies in the inflorescence bracts of four *Phalaris* species with their possible relevance to carcinogenesis. *New Phytol.* **93**: 105.

Selikoff, I.J. and D.H.K. Lee. 1980. *Asbestos and disease.* Academic Press, New York.

Simpson, T.L. and B.E. Volcani. 1981. *Silica and siliceous structure in biological systems.* Springer Verlag, New York.

Slaga, T.J., S.M. Fischer, K. Nelson, and G.L. Gleason. 1980. Studies on the mechanisms of skin tumor promotion: Evidence for several stages in promotion. *Proc. Natl. Acad. Sci. U.S.A.* **77**: 3659.

Stanton, M.F., M. Layard, A. Tegeris, E. Miller, M. May, and E. Kent. 1977. Carcinogenicity of fibrous glass: Pleural response in relation to fiber dimensions. *J. Natl. Cancer Inst.* **58**: 587.

Stanton, M.F., M. Layard, A. Tegeris, E. Miller, M. May, E. Morgan, and A. Smith. 1981. Relation of particle dimension to carcinogenicity in amphibole asbestos and other fibrous materials. *J. Natl. Cancer Inst.* **67**: 965.

Wagner, J.C. 1984. Mineral fiber carcinogenesis. In *American Chemical Society monograph 182: Chemical carcinogens* (ed. C.E. Searle), 2nd ed., vol. 1, p. 631. American Chemical Society, Washington, D.C.

Wagner, J.C. and G. Berry. 1980. Carcinogenesis and mineral fibres. *Br. Med. Bull.* **36**: 53.

Wagner, J.C., M. Chamberlain, R.C. Brown, G. Berry, F.D. Pooley, R. Davies, and D.M. Griffiths. 1982. Biological effects of tremolite. *Br. J. Cancer* **45**: 352.

COMMENTS

ROE: We did an old-fashioned experiment, applying 300 μg of DMBA in acetone to the skin of mice followed either by acetone only or by croton oil dissolved in acetone. All treatments were applied in volumes of 0.2 ml or 0.3 ml to the entire dorsal skin after removal of the hair by clipping. In the group given DMBA in acetone followed by just acetone, we observed virtually no tumors on the treated dorsal skin. However, we did obtain a high incidence of tumors on the head, very similar to those which you have just described. In contrast, animals that received DMBA followed by croton oil developed lots of tumors on their backs, but very few on their heads. These results were published in the *British Journal of Cancer* (1956, *10,* 61–69). I cannot give you any explanation for these findings.

COOMBS: Were the latent periods of the tumors similar for the two types of tumors?

ROE: No. In animals that received an application of DMBA and then 18 once-weekly applications of croton oil, benign tumors began to appear in the treated dorsal skin after about 4 or 5 weeks. After the cessation of croton oil treatment, most of these dorsally located tumors regressed and very few of these mice went on to develop facial tumors. In contrast, mice exposed to DMBA and then only to acetone for 18 weeks began to develop facial papillomas after 30 weeks.

COOMBS: That is a most interesting result.

CERUTTI: Is there an inflammatory response in the dermis after application of these fibers?

COOMBS: Yes. We have been trying to cut sections. Of course, silica, which is about the hardest thing known, won't cut; so it just gets pushed out of the way. It has been very difficult to prove, in fact, that there is any silica in the tumors that we are looking at. We started embedding in epoxy resin and we are beginning to see that there is a certain amount of silica there. But, the problem all along has been to actually identify the silica in the skin.

CERUTTI: I don't mean in the tumor; in the treated skin.

COOMBS: Yes.

SLAGA: Is there hyperplasia, or do you get any alteration in morphology?

COOMBS: There is a certain amount of reddening of the area when you rub; and it is very irritating if you get it onto your own skin.

DI GIOVANNI: Did you ever do any controls where you just rubbed sand or some other kind of abrasive-type substance?

COOMBS: What we did was simply take the mouse and rub with the gloved finger. We held the mouse by the tail and gave it ten forward strokes with moderately firm pressure. We also did this to the control groups, and they produced nothing at all.

DI GIOVANNI: I was thinking more in terms of something that might produce a low level of abrasion.

COOMBS: I don't really think this produces abrasion. It's a lovely soft white powder, rather like talcum powder, when you produce it.

DI GIOVANNI: If you do histological evaluations from the back of the mouse where you can see these fibers, are cells attached to them as you observed in your culture?

COOMBS: It has been difficult to do this histology because we can't cut through the fibers; so, unless by chance you actually cut sort of parallel to the fiber, the thing gets pushed out of the way. This has been the trouble up to now. They are continuing trying to do this.

REITZ: What do you know about the health of the workers in Australia that work in this environment?

COOMBS: I think there are too few people involved to do very much in the way of statistics. We don't know about this. But, obviously, they have had trouble in preparing this material, and they have gone to the trouble of actually putting fans in to get all the dust into bags and out of the way.

BUTTERWORTH: How much preening do the animals do?

ROE: A lot. But this does not explain why the animals that were exposed to DMBA only developed more facial tumors than those that had croton oil as well.

COOMBS: Yes, that's difficult to understand.

SWENBERG: I was just going to say that a technique that you might find useful would be something like scanning electron microscopy with energy dispersive X-ray analysis. You would be able to pick your silicon up very nicely.

COOMBS: Yes. We have been doing that. Unfortunately, the electron beam does not penetrate very far into the skin; so we still have to use sections.

SIVAK: Seeing your figure of the cells growing around the fiber recalls some findings in the cell transformation area where we are looking at BALB/c-3T3 cells. Every once in awhile, we would see "spontaneous" transformed foci in dishes. Some fraction of these would, in fact, be around a piece of the silica or the cotton that came from the pipette when the medium was put into the dish. This event did not happen very frequently, but it has happened often enough to note it. In fact, there is a very severe geographical alteration of cells growing in culture when their environment is perturbed by a solid object, and so much so that the focus that derives from the cells that have attached to that piece of glass or fiber are indistinguishable from those that result from carcinogen treatment.

Bladder Stones and Bladder Cancer: A Review of the Toxicology of Terephthalic Acid

HENRY d'A. HECK
Department of Biochemical Toxicology and Pathobiology
Chemical Industry Institute of Toxicology
Research Triangle Park, North Carolina 27709

OVERVIEW

Ingestion of large doses of terephthalic acid (TPA) or dimethyl terephthalate (DMT) by rats results in the formation of bladder calculi, which are composed primarily of CaTPA. Rats exposed chronically to TPA developed calculi and bladder cancer. TPA does not appear to be mutagenic and is not metabolized by rats, suggesting that TPA is not genotoxic. Calculi injure the bladder wall and induce cell proliferation, which is probably a critical factor in the induction of bladder neoplasia by TPA. Since bladder calculi cannot occur unless the solubility of the stone components is exceeded (i.e., unless the product of the concentrations of Ca^{++} and TPA^{--} in urine exceeds the solubility product of CaTPA), the formation of calculi and the toxic responses that result from calculus formation are threshold effects. Therefore, a linear low-dose extrapolation model is inappropriate for risk assessment. A safety factor approach based on the solubility of bladder stone components is conservative and scientifically justifiable.

INTRODUCTION

A number of chemicals, including diethylene glycol (Weil et al. 1965), 4-ethyl-sulfonylnaphthalene-1-sulfonamide (Clayson 1974), nitrilotriacetate (Anderson and Kanerva 1978), saccharin (Munro et al. 1975), TPA and DMT (Chin et al. 1981), and melamine (Melnick et al. 1984), have been found to induce crystalluria or calculi in the bladders of experimental animals. Many of these compounds also induced bladder cancer during chronic feeding studies (Weil et al. 1967; Clayson 1974; Gross 1974; Arnold et al. 1983; Melnick et al. 1984; Anderson et al. 1985).

Calculi can significantly influence the outcome of a carcinogenesis bioassay. Several studies, both in experimental animals and in humans, have provided evidence that bladder calculi increase the incidence of bladder cancer. The implantation of inert solids (glass beads or paraffin wax) in the bladders of rats and mice produced bladder tumors (Weil et al. 1967; Jull 1979). Epidemiology studies suggest a link between the occurrence of bladder stones and bladder cancer in humans (Kantor et al. 1984). The association between calculi and cancer was

Banbury Report 25: Nongenotoxic Mechanisms in Carcinogenesis
© Cold Spring Harbor Laboratory. 0-87969-225-1/87. $1.00 + .00

apparently not due to urinary tract infection, which is also a risk factor for bladder cancer in humans. Kantor et al. (1984) concluded that "factors associated with inflammation of the bladder, or bladder stone formation, are etiologically relevant."

The formation of urinary tract calculi is well understood in physicochemical terms (Finlayson 1977). The fundamental requirement for stone formation is that urine must be supersaturated with respect to the stone components. Kinetic factors, such as the rates of nucleation and growth of stones, determine whether calculi actually form in supersaturated urine. Biological parameters, such as the age and sex of experimental animals, markedly affect the incidence and quantity of stones produced, as well as their retention in the bladder (Weil et al. 1965; Teelmann and Niemann 1979; Chin et al. 1981).

The mechanism by which inert solids enhance bladder cancer is not well understood. The normal bladder epithelium is known to have a very low level of mitotic activity (Hicks et al. 1975). Calculi injure the bladder wall, usually inducing epithelial cell hyperplasia and causing an increase in the mitotic index (Clayson 1974). It is possible that the increase in cell replication may result in damage to the DNA by endogenous mutagens or may lead to the activation of oncogenes. The details of this process are unclear, but from the work with inert solids, it seems very likely that the increase in cell replication is a critical factor in carcinogenesis.

Several years ago, studies of urolithiasis induction by TPA and dimethyl terephthalate DMT were begun at the Chemical Industry Institute of Toxicology (CIIT). The aims of the studies were (1) to investigate the chronic toxicity and carcinogenicity of TPA, (2) to study the tissue distribution and metabolism of TPA and DMT, (3) to determine the composition of bladder stones and the concentrations of stone components in urine, (4) to relate the presence of stones to various forms of bladder pathology, and (5) to investigate the solubility of stone-forming materials and to utilize the solubility data for risk assessment. The results of these investigations have been published (Heck and Kluwe 1980; Chin et al. 1981; Heck 1981; Wolkowski-Tyl et al. 1982a; Heck and Tyl 1985). Because bladder stones have played an important role in some carcinogenesis bioassays, it seems appropriate to review these data in the context of the information presented in this volume.

RESULTS

Distribution and Metabolism of TPA and DMT

Following oral or intravenous administration of [^{14}C]TPA to rats, the compound is rapidly distributed and excreted unchanged into the urine ($t_{1/2} \simeq 60\text{–}100$ min) (Hoshi and Kuretani 1968; Wolkowski-Tyl et al. 1982a). Urinary metabolites of [^{14}C]TPA were not detected, either by thin-layer chromatography (Hoshi and

Kuretani 1968) or by paired-ion high-performance liquid chromatography (Wolkowski-Tyl et al. 1982a); hence, TPA does not appear to be metabolized by rats.

Owing to its low solubility in both aqueous and organic solvents, the absorption of [^{14}C]TPA following oral administration of the compound to rats is incomplete (Moffitt et al. 1975). In contrast, the absorption of [ring-^{14}C]DMT appears to be nearly complete following an oral dose (Moffitt et al. 1975). Metabolism of [ring-^{14}C]DMT by F344 rats results in the almost total conversion of DMT to TPA (Heck and Kluwe 1980). Only trace amounts of monomethyl [^{14}C]terephthalate and no [^{14}C]DMT were detected in rat urine. Thus, the metabolism of DMT appears only to involve hydrolysis of the ester groups.

Genotoxicities of TPA and DMT

The ability of TPA and DMT to induce mutations in bacteria was tested using *Salmonella typhimurium* strains TA98, TA100, TA1535, and TA1537 in the presence and absence of liver S-9 activating systems from Aroclor 1254-induced rats and hamsters (Zeiger et al. 1982). The results were negative for both compounds. Other laboratories have also tested TPA and DMT with negative results (for review, see Heck and Tyl 1985). Thus, neither compound appears to be genotoxic under the conditions of the Ames test. There were no reports indicating that either compound has been examined using other genotoxicity tests.

Chronic Toxicities of TPA and DMT

The chronic toxicity and carcinogenicity of TPA have been tested in two laboratories. The first study was carried out at the Hebrew University-Hadassah Medical School, Department of Experimental Medicine and Cancer (Jerusalem, Israel), under the auspices of the U.S. Department of Agriculture (Gross 1974). Rats of the Wag-Rij (Wistar-derived) strain were administered TPA in the diet at concentrations of 1%, 2%, or 5% for 2 years. Rats in the highest dosage group developed a high incidence of urinary tract calculi, with much lower incidences occurring in the other two dosage groups (Table 1). Malignant tumors of the bladder were detected only in the highest dosage group.

The final report of the Israeli study did not provide details on the occurrence of stones and tumors in individual animals. For this reason, the tissue sections were reviewed in 1978 by H.F. Sherman (E.I. du Pont de Nemours and Co.) together with J. Gross, the study director. According to H.F. Sherman (pers. comm.), the classification of "tumors" in the Israeli study was incomplete, since hyperplasia, papilloma, and cancer were all labeled as tumors. The incidences of bladder cancer presented in Table 1 were obtained by H.F. Sherman (pers. comm.).

The second study of the chronic toxicity of TPA was carried out for CIIT at the Illinois Institute of Technology Research Institute (Chicago, Illinois) (Chemical

Table 1

Induction of Bladder Calculi and Bladder Cancer in Rats by Terephthalic Acid

Strain/Dose	Bladder calculi		Bladder cancer[a]	
	males	females	males	females
Wag–Rij strain[b]				
(dietary %)				
0	0/45 (0%)	0/46 (0%)	0/45 (0%)	0/46 (0%)
1	0/48 (0%)	1/48 (2%)	0/43 (0%)	0/48 (0%)
2	0/50 (0%)	2/50 (4%)	0/48 (0%)	0/47 (0%)
5	44/47 (94%)	36/42 (86%)	7/37[c] (19%)	3/34[c] (9%)
F344 strain[d]				
(mg/kg/day)				
0	0/87 (0%)	0/83 (0%)	0/85 (0%)	1/71 (1%)
20	0/82 (0%)	0/76 (0%)	0/82 (0%)	0/76 (0%)
142	0/82 (0%)	0/70 (0%)	0/82 (0%)	0/70 (0%)
1000	0/82 (0%)	11/86 (13%)	0/80 (0%)	11/73[e] (15%)

[a]Includes adenomas and carcinomas but excludes hyperplasia and papillomas.
[b]Bladder cancer data from H.F. Sherman (pers. comm.).
[c]All rats (100%) with bladder neoplasms had bladder stones.
[d]Data from Chemical Industry Institute of Toxicology (1983).
[e]Eight of 11 rats (73%) with bladder neoplasms had bladder stones.

Industry Institute of Toxicology 1983). F344 rats were administered dietary TPA at doses of 20, 142, and 1000 mg/kg/day for 2 years. The results of this study are summarized in Table 1. A low incidence of calculi was produced, which can be explained by the relatively low doses of TPA administered to the animals. The highest dose corresponds to an approximate dietary concentration of 2.0–2.8% in adult F344 rats. Calculi were found only in female rats, and bladder cancer occurred only in animals of this sex.

In both chronic studies of TPA, a strong correlation was found between the occurrence of bladder stones and cancer. In the Israeli study, 100% of the animals with bladder cancer had bladder stones. In the CIIT study, 73% (8/11) of the female rats with bladder cancer were found to have calculi. The possibility that small calculi were passed (Teelman and Niemann 1979) or were lost during processing of tissues for microscopic examination (Heck and Tyl 1985) could explain the absence of stones from some of the neoplastic bladders.

The carcinogenicity of DMT has been tested in F344 rats and B6C3F$_1$ mice (National Cancer Institute). The dietary concentrations used (0.25% and 0.5%) were too low to induce bladder calculi (see below). A renal calculus was noted in only 1 of 50 high-dose female rats. Uroliths were not detected in any other group. It was concluded that at these doses, DMT ''had no appreciable effect on the mean body weights of the rats or mice of either sex . . . and . . . no tumors occurred at incidences that clearly were related to administration of the test chemical'' (National Cancer Institute 1979).

Calculus Induction by TPA and DMT in Weanling Rats and Its Pathologic Sequelae

The weanling rat is a useful model for the study of urolithiasis, owing to the relatively large amount of food consumed per unit of body weight, which results in the ingestion of relatively large doses of test agents (Weil et al. 1965; Wolkowski-Tyl et al. 1982b). Calculi were rapidly and reproducibly induced in weanling (28-day-old) F344 rats exposed for 2 weeks to selected dietary concentrations of either TPA or DMT (Chin et al. 1981). These animals were used to investigate the toxicologic characteristics of bladder stone formation by TPA and DMT.

Calculus formation in weanling rats was characterized by a very steep concentration-response curve (Fig. 1). Of the male rats exposed to TPA, 93.3% (28/30) developed stones at the highest dietary concentration (5%), whereas no calculi were detected in rats ingesting 1.5% dietary TPA. Of male rats exposed to DMT, 100% (18/18) developed calculi in the highest dosage group (3%), whereas calculi were not induced at 1% DMT. The incidence of calculi in female rats was lower than in male rats at all dietary doses. This sex difference in susceptibility to calculus formation is probably anatomic in origin. The female mouse has been shown to be more capable than the male mouse of eliminating implanted foreign bodies from the bladder (Teelmann and Niemann 1979).

Analyses of calculi showed that TPA-induced calculi were composed primarily of CaTPA and CaHPO$_4$. DMT-induced calculi were composed largely of CaTPA, with very little phosphate present in the stones (Chin et al. 1981). The greater potency of DMT than of TPA as a calculus inducer (Fig. 1) is consistent with the fact that DMT is absorbed more efficiently than TPA (Moffitt et al. 1975) and is biotransformed almost entirely to TPA by F344 rats (Heck and Kluwe 1980).

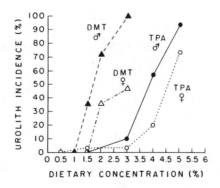

Figure 1

Incidence of urolithiasis in weanling F344 rats ingesting dietary TPA or DMT for 14 days. (Reprinted, with permission, from Heck and Tyl 1985.)

Specific changes in several urinary ion concentrations were noted in rats ingesting high doses of TPA and DMT. Urinary acidity and urinary Ca^{++} concentrations were significantly increased by both compounds (Table 2). The concentration of TPA in rat urine that induced calculi in approximately 50% of the male rats was about 80–120 mM (Table 2). TPA did not significantly change the concentration of urinary phosphate, but DMT significantly decreased the concentration of this electrolyte in urine (Table 2). The decreased phosphate concentration in urine from DMT-treated rats is in agreement with the stone analyses, which indicated an absence of $CaHPO_4$ in DMT-induced calculi. However, the mechanism responsible for the decrease in urinary phosphate by DMT is not known.

The histologic lesions observed in the bladders of weanling rats ingesting dietary TPA were dependent on the presence of stones (Chin et al. 1981). The bladders of four rats that ingested 4% dietary TPA for 2 weeks but did not develop calculi appeared normal histologically, including a normal transitional epithelial lining. In

Table 2

Urinary Electrolyte and Metabolite Concentrations in Weanling F344 Rats Ingesting TPA or DMT

Urine component	Sex	Dietary TPA concentration			
		0% (18M, 10F)	0.5% (9M, 14F)	3% (17M, 10F)	4% (19M, 13F)
pH[a]	M	6.35 ± 0.11	5.79 ± 0.04[**]	5.75 ± 0.03[**]	5.74 ± 0.02[**]
	F	6.19 ± 0.12	5.73 ± 0.03[**]	5.65 ± 0.03[**]	5.78 ± 0.04[**]
Ca[a]	M	5.6 ± 0.7	11.7 ± 1.3	22.5 ± 2.2[**]	22.4 ± 2.0[**]
	F	4.9 ± 0.7	11.0 ± 1.5	25.0 ± 1.2[**]	22.4 ± 3.1[**]
PO$_4$[a]	M	92 ± 13	71 ± 11	88 ± 11	113 ± 11
	F	107 ± 19	59 ± 5[*]	108 ± 6	121 ± 12
TPA[b]	M	—	44 ± 3	68 ± 7	83 ± 6
	F	—	37 ± 4	81 ± 2	101 ± 9
		Dietary DMT concentration			
		0% (24M, 13F)	0.5% (11M, 7F)	1.5% (13M, 8F)	2% (13M, 9F)
pH[a]	M	6.41 ± 0.10	5.94 ± 0.06[**]	5.84 ± 0.05[**]	5.95 ± 0.07[**]
	F	6.22 ± 0.10	6.11 ± 0.11	5.72 ± 0.05[**]	5.72 ± 0.03[**]
Ca[a]	M	5.2 ± 0.5	10.7 ± 1.5[*]	22.5 ± 1.9[**]	15.1 ± 1.9[**]
	F	4.7 ± 0.6	10.1 ± 2.8	27.3 ± 3.9[**]	25.4 ± 3.4[**]
PO$_4$[a]	M	101 ± 13	71 ± 14	60 ± 16	16 ± 2[**]
	F	111 ± 14	50 ± 9[**]	62 ± 12[*]	22 ± 4[**]
TPA[b]	M	—	46 ± 9	105 ± 16	103 ± 17
	F	—	23 ± 7	116 ± 20	127 ± 16

All concentrations, except for pH, are millimolar; values shown are the mean ± s.e. Data adapted from Heck (1981).

[a]Dunnett's procedure (Steel and Torrie 1960) was used to test for significant deviations from controls. Single asterisk indicates $0.05 > p > 0.01$; double asterisk indicates $0.01 > p$.

[b]Student-Newman-Keuls' test (Steel and Torrie 1960) was used to examine deviations among treatment means. Underlined values are not significantly different.

contrast, six animals that developed calculi under the same dosage regimen exhibited a variety of histologic lesions, varying in severity from animal to animal. The transitional epithelium was diffusely hyperplastic throughout the bladder lining. In some instances, the thickened transitional epithelial layer extended into the lamina propria and muscular wall, and even into the serosa of the bladder wall (Chin et al. 1981). Small calculi were occasionally noted in the hyperplastic epithelium (Fig. 2). Mitotic figures were numerous.

The transitional cell proliferative lesion induced by TPA was considered hyperplastic rather than neoplastic (Chin et al. 1981). The cells lacked pleomorphism, anaplasia, or dysplasia. Additional time sequence studies are required to characterize the ability of the lesion to regress or perhaps progress to neoplasia.

Solubility of CaTPA in Relation to Risk Assessment

The extremely steep dose-response curves for TPA- and DMT-induced urolithiasis are indicative of a threshold effect. A threshold is expected in this case, because calculus formation cannot occur unless the concentration product of Ca^{++} and TPA^{--} in rat urine exceeds the solubility product, K_{sp}, of CaTPA. Therefore, by determining the solubility of CaTPA, the minimum concentration of TPA in

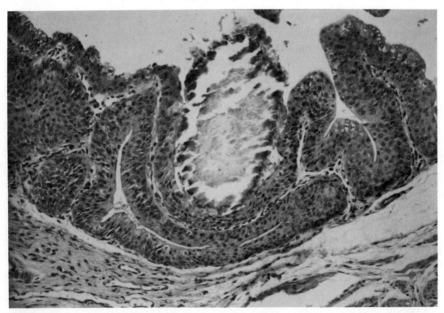

Figure 2

Microcalculus embedded in the hyperplastic surface epithelium of a 42-day-old male rat exposed for 2 weeks to 4% dietary TPA. (Reprinted, with permission, from Chin et al. 1981.)

rat or human urine that would be required to induce stones can be calculated (Heck 1981).

The solubility of CaTPA at 37°C was investigated in a variety of different salt solutions at ionic strengths as high as 1.44 M (Heck 1981; Heck and Tyl 1985). Since the ionic strength of rat urine ranges from approximately 0.6 M to 1.2 M (Heck and Kluwe 1980) and that of human urine is about 0.3 M (Elliot 1964), these studies permitted the solubility properties of CaTPA to be determined at salt concentrations in the physiological range.

The solubility product of CaTPA, defined as $K_{sp} = [Ca^{++}][TPA^{--}]$, is equal to $(1.02 \pm 0.18) \times 10^{-6} M^2$ at zero ionic strength and 37°C; i.e., the solubility of CaTPA in pure water is about 1.0 mM at this temperature (Heck 1981). The solubility of CaTPA in aqueous solutions of NaCl, KCl, KNO_3, NH_4Cl, or $MgCl_2$ increases with increasing ionic strength, reaching a maximum (~ 10–12 mM) at ionic strengths normally occurring in rat urine (Heck 1981; Heck and Tyl 1985). The increased solubility of CaTPA with increasing ionic strength is due to electrostatic shielding and is in accordance with theoretical predictions (Pitzer 1977).

From the calculated values of the urinary ionic strength, the corresponding values of K_{sp}, and the measured concentrations of urinary Ca^{++}, the concentrations of TPA^{--} required to saturate urine with respect to CaTPA were estimated (Heck 1981). The values obtained (11–22 mM) represent a conservative estimate of the urinary TPA^{--} concentration required for the formation of calculi, because calculus formation can only occur in urine that is supersaturated with respect to the stone components. Calculus formation did not occur in rats until the concentration of TPA^{--} in urine was at least 70 mM (Chin et al. 1981); i.e., the minimum urinary concentration of TPA^{--} required to induce stones was three- to sixfold higher than the concentration required for saturation.

Similar calculations were made for human urine (Heck 1981). The results indicated that human urine would become saturated with respect to CaTPA at TPA^{--} concentrations in the range of 8–16 mM. Assuming that humans excrete about 1.5 liters of urine per day, that TPA is not metabolized by humans, and that DMT is metabolized entirely to TPA, the amount of TPA (DMT) that would have to be absorbed in order to produce the minimum saturating concentration of TPA^{--} (8 mM) was estimated. The calculation indicated that at least 2.0 g/day of TPA (2.4 g/day of DMT) would have to be absorbed (Heck 1981). It is improbable that workplace exposures could result in the absorption of such large quantities. However, monitoring the urines of exposed individuals could readily verify that the urinary concentration of TPA^{--} remained well below the saturation limit.

CONCLUSIONS

Since TPA-induced calculi cannot be formed unless the product of the concentrations of Ca^{++} and TPA^{--} in urine exceeds the value of K_{sp}, the formation of calculi and the toxic responses that result therefrom are threshold effects. The manner in which thresholds can be incorporated into carcinogenic risk assessments has not been defined. This is perhaps one reason for the wide use of the linear model to estimate risks, even in the case of urolithiasis (Environmental Protection Agency 1984). If risk assessment is to become scientifically credible, mechanistic data that suggest a threshold or a nonlinearity in a carcinogenesis dose-response curve should not be excluded from risk estimations, which can have important societal and economic implications.

A scientifically justifiable method for the setting of exposure limits in the case of chemicals that involve a threshold is the safety factor approach. The safety factor method is consistent with the mechanistic data and is therefore more plausible than the linear model, which does not admit the existence of a threshold. Hence, the exposure limits defined by the safety factor method would be expected to be based more closely on actual risks than is the case for the linear model.

The induction of bladder cancer by bladder stones provides a good example of carcinogenesis associated with exposure to an apparently nongenotoxic compound. The bladder stones were central to the toxicity of TPA, but it is unlikely that calculi are sufficient to induce bladder cancer, since a number of animals with calculi did not develop tumors. Other factors that may be required for the induction of bladder neoplasia by lithogenic chemicals include exogenous carcinogens present as impurities, or perhaps more likely, endogenous mutagens present in the urine or generated within the proliferating epithelial cells. The ability of these factors to induce bladder cancer is probably dependent on the rate of cell proliferation and thus is likely to be affected by the presence of calculi. Hence, in this case as in several others reported elsewhere in this volume, forced cell proliferation appears to be an essential component of the carcinogenic process.

REFERENCES

Anderson, R.L. and R.L. Kanerva. 1978. Hypercalcinuria and crystalluria during ingestion of dietary nitrilotriacetate. *Food Cosmet. Toxicol.* **16:** 569.

Anderson, R.L., W.E. Bishop, and R.L. Campbell. 1985. A review of the environmental and mammalian toxicology of nitrilotriacetic acid. *CRC Crit. Rev. Toxicol.* **15:** 1.

Arnold, D.L., D. Krewski, and I.C. Munro. 1983. Saccharin: A toxicological and historical perspective. *Toxicology* **27:** 179.

Chemical Industry Institute of Toxicology (CIIT). 1983. *Chronic dietary administration of terephthalic acid.* CIIT, Research Triangle Park, North Carolina.

Chin, T.Y., R.W. Tyl, J.A. Popp, and H.d'A. Heck. 1981. Chemical urolithiasis. 1. Characteristics of bladder stone induction by terephthalic acid and dimethyl terephthalate in weanling Fischer-344 rats. *Toxicol. Appl. Pharmacol.* **58:** 307.

Clayson, D.B. 1974. Bladder carcinogenesis in rats and mice: Possibility of artifacts. *J. Natl. Cancer Inst.* **52:** 1685.

Elliot, J.S. 1964. The urinary excretion of inorganic salts. *Invest. Urol.* **1:** 582.

Environmental Protection Agency (EPA). 1984. Cyromazine: Proposed tolerance. *Fed. Regist.* **49:** 18120.

Finlayson, B. 1977. Calcium stones: Some physical and clinical aspects. In *Calcium metabolism in renal failure and nephrolithiasis* (ed. D.S. David), p. 337. Wiley, New York.

Gross, J. 1974. *The effects of prolonged feeding of terephthalic acid (TPA) to rats*, project FG-Is-175. Agricultural Research Service, U.S. Department of Agriculture, Washington, D.C.

Heck, H.d'A. 1981. Chemical urolithiasis. 2. Thermodynamic aspects of bladder stone induction by terephthalic acid and dimethyl terephthalate in weanling Fischer-344 rats. *Fundam. Appl. Toxicol.* **1:** 299.

Heck, H.d'A. and C.L. Kluwe. 1980. Microanalysis of urinary electrolytes and metabolites in rats ingesting dimethyl terephthalate. *J. Anal. Toxicol.* **4:** 222.

Heck, H.d'A. and R.W. Tyl. 1985. The induction of bladder stones by terephthalic acid, dimethyl terephthalate, and melamine (2,4,6-triamino-*s*-triazine) and its relevance to risk assessment. *Regul. Toxicol. Pharmacol.* **5:** 294.

Hicks, R.M., J. St. J. Wakefield, and J. Chowaniec. 1975. Evaluation of a new model to detect bladder carcinogens or co-carcinogens: Results obtained with saccharin, cyclamate, and cyclophosphamide. *Chem. Biol. Interact.* **11:** 225.

Hoshi, A. and K. Kuretani. 1968. Distribution of terephthalic acid in tissues. *Chem. Pharm. Bull.* **16:** 131.

Jull, J.W. 1979. The effect of time on the incidence of carcinomas obtained by the implantation of paraffin wax pellets into mouse bladder. *Cancer Lett.* **6:** 21.

Kantor, A.F., P. Hartge, R.N. Hoover, A.S. Narayana, J.W. Sullivan, and J.F. Fraumeni, Jr. 1984. Urinary tract infection and risk of bladder cancer. *Am. J. Epidemiol.* **119:** 510.

Melnick, R.L., G.A. Boorman, J.K. Haseman, R.J. Montall, and J. Huff. 1984. Urolithiasis and bladder carcinogenicity of melamine in rodents. *Toxicol. Appl. Pharmacol.* **72:** 292.

Moffitt, A.E., Jr., J.J. Clary, T.R. Lewis, M.D. Blanck, and V.B. Perone. 1975. Absorption, distribution and excretion of terephthalic acid and dimethyl terephthalate. *Am. Ind. Hyg. Assoc. J.* **36:** 633.

Munro, I.C., C.A. Moodie, D. Krewski, and H.C. Grice. 1975. A carcinogenicity study of commercial saccharin in the rat. *Toxicol. Appl. Pharmacol.* **32:** 513.

National Cancer Institute (NCI). 1979. *Bioassay of dimethyl terephthalate for possible carcinogenicity*, NIH publ. no. 79-1376. Carcinogenesis Testing Program, National Cancer Institute, National Institutes of Health, Bethesda, Maryland.

Pitzer, K.S. 1977. Electrolyte theory—Improvements since Debye and Hückel. *Acc. Chem. Res.* **10:** 371.

Steel, R.G.D. and J.H. Torrie. 1960. *Principles and procedures of statistics*, p. 110. McGraw-Hill, New York.

Teelmann, K. and W. Niemann. 1979. The short term fate of dischargeable glass beads implanted surgically in the mouse urinary bladder. *Arch. Toxicol.* **42:** 51.

Weil, C.S., C.P. Carpenter, and H.F. Smyth, Jr. 1965. Urinary bladder response to diethylene glycol. *Arch. Environ. Health* **11:** 569.

———. 1967. Urinary bladder calculus and tumor response following either repeated feeding of diethylene glycol or calcium oxalate stone implantations. *Ind. Med. Surg.* **36:** 55.

Wolkowski-Tyl, R., T.Y. Chin, and H.d'A. Heck. 1982a. Chemical urolithiasis. III. Pharmacokinetics and transplacental transport of terephthalic acid in Fischer-344 rats. *Drug Metab. Dispos.* **10:** 486.

Wolkowski-Tyl, R., T.Y. Chin, J.A. Popp, and H.d'A. Heck. 1982b. Urolithiasis: Chemically induced urolithiasis in weanling rats. *Am. J. Pathol.* **107:** 419.

Zeiger, E., S. Haworth, W. Speck, and K. Mortelmans. 1982. Phthalate ester testing in the National Toxicology Program's environmental mutagenesis test development program. *Environ. Health Perspect.* **45:** 99.

COMMENTS

ROE: Did you say that in your TPA-treated animals the amount of calcium in the urine, as distinct from stones, was increased?

HECK: Yes.

ROE: Where did this calcium come from? Does this mean that there was increased calcium absorption?

HECK: Yes. The calcium came from increased absorption from the gut.

ROE: Do you know whether any increased absorption occurs in humans, because in the case of lactose and various polyols, the increase in calcium absorption is very much less in humans than in rodents. The maintenance of calcium balance is seemingly quite different in rodents than in humans. Therefore, if one proposes to make a risk assessment using a calcium-linked parameter as one of the risk factors and then to extrapolate from rats to humans, there are many other things that have to be taken into account, particularly species differences in calcium absorption.

HECK: That would be presuming that exposure to TPA causes an increased calcium absorption in humans.

ROE: This is measurable.

SIVAK: I noted that in the DMT group there was a substantial reduction in the phosphate. Is there any explanation for why it happened with the dimethylteraphthalate and not the phthalate? Is there some physiological mechanism, or is it physical, or what?

HECK: We don't know why that occurred. When we gave very high doses of DMT to adult rats (these were weanling rats) we did not see a decrease in urinary phosphate.

SIVAK: One would expect that low-phosphate calculi would be very unusual.

COHEN: Those invasive lesions you've described are diverticuli, which are much more commonly seen in mice than in rats, but are not tumors. Are the teraphthalate-induced tumors squamous cell or transitional cell? In humans, calculus-related tumors of the bladder and urothelial tract tend to be squamous cell rather than transitional cell.

HECK: These were transitional cell tumors.

SWENBERG: I might just point out that the regulatory agencies are using this kind of an approach. Melamine was found to be carcinogenic in the National Toxicology Program study and the Environmental Protection Agency decided not to regulate it on the basis that it was secondary to calculus formation.

HECK: A risk assessment was done for melamine on the basis of a linear low-dose extrapolation.

SWENBERG: Yes, but I believe that Jack Moore overruled that and said that it was inappropriate. The agency went on not to regulate it.

ROE: It is not true that there is *no* risk of urinary tract cancer in humans from calculi. Maybe there is not much risk because humans have stones removed from the bladder because they give rise to unpleasant symptoms. However, higher up the urinary tract, stones may reside silently in the renal pelvis for prolonged periods, and at this site, a clear-cut relationship exists between stones and cancers. A perennial question is, Which comes first, the stone or the cancer? However, the increased risk of cancer of the renal pelvis in cysteinuric patients establishes beyond reasonable doubt that the stones predispose to the cancer.

Session 5:
Examples of Nongenotoxic Carcinogens

TCDD: Mechanisms of Altered Growth Regulation in Human Epidermal Keratinocytes

WILLIAM F. GREENLEE, ROSEMARIE OSBORNE, KAREN M. DOLD,
LISA ROSS, AND JON C. COOK
Department of Cell Biology
Chemical Industry Institute of Toxicology
Research Triangle Park, North Carolina 27709

OVERVIEW

The use of various in vitro models has increased our understanding of the biochemical and molecular bases for the adverse actions of 2,3,7,8-tetra-chlorodibenzo-p-dioxin (TCDD or dioxin) on the growth and differentiation of human keratinocytes. Normal and transformed keratinocytes possess a specific receptor protein (the Ah receptor) for TCDD (Hudson et al. 1983; Osborne and Greenlee 1985). The available data indicate that the human epidermal Ah receptor has many functional properties in common with its murine counterpart, specifically, the regulation of inducible xenobiotic metabolizing enzymes (Hudson et al. 1983), the mediation of hyperkeratinization, and, in certain lines, hyperproliferative responses to TCDD (Greenlee et al. 1987). These abnormal growth patterns result, in part, from regulatory actions on the receptor systems for at least three of the physiologic mediators of keratinocyte proliferation: epidermal growth factor (EGF), glucocorticoids, and cyclic AMP (cAMP). Studies of TCDD action in these keratinocyte models should result in the elucidation of the molecular (genetic) basis for potential interindividual differences in sensitivity to TCDD and provide a relevant data base for assessing the oncogenic potential of dioxin-like compounds for human skin and possibly other epithelial tissues.

INTRODUCTION

TCDD is the prototype for several classes of structurally related halogenated aromatic compounds (Poland et al. 1979; Goldstein 1980; Poland and Knutson 1982). In humans and a limited number of animal species, TCDD and isosteric compounds produce a pattern of skin lesions (chloracne) characterized by the appearance of keratinaceous cysts and comedones (Kimmig and Shulz 1957; Crow 1970). These lesions result from the reprogramming of the differentiation of sebaceous acinar base cells. These cells normally differentiate into sebum- or lipid-producing cells but are induced by TCDD and other chloracneogens to differentiate into keratinizing squamous epithelium (Suskind 1985). Plugging of the hair follicles occurs concomitantly

Banbury Report 25: Nongenotoxic Mechanisms in Carcinogenesis
© Cold Spring Harbor Laboratory. 0-87969-225-1/87. $1.00 + .00

with the sebaceous gland hyperkeratinization. Follicular atrophy and keratinization can be accompanied by interfollicular epidermal hyperplasia (acanthosis) and hyperkeratinization (Taylor et al. 1977; Kimbrough 1980).

Ah Receptor: Role in Enzyme Induction and Toxicity

The actions of TCDD on skin target cells are mediated by a specific receptor protein, designated the *Ah* receptor (Poland and Knutson 1982; Greenlee et al. 1985, 1987). This protein was identified and characterized originally in livers from inbred murine strains as the induction receptor for cytochrome P_1-450 and other enzymes involved in xenobiotic metabolism (Poland et al. 1976, 1979; Poland and Knutson, 1982). Several of the toxic responses in animals to TCDD also appear to be mediated by the *Ah* receptor (Poland and Knutson 1982). Genetic analysis of TCDD-induced epidermal hyperplasia in HRS/J hairless (*hr/hr*) mice indicate the involvement of at least two regulatory genes, *Ah* (the putative structural gene for the *Ah* receptor) and *hr* (Knutson and Poland 1982). The *Ah* locus determines sensitivity and the *hr* locus determines the extent of the response regulated by the *Ah* locus (Poland and Knutson 1982).

Modulation of Keratinocyte Proliferation and Differentiation In Vitro

TCDD enhances stratification and induces hyperkeratinization in murine XB cells (Knutson and Poland 1980). In early passage, normal human epidermal cells at confluence and in at least one human squamous cell carcinoma (SCC) line (SCC-12F), TCDD enhances the commitment of proliferating basal cells to terminal differentiation (Osborne and Greenlee 1985; Hudson et al. 1985, 1986). This response is similar morphologically to hyperkeratinization in vivo (Fig. 1). In another human SCC line (SCC-9), TCDD potentiates glucocorticoid-dependent cell proliferation (Rice and Greenlee 1982; Greenlee et al. 1985).

The abnormal growth patterns induced by TCDD in human epidermal cells in culture result, in part, from regulatory actions by the TCDD-*Ah* receptor complex on the receptor systems for at least three of the physiologic mediators of keratinocyte proliferation: EGF, glucocorticoids, and cAMP (Greenlee et al. 1987). This report summarizes studies on the mechanisms of regulation of the EGF and glucocorticoid receptors. The relevance of increased understanding of the molecular mechanisms of action of TCDD in human epidermal keratinocytes to the assessment of the human oncogenic potential of TCDD is discussed below.

RESULTS

Regulation of EGF-receptor-binding Activity

Studies on the regulation of EGF receptor binding by TCDD have been carried out in normal human epidermal cells (Osborne and Greenlee 1985) and in the

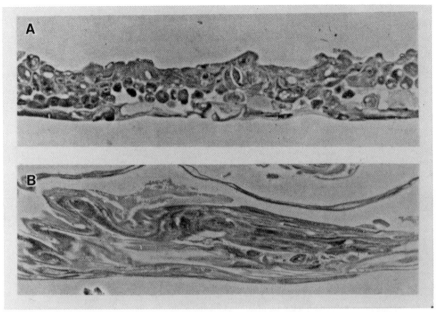

Figure 1

Enhanced stratification in confluent cultures of normal human epidermal cells treated with TCDD. Cultures were treated for 4 days with solvent vehicle (*A*) or 10 nM TCDD (*B*). Histologic analysis was performed as described previously (Osborne and Greenlee 1985). The cell layer adjacent to the plastic culture dish (basal cell layer) is toward the bottom of each panel. (Reprinted, with permission, from Osborne and Greenlee 1985.)

nontumorigenic human keratinocyte cell line SCC-12F (Hudson et al. 1985, 1986). Both cell types display a marked increase in terminal differentiation in the presence of TCDD (Fig. 1 and Table 1). This response is associated with a decrease in high-affinity EGF-receptor-binding sites (Fig. 2) mediated by the TCDD-*Ah* receptor complex. Analyses of the actions of TCDD on SCC-12F cells in reduced (50 μM)-calcium medium (conditions selective for basal cells) and in other SCC lines indicate that (1) the regulation of EGF binding is a direct response to TCDD occurring in the basal population, (2) enhanced differentiation is a consequence of the modulatory actions on EGF receptor binding, and (3) in at least one SCC line (SCC-9), modulation of EGF binding and terminal differentiation by TCDD is suppressed by glucocorticoids (Table 1) (Hudson et al. 1986).

Two characteristics distinguish the regulation of EGF receptor binding by TCDD versus the actions of EGF and other endogenous peptides, or xenobiotics such as phorbol esters and polycyclic aromatic hydrocarbons: (1) Suppression of high-affinity EGF binding is delayed, with a time course similar to that for EGF receptor turnover (Fig. 3), and (2) the response is sustained (reduced EGF binding is

Table 1
Modulation of EGF Binding and Terminal Differentiation by TCDD in Various SCC Lines

Cell line	Dexamethasone	Relative EGF binding (%)	Differentiation
SCC–12F	–	40	+ +
	+	48	+ +
SCC–9	–	58	+
	+	95	–
SCC–4	–	56	–
	+	83	–

All SCC lines were grown in complete DMEM in the presence or absence of 10 nM dexamethasone and then treated with 100 nM TCDD for 72 hr (Hudson et al. 1986). EGF binding (Hudson et al. 1985) and differentiation (Osborne and Greenlee 1985) were assayed as described. Data taken from Hudson et al. (1986).

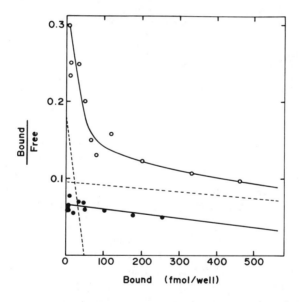

Figure 2
Scatchard analysis of EGF-specific binding in control and TCDD-treated SCC-12F cells. Confluent cultures were treated with solvent vehicle (○) or 100 nM TCDD (●) for 72 hr. EGF binding was measured as described previously (Hudson et al. 1985). Computer resolution of the Scatchard plot from control cultures indicated two binding components: (1) K_d = 0.28 nM, n = 2.3 × 10^4 sites/cell and (2) K_d = 46 nM, n = 2 × 10^6 sites/cell. A single low-affinity binding component (K_d = 15 nM, n = 5 × 10^5 sites/cell) was observed in the TCDD-treated cultures. Data taken from Hudson et al. (1985).

observed up to 10 days after treatment with TCDD) (Hudson et al. 1985, 1986). These observations are consistent with the hypothesis that TCDD inhibits the synthesis of the EGF receptor. However, analysis of the transcriptional activity of the EGF receptor structural gene in SCC-12F cells treated with TCDD indicated no change in the amount or processing of total RNA for the EGF receptor (W.F. Greenlee, unpubl.). Studies in progress are examining EGF receptor turnover in control and TCDD-treated cells to assess adverse actions on potential post-transcriptional and/or posttranslational regulatory mechanisms, including receptor glycosidation and phosphorylation.

Regulation of Glucocorticoid-receptor-binding Activity

Hydrocortisone promotes the proliferation of normal human epidermal cells (Rheinwald and Green 1975), and in certain human SCC lines, TCDD acts like a synergist for glucocorticoid-dependent cell growth (Rice and Greenlee 1982). The actions of glucocorticoids on epidermal and other target cells are mediated by specific intracellular receptors (Slaga et al. 1977; Ponec et al. 1981; Ringold 1985). The potentiation of glucocorticoid-dependent cell proliferation by TCDD in SCC-9 cells appears to result from the regulation of glucocorticoid-receptor-binding activity by the TCDD-*Ah* receptor complex (Hudson 1985).

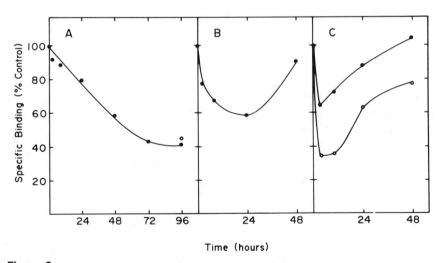

Figure 3

Kinetics of inhibition of EGF-specific binding by (*A*) TCDD, (*B*) benzo(a)pyrene, or (*C*) EGF. Confluent cultures of SCC-12F cells were treated with TCDD (100 nM), benzo(a)pyrene (1 μM), or EGF (●, 1 ng/ml; ○, 10 ng/ml) for the times indicated prior to the determination of EGF-specific binding. Data taken from Greenlee et al. (1987) and in part from Hudson et al. (1985).

Scatchard analysis and sucrose density gradient analysis of dexamethasone (a synthetic glucocorticoid)-specific binding to cytosol fractions from control and TCDD-treated SCC-9 cells suggest that the glucocorticoid receptor is inducible by TCDD (Hudson 1985). This hypothesis is supported by the inhibition of TCDD-stimulated glucocorticoid receptor binding by actinomycin D and cycloheximide; however, no change in the total RNA for the glucocorticoid receptor is observed after treatment of SCC-9 cells with 10 nM TCDD for 6 hours and 24 hours, respectively (W.F. Greenlee, unpubl.). Preliminary data suggest that the TCDD-Ah receptor complex regulates the binding activity of the glucocorticoid receptor through stimulation of receptor phosphorylation. If substantiated by studies in progress, regulation of phosphorylation activities may represent an important mechanism for the Ah-receptor-dependent control of other receptor systems as well.

DISCUSSION

Chloracne and the accompanying proliferative changes in the interfollicular epidermis are the most sensitive and widely expressed toxic responses to TCDD observed in humans (Crow 1970). The research described in this report on the actions of TCDD on human keratinocytes in culture suggests that regulation of the receptor systems for EGF and glucocorticoids by the TCDD-Ah receptor complex may be a determinant of the adverse growth responses observed in the interfollicular epidermis.

Elucidation of the molecular mechanisms of toxicity of TCDD to human keratinocytes in culture is providing the basis for detailed understanding of the genetic determinants of human susceptibility to TCDD and other dioxin-like compounds. Human epidermal cell strains differ in their sensitivity to Ah-receptor-dependent toxic responses (Osborne et al. 1985). These cells are being characterized for differences in the expression of the Ah receptor and for Ah-receptor-dependent regulation of EGF and glucocorticoid receptor activities. Genetic analysis of identified Ah receptor variants should result in the identification of other regulatory genes required for the expression of TCDD-induced adverse growth responses.

TCDD is an animal carcinogen (Kociba et al. 1978) and an extraordinarily potent tumor promoter (Pitot et al. 1980; Poland et al. 1982; Abernethy et al. 1985). TCDD promotes the formation of transformed foci in N-methyl-N'-nitro-N-nitrosoguanidine (MNNG)-initiated C3H/10T1/2 cells (Abernethy et al. 1985) and the formation of papillomas in MNNG-initiated skin of HRS/J hairless mice (Poland et al. 1982). At this time, no definitive evidence exists implicating TCDD as a human carcinogen. The molecular and biochemical bases for interspecies differences in the toxic and carcinogenic potential of TCDD are not known. Detailed study of the actions of TCDD on initiated human and murine keratinocytes in culture should provide data useful for the assessment of the promoting potential of TCDD in human skin and should help to elucidate the molecular basis for interspecies differences in the responsiveness of epidermal cells to TCDD and related halogenated aromatic compounds.

REFERENCES

Abernethy, D.J., W.F. Greenlee, J.C. Huband, and C.J. Boreiko. 1985. 2,3,7,8-Tetrachlorodibenzo-p-dioxin (TCDD) promotes the transformation of C3H10T1/2 cells. *Carcinogenesis* **6**: 651.

Crow, K.D. 1970. Chloracne. A critical review including a comparison of two series of cases of acne from chlornaphthalene and pitch fumes. *Trans. St. Johns Hosp. Dermatol. Soc.* **56**: 79.

Goldstein, J.A. 1980. Structure-activity relationships for the biochemical effects and relationships to toxicity. In *Halogenated biphenyls, terphenyls, naphthalenes, dibenzodioxins, and related products* (ed. R.D. Kimbrough), p.151. Elsevier/North Holland, New York.

Greenlee, W.F., R. Osborne, K.M. Dold, L.G. Hudson, and W.A. Toscano, Jr. 1985. Toxicity of chlorinated aromatic compounds in animals and humans: *In vitro* approaches to toxic mechanisms and risk assessment. *Environ. Health Perspect.* **60**: 69.

Greenlee, W.F., R. Osborne, K.M. Dold, L.G. Hudson, M.J. Young, and W.A. Toscano, Jr. 1987. Altered regulation of epidermal cell proliferation and differentiation by 2,3,7,8-tetrachlorodibenzo-p-dioxin (TCDD). In *Reviews in biochemical toxicology* (ed. E. Hodgson et al.), vol. 8, p. 1. Elsevier/North Holland, New York.

Hudson, L.G. 1985. *Regulation of human epithelial cell proliferation and differentiation by 2,3,7,8-tetrachlorodibenzo-p-dioxin.* Ph.D. Thesis, Harvard University, Boston, Massachusetts.

Hudson, L.G., W.A. Toscano, Jr., and W.F. Greenlee. 1985. Regulation of epidermal growth factor binding in a human keratinocyte cell line by 2,3,7,8-tetrachlorodibenzo-p-dioxin (TCDD). *Toxicol. Appl. Pharmacol.* **77**: 251.

———. 1986. 2,3,7,8-Tetrachlorodibenzo-p-dioxin (TCDD) modulates epidermal growth factor (EGF) binding to basal cells from a human keratinocyte cell line. *Toxicol. Appl. Pharmacol.* **82**: 481.

Hudson, L.G., R. Shaikh, W.A. Toscano, and W.F. Greenlee. 1983. Induction of 7-ethoxycoumarin O-deethylase activity in cultured human epithelial cells by 2,3,7,8-tetrachlorodibenzo-p-dioxin (TCDD): Evidence for TCDD receptor. *Biochem. Biophys. Res. Commun.* **115**: 611.

Kimbrough, R.D. 1980. Occupational exposure. In *Halogenated biphenyls, terphenyls, naphthalenes, dibenzodioxins and related products* (ed. R.D. Kimbrough), p.373. Elsevier/North Holland, New York.

Kimmig, J. and K.H. Schulz. 1957. Chlorinated aromatic cyclic ethers as the cause of chloracne. *Naturwissenschaften* **44**: 337.

Knutson, J.C. and A. Poland. 1980. Keratinization of mouse teratoma cell line XB produced by 2,3,7,8-tetrachlorodibenzo-p-dioxin: An *in vitro* model of toxicity. *Cell* **22:** 27.

———. 1982. Response of murine epidermis to 2,3,7,8-tetrachlorodibenzo-p-dioxin: Interaction of the *Ah* and *hr* loci. *Cell* **30:** 225.

Kociba, R.J., D.G. Keyes, J.E. Beyer, R.M. Carreon, C.E. Wade, D.A. Dittenber, R.P. Kalnins, L.E. Frauson, C.N. Park, S.D. Barnard, R.A. Hummel, and C.G. Humiston. 1978. Results of a two-year chronic toxicity and oncogenicity study of 2,3,7,8-tetrachlorodibenzo-p-dioxin in rats. *Toxicol. Appl. Pharmacol.* **46:** 279.

Osborne, R. and W.F. Greenlee. 1985. 2,3,7,8-Tetrachlorodibenzo-p-dioxin (TCDD) enhances terminal differentiation of cultured human epidermal cells. *Toxicol. Appl. Pharmacol.* **77:** 434.

Osborne, R., K.M. Dold, and W.F. Greenlee. 1985. Strain differences in sensitivityof human epidermal cells to 2,3,7,8-tetrachlorodibenzo-p-dioxin. *Fed. Proc.* **44:**8358.

Pitot, H.C., T. Goldsworthy, H.A. Campbell, and A. Poland. 1980. Quantitative evaluation of the promotion by 2,3,7,8-tetrachlorodibenzo-p-dioxin of hepatocarcinogenesis from diethylnitrosamine. *Cancer Res.* **40:** 3616.

Poland, A. and J.C. Knutson. 1982. 2,3,7,8-Tetrachlorodibenzo-p-dioxin and related halogenated aromatic hydrocarbons: Examination of the mechanism of toxicity. *Annu. Rev. Pharmacol. Toxicol.* **22:** 517.

Poland, A., E. Glover, and A.S. Kende. 1976. Stereospecific, high affinity binding of 2,3,7,8-tetrachlorodibenzo-p-dioxin by hepatic cytosol. Evidence that the binding species is receptor for induction of aryl hydrocarbon hydroxylase. *J. Biol. Chem.* **251:** 4936.

Poland, A., W.F. Greenlee, and A.S. Kende. 1979. Studies on the mechanism of action of the chlorinated dibenzo-p-dioxins and related compounds. *Ann. N.Y. Acad. Sci.* **320:** 214.

Poland, A., D. Palen, and E. Glover. 1982. Tumour promotion by TCDD in skin of HRS/J mice. *Nature* (Lond.). **300:** 271.

Ponec, M., J.A. Kempenaar, and E.R. De Kloet. 1981. Corticoids and cultured human epidermal keratinocytes: Specific intracellular binding and clinical efficacy. *J. Invest. Dermatol.* **76:** 211.

Rheinwald, J.G. and H. Green. 1975. Serial cultivation of strains of human epidermal keratinocytes: The formation of keratinizing colonies from single cells. *Cell* **6:** 331.

Rice, R.H. and W.F. Greenlee. 1982. Effects of 2,3,7,8-tetrachlorodibenzo-p-dioxin in cultured human epithelial target cells: Modulation by hydrocortisone. *Toxicologist* **2:** 463.

Ringold, G.M. 1985. Steroid hormone regulation of gene expression. *Annu. Rev. Pharmacol. Toxicol.* **25:** 529.

Slaga, T., S. Thompson, and J. Schwartz. 1977. Binding of dexamethasone by the subcellular fractions of mouse epidermis and dermis. *J. Invest. Dermatol.* **68:** 307.

Suskind, R.R. 1985. Chloracne, "the hallmark of dioxin intoxication." *Scand. J. Work Environ. Health* **11:** 165.

Taylor, J.S., R.C. Wuthrich, K.M. Lloyd, and A. Poland. 1977. Chloracne from manufacture of a new herbicide. *Arch. Dermatol.* **113:** 616.

COMMENTS

BARRETT: With the increased kinase activity you observed, do you know which amino acid residues were phosphorylated?

GREENLEE: No.

SLAGA: Did you do any studies with the squamous cell carcinoma cells in terms of EGF receptor and the glucocorticoid receptor and the effects of TCDD on them?

GREENLEE: Our studies are carried out in both normal human epidermal cells and human SCC lines. Two SCC lines have been identified which display predominantly either a hyperdifferentiation (SCC-12F) or hyperproliferative (SCC-9) response to TCDD. These lines have been used as prototypes to study the regulation of EGF and glucocorticoid receptor binding activities by the TCDD-*Ah* receptor complex. The responses observed in SCC-12F cells are also seen in most of the normal human epidermal cell strains examined in culture.

Genetic Toxicology
of Di(2-ethylhexyl)phthalate

BYRON E. BUTTERWORTH
Department of Genetic Toxicology
Chemical Industry Institute of Toxicology
Research Triangle Park, North Carolina 27709

OVERVIEW

Di(2-ethylhexyl)phthalate (DEHP) is among the most widespread of synthetic environmental chemicals. The observation that lifetime bioassays with massive doses of DEHP yielded tumors in mouse and rat livers has raised serious concerns as to the hazard of this agent to humans. Numerous cell culture assays for mutagenicity and other genotoxic endpoints consistently show no DNA reactivity for DEHP or its metabolites. Summaries of the profile of genotoxic activity for DEHP that focus on what appear to be a few spurious positive results for isolated tests illustrate the serious credibility crisis in the field of genetic toxicology. For any known carcinogen, additional weight is often given to any positive short-term test at the expense of a more objective view of all the data, even if it appears that the mechanism of action in the cell culture system may not be relevant to the mechanisms of toxicity and carcinogenesis that are taking place in the whole animal. It may be felt by some that in order to protect the public, this stand is justified to assure the use of the conservative hypothetical mathematical models for risk assessment that rely on assumptions of irreversible genetic events. Unfortunately, the perception now exists that if one examines enough tests and test conditions, it will be possible to generate at least one report of a positive genotoxicity response for any chemical.

Results in the C3H/10T1/2 cell transformation assay show no initiating or promoting activity with DEHP. However, activity is seen in the Syrian hamster embryo (SHE) cell transformation assay, which appears to be measuring events early in the transformation process. Consistent with this are indications of activity with DEHP in some assays for aneuploidy; however, the exact role of aneuploidy induction in chemical carcinogenesis is still being defined and the detergent effects of DEHP on cells in culture are of unknown relevance at physiological concentrations.

DEHP is similar to other hypolipidemic carcinogens that induce liver hyperplasia and peroxisomal proliferation in the treated animal. One suggestion is that increased active oxygen species produced as a result of peroxisomal proliferation may damage the DNA in the intact animal. Yet, numerous studies in which animals were administered DEHP sufficient to cause peroxisomal proliferation failed to show any focal hepatic proliferative lesion (FHPL)-initiating activity or any DNA-binding or

Banbury Report 25: Nongenotoxic Mechanisms in Carcinogenesis
© Cold Spring Harbor Laboratory. 0-87969-225-1/87. $1.00 + .00

DNA-damaging activity. Studies to examine the FHPL-promoting action of DEHP show activity in mice but not in rats.

One activity that does appear to correlate with tumorigenic potency for the hypolipidemic agents is induced hepatic hyperplasia. Although some feedback mechanism eventually inhibits uncontrolled growth of the liver, it is possible that key genes related to the regulation of cellular growth and cancer remain stimulated during the continued administration of the chemical.

Knowledge of the mechanism of action of DEHP is not simply an academic exercise. Many manufacturers are already switching to substitutes for DEHP for which there are no cancer data at all. If one knew why DEHP is carcinogenic, one could make a more intelligent decision for a safe substitute. If it should turn out that induced hyperplasia is important and is mediated through species-specific cellular receptors, then activity in the rodent may be of little relevance to human beings. It is less than comforting to hear that justification for using a particular substitute for DEHP was that it was negative in the Ames test.

INTRODUCTION

DEHP is widely used as a plasticizer to impart flexibility in many consumer plastic products and medical devices. Some formulations can contain as much as 30% of the compound. With an estimated 2 billion pounds produced annually worldwide, DEHP is among the most widespread of synthetic environmental chemicals (Thomas and Thomas 1984). DEHP can be hydrolized in the environment to produce mono(2-ethylhexyl)phthalate (MEHP) and 2-ethylhexanol (2-EH). Pharmacokinetic studies indicate rapid conversion of DEHP in the body to MEHP and 2-EH, so that plasma levels of MEHP are much higher than the levels of DEHP. Thus, both DEHP and MEHP are considered in this discussion.

A chronic study with 4000 ppm (300 mg/kg/day) DEHP administered in the diet to Sherman rats for 2 years yielded no tumors (Carpenter et al. 1953). No tumors were observed in Wistar rats given 5000 ppm (375 mg/kg/day) DEHP in the diet for 2 years (Harris et al. 1956). The information from these studies was limited because of low numbers of exposed animals or limited pathology. No tumors were reported in rats treated for 2 years with 20,000 ppm (1500 mg/kg/day) DEHP in the diet (Ganning et al. 1984). A more rigorous carcinogenesis bioassay was conducted in which F344 rats were given 6000 and 12,000 ppm DEHP and B6C3F$_1$ mice were given 3000 and 6000 ppm DEHP in the diet for 2 years (National Toxicology Program 1983). In this study, statistically significant increases in hepatocellular carcinomas were observed in the female rats receiving 12,000 ppm DEHP, in the male mice receiving 6000 ppm DEHP, and in the female mice receiving 3000 and 6000 ppm DEHP (Table 1). Interestingly, the incidence of several tumor types was decreased in those animals administered DEHP relative to controls (Table 2). In light of the widespread human exposure to DEHP, the borderline carcinogenic

Table 1

Percentage of Animals with Hepatocellular Carcinoma following Treatment with DEHP in the Diet for 2 Years

| Species | Sex | Control | Treated animals | | | DEHP intake at highest dose (mg/kg/day) |
			3000 ppm	6000 ppm	12,000 ppm	
Rat	male	2%		2%	10%	674
Rat	female	0%		4%	16%	774
Mouse	male	18%	29%	38%		1325
Mouse	female	0%	14%	34%		1821

Data from National Toxicology Program (1983).

response obtained with this chemical has been the impetus for much research to determine the potential human risk and mechanism of action of DEHP.

A key step in the complex process of carcinogenesis appears to be alteration of the information coded in the DNA, and many carcinogens have been shown to be genotoxic (McCann et al. 1975). The process of correlating results in short-term tests for genotoxicity with results from cancer studies has acquired the name of validation studies. Genetic toxicology assays have somehow been placed in the untenable position of perfect correlation with cancer studies. It is common when dealing with a known carcinogen to look for and give weight to any positive genotoxicity result at the expense of a more objective overview of all the data. Assays are often pushed to extreme limits just to get the ''correct'' response. In many cases, the ''right'' answer is obtained, but by a mechanism unrelated to the one producing tumors in the animal. With so much genetic toxicology testing being done in such a variety of systems, it would appear that if one looks long and hard enough, one can find an assay or conditions such that any compound will be positive in at least one short-term test. To retain credibility, the field of genetic toxicology must recognize that there are nongenotoxic carcinogens that may be acting by means other than direct reactivity of the chemical or its metabolites with the DNA. DEHP

Table 2

Percentage of Male Rats with Tumors following Treatment with DEHP in the Diet for 2 Years

| Tumor | Untreated animals | Treated animals | |
		6000 ppm	12,000 ppm
Hepatocellular carcinoma	2%	2%	10%
Pituitary adenoma	9%	12%	2%
Thyroid C-cell carcinoma	8%	2%	
Testicular interstitial-cell tumor	96%	95%	23%

Data from National Toxicology Program (1983).

is an interesting test case. A massive amount of genotoxicity data now exists for DEHP. If it is not possible to conclude that this chemical is at least not mutagenic, then it is the field of genetic toxicology that is in trouble.

RESULTS AND DISCUSSION

Cell Culture Genotoxicity Assays

Studies in numerous laboratories with DEHP and its principal metabolites, MEHP and 2-EH, have consistently failed to show mutagenic activity in a variety of sensitive bacterial mutagenesis assays (Chemical Manufacturers Association 1982; Kozumbo et al. 1982; Seed 1982; Zeiger et al. 1982, 1985; Kirby et al. 1983; Yoshikawa et al. 1983). DEHP was one of the chemicals chosen in a very large collaborative study, sponsored by the International Programme on Chemical Safety (IPCS), that provided some 90 individual sets of experimental data on the activity of DEHP in various short-term tests (Ashby et al. 1985). In the IPCS study, all five assays for mutagenesis in *Salmonella* were negative (Ashby et al. 1985). There is one report that DEHP and MEHP were mutagenic in the Ames test (Tomita et al. 1982), in contradiction to all of the above reports. In the IPCS study, DEHP was reported as negative in five out of six assays for yeast gene mutation and negative for all three assays for mutagenesis in somatic cells in *Drosophila* (Ashby et al. 1985). Neither DEHP, MEHP, nor 2-EH were mutagenic in the L5178Y mouse lymphoma mutagenesis assay (CMA 1982; Kirby et al. 1983) or in the Chinese hamster ovary (CHO) mutagenesis assay (Phillips et al. 1982). In the IPCS study, DEHP was negative in five out of six mammalian cell gene mutation assays (Ashby et al. 1985).

In the IPCS study, all three assays for chromosomal aberrations and both assays for sister chromatid exchange (SCE) induction in mammalian cell cultures were negative (Ashby et al. 1985). DEHP did not yield chromosome damage in human lymphocytes or in human fetal lung cells (Stenchever et al. 1976). No increase in chromosome aberrations was observed in CHO cells (Abe and Sasaki 1977). The same study reported a slight increase in the SCE frequency of cells treated with DEHP, but the authors concluded that the response was not enough to classify the chemical as an SCE-inducing agent. There is one report that MEHP but not DEHP was clastogenic at high concentrations in CHO cells (Phillips et al. 1982). The same study reported both compounds as negative in the CHO SCE assay. These results are curious because the SCE assay is usually the more sensitive cytogenic endpoint. More information was recently presented which may clarify this paradox (Phillips et al. 1986). It was found that the CHO cultures were not viable in the presence of 0.7 mM MEHP as measured by trypan blue exclusion and plating efficiency, while the chromosomal effects were only seen above 1.0 mM MEHP. Furthermore, it was shown that MEHP had detergent activity, as one would predict from its structure, and could lyse red blood cells. One must be cautious in interpreting results in sensitive cell culture systems where the concentrations of the compounds are so high as to physically alter the cells or to produce severe toxicity. Tomita et al. (1982) reported that MEHP induced SCE in CHO cells at excessively high doses, but no cytotoxicity information was provided.

Neither DEHP, MEHP, nor 2-EH induced DNA repair in metabolically competent primary rat or mouse hepatocyte cultures (CMA 1982; Hodgson et al. 1982; Butterworth et al. 1984; Kornbrust et al. 1984; Smith-Oliver and Butterworth 1987). Similarly, no activity was seen with DEHP or MEHP in the primary human hepatocyte DNA repair assay (Butterworth et al. 1984). In the IPCS study, DEHP was negative in all three of the DNA-repair assays done by autoradiography (Ashby et al. 1985). One assay in the IPCS study reported a positive response in the rat hepatocyte DNA-repair assay with scintillation counting. Scintillation counting methods, however, are inappropriate for DNA-repair studies because one cannot distinguish a general DNA-repair response from a slight stimulation of the number of cells in S phase (Doolittle et al. 1983). In fact, other hypolipidemic agents have indeed been shown to stimulate S-phase DNA synthesis in primary hepatocyte cultures (Bieri et al. 1984). There is one report that the hypolipidemic agents Wy-14,643 and BR-931 induced DNA repair in primary rat hepatocyte cultures treated with hydroxyurea to inhibit S phase, as judged by scintillation counting techniques (Glauert et al. 1984). Experiments using quantitative autoradiography did not detect any DNA-repair activity for these compounds (Cattley et al. 1986); however, incomplete inhibition of replicative DNA synthesis by hydroxyurea was noted. It is clear that DEHP and its principal metabolites MEHP and 2-EH do not directly interact with, or alter the primary structure of, the DNA in cell culture models.

Whole Animal Genotoxicity Assays

DEHP induces several functional changes in the liver, including hepatomegaly and peroxisomal proliferation (Miyazawa et al. 1980), in a manner similar to that of hypolipidemic drugs such as clofibrate. An attractive hypothesis put forth by J.K. Reddy is that peroxisomal proliferating agents constitute a novel class of carcinogens (Reddy and Lalwani 1983). Although these agents are not directly genotoxic themselves, it is proposed that following peroxisomal proliferation, genotoxic activity results from an increase in the production of DNA-damaging reactive oxygen species (Warren et al. 1982; Cerutti 1985). It is therefore mandatory to examine potential mechanisms for genotoxicity that may be operative in the whole animal that would not be expressed in cells in culture.

No activity was seen in a mouse bone marrow micronucleus assay with DEHP, MEHP, or 2-EH (CMA 1982) or in a rat bone marrow cytogenetics assay (Putman et al. 1983).

The ability of DEHP to induce DNA repair was examined in the in vivo hepatocyte DNA-repair assay (Mirsalis and Butterworth 1980). In this system, the compound is administered to the animal, primary cell cultures are prepared and incubated with [^{3}H]thymidine, and DNA repair, as unscheduled DNA synthesis, is quantitated by autoradiography. In addition, DNA damage was measured by alkaline elution of cellular DNA from the same cultures (Bermudez et al. 1982). Treatments were as follows: (1) female rats, 12,000 ppm DEHP in the diet for 30 days; (2) female rats, 12,000 ppm DEHP in the diet for 30 days, followed by 500 mg/kg DEHP by gavage 2 hours before sacrifice; (3) male rats, 500 mg/kg DEHP by gavage 2, 12, 24, or 48 hours before sacrifice; and (4) male rats, 150 mg/kg/day DEHP by gavage for 14 days. No chemically induced DNA damage or repair was seen under any of the conditions employed (Butterworth et al. 1984). In a similar study, male Sprague-Dawley rats were given a single dose of 5000 mg/kg DEHP or fed a diet containing 20,000 ppm DEHP for up to 8 weeks and genotoxicity was evaluated in the in vivo hepatocyte DNA-repair assay. No chemically induced DNA repair was observed, even with animals pretreated with 3-amino-1,2,4-triazole to inhibit catalase activity and thus attempt to maintain any elevated peroxide levels that might have existed (Kornbrust et al. 1984). These studies indicate that neither the parent compound nor its metabolites bound to the DNA to elicit the DNA-repair response. Similarly, no covalent binding to the DNA was observed in rats administered DEHP (Lutz 1986).

The alkaline elution assay detected no significant DNA strand breaks in the cells from the treated animals (Butterworth et al. 1984). Further studies confirmed these observations. Rats were treated for up to 1 month with DEHP, MEHP, methyl-clofenapate, or clofibrate. Although there was marked peroxisome proliferation, no increased lipid peroxidation (malondialdehyde production) or DNA strand breaks (alkaline elution) were observed in the livers of the treated animals (Elliott and Elcombe 1985).

Administration of DEHP in the range of 500–5,000 ppm in the diet of male Sprague-Dawley rats caused large increases in carnitine palmitoyltransferase, carnitine acetyltransferase, and β-oxidation capacity (Morton 1979). Similar increases have been observed in F344 rats (Butterworth et al. 1984). Therefore, in all probability, the animals fed 6000 ppm DEHP in the long-term bioassay must have had significant peroxisomal proliferation, and yet neither the female nor the male rats developed an increase in hepatocellular carcinomas at that dose. Similarly, di(2-ethylhexyl)adipate (DEHA) is a peroxisome proliferator in rodents (Reddy and Lalwani 1983) but produced no tumors in F344 rats given 25,000 ppm DEHA in the diet for 2 years (NTP 1982). DEHA, however, did produce tumors in mice at the same dose. Furthermore, DEHP is more effective in inducing peroxisomal enzymes in male Sprague-Dawley rats than in female Sprague-Dawley rats (Osumi and Hashimoto 1978) and F344 rats (CMA 1982; Mitchell et al. 1984; Lington et al. 1985). Yet, it was the female and not the male rats that exhibited the increased rate of liver tumors (NTP 1983). Furthermore, lipid peroxidation measured in animals given 20,000 ppm DEHP in the diet for 6 weeks plus a single dose of 5 g/kg body weight (bw) by gavage of DEHP did not differ from that of controls (Kornbrust et al. 1984). However, co-administration of antioxidants did reduce the tumorigenic response of ciprofibrate, suggesting a possible role of active oxygen in the carcinogenic process for that potent agent (Rao et al. 1984a).

There are several models for initiation and promotion in the rodent liver in which one treats with a single dose of initiator followed by an extended period of treatment with promoter. The endpoints generally observed are focal hepatocellular proliferative lesions (FHPL) such as gamma glutamyl transpeptidase (GGT)-positive foci. Although it has never rigorously been shown that GGT-positive foci are actual precursors to liver tumors, the evidence taken as a whole indicates that these assays reflect initiating and promoting events. Studies in which female F344 rats were given a single dose of 10 mg/kg bw DEHP or 12,000 ppm DEHP in the diet for 12 weeks as an initiator, followed by a growth selection regimen to express initiated sites, failed to demonstrate any initiating activity of the compound (Garvey et al. 1986). As with rats, DEHP was found to have no initiating activity in B6C3F$_1$ mice, consistent with the conclusion that the compound and its metabolites are not genotoxic (Ward et al. 1983).

Although evidence exists that in subcellular preparations of peroxisomal enzymes it is possible to generate hydrogen peroxide and hydroxyl radicals, no evidence of these species damaging the DNA in the intact animal has been reported (Fahl et al. 1984; Elliott et al. 1986). The very large body of evidence presented above on the activity of DEHP in the whole animal does not support a direct link between peroxisomal proliferation and the initiation of liver cancer.

Promotion

Promoters are compounds that have the ability to enhance tumor formation from initiated cells. They differ from initiators in that they do not always appear to directly alter the DNA, prolonged exposure is required, and the effects may be reversible. There are examples of potent carcinogens, such as 2,3,7,8-tetrachlorodibenzo-p-dioxin (TCDD), that appear to possess only promoting activity (Pitot et al. 1980; Abernethy et al. 1985). Promotional activity became a plausible hypothesis for the mechanism of action of DEHP in light of its lack of genotoxic action. Rats initiated with diethylnitrosamine (DEN) followed by 12,000 ppm DEHP in the diet for 6 months as a promoter showed no increase in enzyme-altered foci, preneoplastic nodules, or liver tumors (Popp et al. 1985). The lack of promoting activity of DEHP has been confirmed in female F344/NCr rats initiated with DEN followed by 14 weeks of promotion with 12,000 ppm DEHP (Ward et al. 1986). In contrast to the results obtained with rats, DEHP given in the diet in concentrations ranging from 3000 to 12,000 ppm was shown to promote FHPL in mouse liver (Ward et al. 1983, 1984). Phenobarbital (PB) is a standard positive control used in these assays with known promoting activity. Whereas PB induced an increase in both the number and size of the FHPL, the effect of DEHP was to increase FHPL size but not number (Ward et al. 1983). Although PB required 168 days of continuous exposure for a promotive effect to be evident, DEHP was an effective promoter after only 28 days (Ward et al. 1984).

It has been proposed that tumor promoters have the ability to disrupt cell-to-cell communication and that this activity may be detected in the Chinese hamster (V79) metabolic cooperation assay (Yotti et al. 1979). Other studies suggest that inhibition of cell-to-cell communication is not a sufficient event for promotion of oncogenic transformation and that caution be used until the assay is tested further (Dorman et al. 1983). Nevertheless, investigators in one laboratory reported that DEHP was negative in the V79 metabolic cooperation assay (Kornbrust et al. 1984), whereas another laboratory reported that DEHP was positive in the same assay (Malcom et al. 1983). Given that, for the induction of FHPL, DEHP is a promoter in the mouse but not in the rat, no conclusion can be drawn as to the mechanistic significance or the predictivity of the V79 metabolic cooperation assay in this case.

In classic skin-painting studies, DEHP displayed very weak complete promoting activity but did show second-stage promoting activity in SENCAR mouse skin. In contrast, the compound was inactive in CD-1 mouse skin-painting experiments (Ward et al. 1986). Although there does appear to be species-specific promoting activity of DEHP in the mouse, the lack of activity in the rat prevents the conclusion that promotional activity provides an adequate answer as to the primary mechanism of action of this chemical.

Cell Transformation

Cell transformation assays appear to measure at least some of the stages in the progress of a cell from the normal to the malignant state. The C3H10T1/2 cell transformation assay is particularly appealing in that it measures both initiating and promoting events (Frazelle et al. 1983). Treatment with DEHP or MEHP did not produce oncogenic transformation, initiate the process of transformation in cultures treated with tumor promoter, or promote the process of transformation in cultures pretreated with a chemical carcinogen (Sanchez et al. 1986). DEHP, MEHP, and 2-EH were negative in the BALB/3T3 cell transformation assay (CMA 1982; Matthews et al. 1985).

The SHE cell transformation assay is sensitive not only to chemicals that affect the primary DNA sequence, but also to agents that cause aneuploidy (changes in chromosome number). In fact, several known carcinogens such as asbestos and diethylstilbestrol (DES), which are negative in traditional mutagenicity tests, are positive in the SHE cell transformation assay (Barrett et al. 1981; Hesterberg and Barrett 1984). Analysis of the action of these agents appears to indicate the induction of aneuploidy (Barrett et al. 1984). DEHP has been shown to have activity in the SHE cell transformation assay in the range of 1.0–100 μg/ml (0.0026–0.26 mM) with reasonable cell survival (Barrett and Lamb 1985; Sanner and Rivedal 1985). It is believed that the SHE cell transformation assay is measuring earlier events in the process of carcinogenesis than measured in the C3H10T1/2 and BALB/3T3 systems.

Interestingly, the only other short-term cell culture tests that indicate any activity for DEHP are those that measure aneuploidy. Two groups in the IPCS study found that DEHP induced aneuploidy in yeast, whereas two other laboratories reported no activity of DEHP in very similar assays (Ashby et al. 1985). One laboratory reported that DEHP induced aneuploidy in Chinese hamster primary liver cells (CH1-L) in culture (Parry 1985); however, the pattern of activity was unusual in that it produced only aneuploidy and no other expected cytogenetic effects. In contrast to DEHP, for example, benzene and DES not only produced aneuploidy, but also exhibited a range of other genetic activities such as clastogenicity and the induction of polyploidy (Ashby et al. 1985). One might predict that if DEHP were inducing aneuploidy with any facility at all, then other cells in the body, in addition to the hepatocytes, would also have been affected. Yet, only weak hepatocarcinogenicity is observed in lifetime studies. Furthermore, even if induction of aneuploidy could be demonstrated in the animal, it does not seem to play an initiating role in FHPL in the liver because DEHP has shown no initiating activity in initiation-promotion studies conducted to date in either the rat or the mouse.

The role of aneuploidy induction in chemical carcinogenesis is still being defined, and we must be cautious in concluding that induction of aneuploidy and cell transformation represent the mechanism of action of DEHP. In the exercise of correlating short-term test results with carcinogenic activity, we must be concerned that the right answer is obtained for the right reason (i.e., that the events measured in culture truly reflect the critical events in the animal). One consideration is that the degree of conversion in the cultures to MEHP was not measured. The detergent properties of this metabolite could well affect cellular organelles such as membranes and mitotic spindles. The detergent effects of DEHP on cells in culture are of unknown relevance at physiological concentrations. Further research to understand the mechanism of action of DEHP in relation to its detergent properties would be of value.

Hyperplasia

It has been proposed that there be a classification of carcinogens that are not directly genotoxic but exert their effects by producing hyperplasia (Loury et al., this volume). One type of agent produces cytotoxicity, resulting in increased regenerative DNA synthesis (Stott et al. 1981). The other type of agent is directly mitogenic with minimal cytotoxicity, resulting in an increased organ-to-body weight ratio (Schulte-Hermann et al. 1983). It is clear that DEHP belongs to the class of toxicants that directly produce a mitogenic response. Cell turnover could result in an increase in the spontaneous mutational frequency and in promotional effects. An advantage of scoring DNA repair by autoradiography is that the number of cells in S phase may be determined as an indication of cell turnover (Mirsalis et al. 1982). One observed action of DEHP in F344 rats was a small, but reproducible, increase in the number of hepatocytes in S phase (Butterworth et al. 1984). This is consistent with the increased liver-to-body weight ratios seen upon prolonged administration of DEHP (Morton 1979; Miyazawa et al. 1980; Mitchell et al. 1984). Similar hepatomegaly and mitogenic stimulation have been seen with the hypolipidemic peroxisomal proliferators (Table 3) (Reddy et al. 1976, 1978, 1979; Moody et al. 1977). In terms of the absolute numbers of animals with tumors, DEHP was more active in the mouse than in the rat (Table 1). If the carcinogenic activity of DEHP were due to promotional effects of cell turnover, one might expect mice to be more susceptible to induction of cell replication. Studies do show that DEHP induces an S-phase response and an increase in liver-to-body weight ratio in mouse liver that is greater in mice than in rats (Table 3) (Smith-Oliver and Butterworth 1987).

One problem with assigning a carcinogenic role to S-phase induction for mitogenic agents like DEHP is that S phase is elevated only for about 1 week during the period of liver enlargement (Cattley and Popp 1985; T. Smith-Oliver and B. Butterworth, in prep.). Nevertheless, one parameter that does correlate with the carcinogenic (NTP 1983) and promotional (Popp et al. 1985; Ward et al. 1986) effects of DEHP is hyperplasia.

Spontaneous tumors and tumors induced by low doses of DEHP occurred far more often in mice than in the rats (NTP 1983). This response is similar to the responses obtained for a variety of other compounds that induce liver tumors in mice, but not in rats, and that appear to be without mutagenic activity (Ward et al. 1979). The stimulation of cellular proliferation may have promoting effects, particularly in mouse liver, which appears to have a significant population of initiated tumor cells (Doull et al. 1983).

It is valuable to contrast the potency of some of the hypolipidemic agents in inducing peroxisomal enzymes with their potency as hepatocarcinogens (Table 3). The first observation, obviously, is that more information is needed. Experiments were done in different animals, at different times, and by different laboratories. Thoughtful experiments in which both peroxisomal proliferation and cell replication are both carefully monitored over time in response to chemical treatment would be of great value. Primary genotoxicity has been omitted from Table 3 because these chemicals are not DNA-reactive. These compounds induce both peroxisomal-specific enzymes and hyperplasia. The degree of the hyperplastic response correlates with the potency of the carcinogenic response as well as, if not better than, the extent of the peroxisomal-specific enzyme induction. DEHP induced about a fourfold increase in palmitoyl-CoA oxidase in female rats at the carcinogenic dose, whereas methyl clofenapate induced about an eightfold increase in the same enzyme at the carcinogenic dose. DEHP is a very weak carcinogen, producing tumors in only 16% of the rats by the end of a lifetime. In contrast, 100% of the rats treated with methyl clofenapate present with severe hepatocellular carcinoma at the end of only 1 year. Note, however, that the methyl clofenapate also caused an approximate tripling of the liver-to-body weight ratio! In general, the more potent carcinogens, such as Wy-14,643, were the most potent mitogens. The parameter that best correlates with carcinogenic potency is increased liver size. The poorest correlation is with genotoxicity.

The molecular signal sent by the hypolipidemic agents is effective in activating all those genes necessary for cell division. Although some feedback mechanism eventually inhibits uncontrolled growth of the liver, it is possible that key genes related to the regulation of cellular growth and cancer remain stimulated during continued administration of the chemical.

CONCLUSION

Numerous mathematical risk-assessment models have been proposed which extrapolate a cancer frequency in the measurable range to the supposed risk at vanishingly small doses of compound. Basing human risk assessment only on the dose of a chemical that caused tumors in a rodent is a simplistic approach. Indeed, the various proposed mathematical models commonly differ by many orders of magnitude in predicting risk (Starr 1983). Yet, in some circles, the reliance on these models has reached the point of dogma. In the interest of better serving the public and regaining credibility, it is important for the field of toxicology to begin to bring mechanistic studies into the risk-assessment process. This is particularly true for nongenotoxic carcinogens, such as DEHP, that require massive lifetime doses to produce a low incidence of rodent tumors.

It would appear at this time that the ability of the hypolipidemic agents to produce hyperplasia and perhaps peroxisomal proliferation are central to their observed hepatocarcinogenic activity. Major differences have been observed in the carcinogenic and cellular and peroxisomal proliferation response between species (Table 3) (Reddy and Lalwani 1983; Elcombe 1985; Rhodes et al. 1986; Elcombe and Mitchell 1987). Microbodies (peroxisomes) were observed in people following long-term administration of the hypolypidemic agent clofibrate, but the effect was less pronounced than observed in rodents (Reddy and Lalwani 1983). Cellular receptors are often species-specific and appear to be playing a role in the mechanism of action of the hypolipidemic agents. Interestingly, studies with primary hepatocyte cultures show that DEHP and the metabolites responsible for peroxisomal proliferation induce peroxisomal enzymes in rat hepatocytes, but not in human, guinea pig, or marmoset hepatocytes (Gray et al. 1982; Elcombe 1985;

Table 3
Comparison of Some Biological Parameters of Hypolipidemic Agents

Chemical treatment	Species/ sex	Liver wt/ body wt (%)	% of Cells in S phase	Palmitoyl-CoA oxidase (% of control)	Incidence of liver cancer (%)	Reference
Control	rat/M	3.5	0.07	100	2	a,b
DEHP 150 mg/kg (2 weeks)	rat/M	4.4	0.50	240		a
DEHP 1000 mg/kg/day (2 weeks)	rat/M	6.2		505		c
DEHP 12,000 ppm 674 mg/kg/day (lifetime)	rat/M				10	b
Control	rat/F	3.0	0.41	100	0	a,b
DEHP 12,000 ppm (1 month)	rat/F	4.8	0.90	430		a
DEHP 12,000 ppm 774 mg/kg/day (lifetime)	rat/F				16	b
Control	mouse/M	4.8	0.4		18	b,d
DEHP 6000 ppm (1 week)	mouse/M		9.2			d
DEHP 6000 ppm (1 month)	mouse/M	8.3	0.3			d
DEHP 6000 ppm 1,325 mg/kg/day (lifetime)	mouse/M				38	b
Gemfibrozil 2500 ppm (4 weeks)	rat/M	5.5		280		e
Gemfibrozil 300 mg/kg/day (lifetime)	rat/M	6.4			10	f

Clofibrate 500 mg/kg/day (2 weeks)	rat/M	6.1		595		c
Clofibrate 5000 ppm (121 weeks)					91	g
Ciprofibrate 200 ppm (30 days)	rat/M	8		1400		h
Ciprofibrate 200 ppm (60 weeks)	rat/M				100	i
Methyl clofenapate 2000 ppm (4 weeks)	rat/M	10.7		1500		e
Methyl clofenapate 1000 ppm (1 year)	rat/M			830	100	j
Wy–14,643 1000 ppm (5 days)	rat/M			600		k
Wy–14,643 1000 ppm (60 weeks)	rat/M				100	l
Control	rat/M	4.08	3.9		0	m
Wy–14,643 1250 ppm (5 days)	rat/M	7.33	27.3			m
Wy–14,643 1000 ppm (16 months)	rat/M				100	m

References: [a]Butterworth et al. (1984); [b]National Toxicology Program (1983); [c]Lake et al. (1984); [d]Smith-Oliver and Butterworth (1987); [e]Lalwani et al. (1983); [f]Fitzgerald et al. (1981); [g]Reddy and Qureshi (1979); [h]Reddy et al. (1986); [i]Rao et al. (1984a); [j]Reddy et al. (1982); [k]R. Cattley (unpubl.); [l] Rao et al. (1984b); [m]Reddy et al. (1979).

Mitchell et al. 1985; Elcombe and Mitchell 1987). It is also possible that some of the very potent hypolipidemic carcinogens may be acting directly with a specific receptor, whereas weak carcinogens such as DEHP may activate the same genes, but through a secondary mechanism. In fact, because of the rodent cancer studies, many manufacturers are already switching to substitutes for DEHP for which there are no cancer data. Knowledge of the primary mechanism of action of these chemicals would provide a valuable basis for selecting a safe substitute.

REFERENCES

Abe, S. and M. Sasaki. 1977. Chromosome aberrations and sister chromatid exchanges in Chinese hamster cells exposed to various chemicals. *J. Natl. Cancer Inst.* **58:** 1635.

Abernethy, D.J., W.F. Greenlee, J.C. Huband, and C.J. Boreiko. 1985. 2,3,7,8-Tetrachlorodibenzo-p-dioxin (TCDD) promotes the transformation of C3H/10T1/2 cells. *Carcinogenesis* **6:** 651.

Ashby, J., F. de Serres, M. Draper, M. Ishidate, Jr., B. Margolin, B. Matter, and M. Shelby, eds. 1985. Evaluation of short-term tests for carcinogenesis. *Prog. Mutat. Res.* **5:** 752.

Barrett, J.C. and P.W. Lamb. 1985. Tests with the Syrian hamster embryo cell transformation assay. *Prog. Mutat. Res.* **5:** 623.

Barrett, C.J., T.W. Hesterberg, and D.G. Thomassen. 1984. Use of cell transformation systems for carcinogenicity testing and mechanistic studies of carcinogenesis. *Pharmacol. Rev.* **36:** 53S.

Barrett, J.C., A. Wong, and J.A. McLachlan. 1981. Diethylstilbestrol induces neoplastic transformation of cells in culture without measurable somatic mutation at two loci. *Science* **212:** 1402.

Bermudez, E., J.C. Mirsalis, and H.C. Eales. 1982. Detection of DNA damage in primary cultures of rat hepatocytes following in vivo and in vitro exposure to genotoxic agents. *Environ. Mutagen.* **4:** 667.

Bieri, F., P. Bentley, F. Waechter, and W. Staubli. 1984. Use of primary cultures of adult rat hepatocytes to investigate mechanisms of action of nafenopin, a hepatocarcinogenic peroxisome proliferator. *Carcinogenesis* **5:** 1033.

Butterworth, B.E., E. Bermudez, T. Smith-Oliver, L. Earle, R. Cattley, J. Martin, J.A. Popp, S. Strom, R. Jirtle, and G. Michalopoulos. 1984. Lack of genotoxic activity of di(2-ethylhexyl)phthalate (DEHP) in rat and human hepatocytes. *Carcinogenesis* **5:** 1329.

Carpenter, C.P., C.S. Weil, and H.F. Smyth. 1953. Chronic oral toxicity of di(2-ethylhexyl)phthalate for rats, guinea pigs, and dogs. *Arch. Ind. Hyg. Occup. Med.* **8:** 219.

Cattley, R. and J. Popp. 1985. Hepatic effects of long-term dietary di(2-ethylhexyl)phthalate (DEHP) in rats. *Proceedings of the 36th annual meeting of the American College of Veterinary Pathologists*, p. 30. Denver, Colorado.

Cattley, R.C., K.K. Richardson, T. Smith-Oliver, J.A.Popp, and B.E. Butterworth. 1986. Effect of peroxisome proliferator carcinogens on unscheduled DNA synthesis in primary rat hepatocytes determined by autoradiography. *Cancer Lett.* **33:** 269.

Cerutti, P.A. 1985. Prooxidant states and tumor promotion. *Science* **227:** 375.

Chemical Manufacturers Association (CMA). 1982. Phthalate esters program panel, voluntary test program. *Health effects testing, phase 1: Validation results* (ed. G.V. Cox and E. J. Moran), vol. 1. Chemical Manufacturers Association, Washington, D.C.

Doolittle, D.J., J.M. Sherrill, and B.E. Butterworth. 1983. Influence of intestinal bacteria, sex of the animal, and position of the nitro group on the hepatic genotoxicity of nitrotoluene isomers in vivo. *Cancer Res.* **43**: 2836.

Dorman, B.H., B.E. Butterworth, and C.J. Boreiko. 1983. Role of intercellular communication in the promotion of C3H/10T1/2 cell transformation. *Carcinogenesis* **4**: 1109.

Doull, J., B.A. Bridges, R. Kroes, L. Golberg, I.C. Munro, O.E. Paynter, H.C. Pitot, R. Squire, G. Williams, and W. Darby. 1983. *The relevance of mouse liver hepatoma to human carcinogenic risk. A report of the International Expert Advisory Committee to the Nutrition Foundation.* The Nutrition Foundation, Washington, D.C.

Elcombe, C.R. 1985. Species differences in carcinogenicity and peroxisome proliferation due to trichloroethylene: A biochemical human hazard assessment. *Arch. Toxicol. Suppl.* **8**: 6.

Elcombe, C.R. and A.M. Mitchell. 1987. Peroxisome proliferation due to di(2-ethylhexyl)phthalate (DEHP) species differences and possible mechanisms. *Environ. Health Perspect.* (in press).

Elliott, B.M. and C.R. Elcombe. 1985. Effects of reactive oxygen species produced by peroxisome proliferation in the livers of rats. *Proc. Am. Assoc. Cancer Res.* **26**: 72.

Elliott, B.M., N.J.F. Dodd, and C.R. Elcombe. 1986. Increased hydroxyl radical production in liver peroxisomal fractions from rats treated with peroxisome proliferators. *Carcinogenesis* **7**: 795.

Fahl, W.E., N.D. Lalwani, T. Watanabe, S. Goel, and J.K. Reddy. 1984. DNA damage related to increased hydrogen peroxide generation by hypolipidemic drug-induced liver peroxisomes. *Proc. Natl. Acad. Sci. U.S.A.* **81**: 7827.

Fitzgerald, J.E., J.L. Sanyer, J.L. Schardein, R.S. Lake, E.J. McGuire, and F.A. de la Iglesia. 1981. Carcinogen bioassay and mutagenicity studies with the hypolipidemic agent gemfibrozil. *J. Natl. Cancer. Inst.* **67**: 1105.

Frazelle, J.H., D.J. Abernethy, and C.J. Boreiko. 1983. Enhanced sensitivity of the C3H/10T1/2 cell transformation system to alkylating and chemotherapeutic agents by treatment with 12-O-tetradecanoylphorbol- 13-acetate. *Environ. Mutagen.* **6**: 81.

Ganning, A.E., U. Brunk, and G. Dallner. 1984. Phthalate esters and their effect on the liver. *Hepatology* **4**: 541.

Garvey, L.K., J.A. Swenberg, T.E. Hamm, Jr., and J.A. Popp. 1986. Di(2-ethylhexyl) phthalate (DEHP): Studies to examine the initiating potential in rat liver. *Toxicologist* **6**: 231.

Glauert, H.P., J.K. Reddy, W.S. Kennan, G.L. Sattler, V.S. Rao, and H.C. Pitot. 1984. Effect of hypolipidemic peroxisome proliferators on unscheduled DNA synthesis in cultured hepatocytes and on mutagenesis in salmonella. *Cancer Lett.* **24**: 147.

Gray, T.J.B., J.A. Beamand, B.G. Lake, J.R. Foster, and S.D. Gangolli. 1982. Peroxisome proliferation in cultured rat hepatocytes produced by clofibrate and phthalate ester metabolites. *Toxicol. Lett.* **10**: 273.

Harris, R.S., H.C. Hodge, E.A. Maynard, and H.J. Blanchet, Jr. 1956. Chronic oral toxicity of 2-ethylhexyl phthalate in rats and dogs. *Arch. Ind. Health* **13**: 259.

Hesterberg, T.W. and C.J. Barrett. 1984. Dependence of asbestos- and mineral duct-induced transformation of mammalian cells in culture on fiber dimension. *Cancer Res.* **44:** 2170.

Hodgson, J.R., B.C. Myhr, M. McKeon, and D.J. Brusick. 1982. Evaluation of di(2-ethylhexyl)phthalate and its major metabolites in the primary rat hepatocyte unscheduled DNA synthesis assay. *Environ. Mutagen.* **4:** 388.

Kirby, P.E., R.F. Pizzarello, T.E. Lawlor, S.R. Haworth, and J.R. Hodgson. 1983. Evaluation of di(2-ethylhexyl)phthalate and its major metabolites in the Ames test and L5178Y mouse lymphoma mutagenicity assay. *Environ. Mutagen.* **5:** 657.

Kornbrust, D.J., T.R. Barfknecht, P. Ingram, and J.D. Shelburne. 1984. Effect of di(2-ethylhexyl)phthalate on DNA repair and lipid peroxidation in rat hepatocytes and on metabolic cooperation in Chinese hamster V-79 cells. *J. Toxicol. Environ. Health* **13:** 99.

Kozumbo, W.J., R. Kroll, and J.R. Rubin. 1982. Assessment of the mutagenicity of phthalate esters. *Environ. Health Perspect.* **45:** 103.

Lalwani, N.D., M.K. Reddy, S.A. Qureshi, C.R. Sirtori, Y. Abiko, and J.K. Reddy. 1983. Evaluation of selected hypolipidemic agents for the induction of peroxisomal enzymes and peroxisome proliferation in the rat liver. *Hum. Toxicol.* **2:** 27.

Lake, B.G., W.R.P. Rijcken, T.J.B. Gray, J.R. Foster, and S.D. Gangolli. 1984. Comparative studies of the hepatic effects of di- and mono-n-octyl phthalates, di-(2-ethylhexyl) phthalate and clofibrate in the rat. *Acta Pharmacol. Toxicol.* **54:** 167.

Lington, A., B. Schneider, E. Moran, M. Stoltz, J. Windels, and M. El-hawari. 1985. Liver and lipid effects of diethylhexyl phthalate (DEHP) and diethylhexyl adipate (DEHA) in Fischer 344 rats. *Toxicologist* **5:** 159.

Lutz, W.K. 1986. Investigation of the potential for binding of di(2-ethylhexyl) phthalate (DEHP) to rat liver DNA in vivo. *Environ. Health Perspect.* **65:** 267.

Malcom, A.R., L.J. Mills, and E.J. McKenna. 1983. Inhibition of metabolic cooperation between Chinese hamster V79 cells by tumor promoters and other chemicals. *Ann. N.Y. Acad. Sci.* **407:** 448.

Matthews, E.J., T. DelBalzo, and J.O. Rundell. 1985. Assays for morphological transformation and mutation to oubain resistance of Balb/c-3T3 cells in culture. *Prog. Mutat. Res.* **5:** 639.

McCann, J., E. Choi, E. Yamasaki, and B.N. Ames. 1975. Detection of carcinogens as mutagens in the Salmonella/microsome test: Assay of 300 chemicals. *Proc. Natl. Acad. Sci. U.S.A.* **72:** 5135.

Mirsalis, J.C. and B.E. Butterworth. 1980. Detection of unscheduled DNA synthesis in hepatocytes isolated from rats treated with genotoxic agents: An in vivo - in vitro assay for potential carcinogens and mutagens. *Carcinogenesis* **1:** 621.

Mirsalis, J.C., C.K. Tyson, and B.E. Butterworth. 1982. Detection of genotoxic carcinogens in the in vivo - in vitro hepatocyte DNA repair assay. *Environ. Mutagen.* **4:** 553.

Mitchell, A.M., J. Lhuguenot, J.W. Bridges, and C.R. Elcombe. 1985. Identification of the proximate peroxisome proliferators derived from di(2-ethylhexyl)phthalate. *Toxicol. Appl. Pharmacol.* **80:** 23.

Mitchell, F.E., S.C. Price, P. Grasso, R.H. Hinton, and J.W. Bridges. 1984. Effects of di(2-ethylhexyl)phthlate on male and female rats. Poster given at the International

Conference on Phthalic Acid Esters, University of Surrey, August 6–7, 1984, Poster Abstracts, p. 10.

Miyazawa, S., S. Furuta, T. Osumi, and T. Hashimoto. 1980. Turnover of enzymes of peroxisomal oxidation in rat liver. *Biochim. Biophys. Acta* **630**: 367.

Moody, D.E., S. Rao, and J.K. Reddy. 1977. Mitogenic effect in mouse liver induced by a hypolipidemic drug, nafenopin. *Virchows Arch. B Cell Pathol.* **23**: 291.

Morton, S.J. 1979. *The hepatic effects of dietary di(2-ethylhexyl)phthalate.* Ph.D. thesis, The Johns Hopkins University, University Microfilms International, Ann Arbor, Michigan.

National Toxicology Program (NTP). 1982. *Carcinogenesis bioassay of di(2-ethylhexyl)adipate (CAS No. 103-23-1) in F344 rats and B6C3F1 mice.* NTP Tech. Rep. Series no. 212. National Institutes of Health, Bethesda, Maryland.

———. 1983. *Carcinogenesis bioassay of di(2-ethylhexyl)phthalate (CAS No. 117-81-7) in F–344 rats and B6C3F1 mice.* NTP Tech. Rep. Series no. 217. National Institutes of Health, Bethesda, Maryland.

Osumi, T. and T. Hashimoto. 1978. Enhancement of fatty acyl-CoA oxidizing activity in rat liver peroxisomes. *J. Biochem.* **83**: 1361.

Parry, E.M. 1985. Tests for effects on mitosis and the mitotic spindle in Chinese hamster primary liver cells (CH1-L) in culture. Evaluation of short-term tests for carcinogenesis. *Prog. Mutat. Res.* **5**: 479.

Phillips, B.J., D. Anderson, and S.D. Gangolli. 1986. Studies on the genetic effects of phthalic acid esters on cells in culture. *Environ. Health Perspect.* **65**: 263.

Phillips, B.J., T.E.B. James, and S.D. Gangolli. 1982. Genotoxicity studies of di(2-ethylhexyl)phthalate and its metabolites in CHO cells. *Mutat. Res.* **102**: 297.

Pitot, H.C., T. Goldsworthy, H.A. Campbell, and A. Poland. 1980. Quantitative evaluation of the promotion by 2,3,7,8-tetrachlorodibenzo-p-dioxin of hepatocarcinogenesis from diethylnitrosamine. *Cancer Res.* **40**: 3616.

Popp, J.A., L.K. Garvey, T.E. Hamm, Jr., and J.A. Swenberg. 1985. Lack of hepatic promotional activity by the peroxisomal proliferating hepatocarcinogen di(2-ethylhexyl)phthalate. *Carcinogenesis* **6**: 141.

Putman, D.L., W.A. Moore, L.M. Schechtman, and J.R. Hodgson. 1983. Cytogenetic evaluation of di(2-ethylhexyl)phthalate and its major metabolites in Fischer 344 rats. *Environ. Mutagen.* **5**: 227.

Rao, M.S., N.D. Lalwani, T.K. Watanabe, and J.K. Reddy. 1984a. Inhibitory effect of antioxicants ethoxyquin and 2(3)-tert-butyl-4-hydroxyanisole on hepatic tumorigenesis in rats fed ciprofibrate, a peroxisome proliferator. *Cancer Res.* **44**: 1072.

Rao, M.S., N.D. Lalwani, and J.K. Reddy. 1984b. Sequential histologic study of rat liver during peroxisome proliferator [4-chloro-6-(2,3-xylidino)-2-pyrimnidinylthio]-acetic acid (Wy-14,643)-induced carcinogenesis. *J. Natl. Cancer Inst.* **73**: 983.

Reddy, J.K. and N.D. Lalwani. 1983. Carcinogenesis by hepatic peroxisome proliferators: Evaluation of the risk of hypolipidemic drugs and industrial plasticizers to humans. *CRC Crit. Rev. Toxicol.* **12**: 1.

Reddy, J.K. and S.A. Qureshi. 1979. Tumorigenicity of the hypolipidaemic peroxisome proliferator ethyl-α-P-chlorophenoxyisobutyrate (clofibrate) in rats. *Br. J. Cancer* **40**: 476.

Reddy, J.K., D.L. Azarnoff, and C.R. Sirtori. 1978. Hepatic peroxisome proliferation:

Induction by BR-931, a hypolipidemic analog of WY-14,643. *Arch. Int. Pharmacodyn. Ther.* **234:** 4.

Reddy, J.K., S. Rao, and D.E. Moody. 1976. Hepatocellular carcinomas in acatalasemic mice treated with nafenopin, a hypolipidemic peroxisome proliferator. *Cancer Res.* **36:** 1211.

Reddy, J.., N.D. Lalwani, M.K. Reddy, and S.A. Qureshi. 1982. Excessive accumulation of autofluorescent lipofuscin in the liver during hepatocarcinogenesis by methyl clofenapate and other hypolipidemic peroxisome proliferators. *Cancer Res.* **42:** 259.

Reddy, J.K., M.S. Rao, D.L. Azarnoff, and S. Sell. 1979. Mitogenic and carcinogenic effects of hypolipidemic peroxisome proliferator. [4-chloro-6-(2,3-xylidino)-2-pyrimidinylthio]acetic acid, in rat and mouse liver. *Cancer Res.* **39:** 152.

Reddy, J.K., M.K. Reddy, M.I. Usman, N.D. Lalwani, and M.S. Rao. 1986. Comparison of hepatic peroxisome proliferative effect and its implication for hepatocarcinogenicity of phthalate esters, di(2-ethylhexyl) phthalate, and di(2-ethylhexyl) adipate with a hypolipidemic drug. *Environ. Health Perspect.* **65:** 317.

Rhodes, C., T.C. Orton, I.S. Pratt, P.L. Batten, H. Bratt, S.J. Jackson, and C.R. Elcombe. 1986. Comparative pharmacokinetics and subacute toxicity of di(2-ethylhexyl) phthalate (DEHP) in rats and marmosets: Extrapolation of effects in rodents to man. *Environ. Health Perspect.* **65:** 299.

Sanchez, J.H., D.J. Abernethy, and C.J. Boreiko. 1986. Lack of di(2-ethylhexyl)phthalate activity in the C3H/10T/1/2 cell transformation system. *Toxicol. In Vitro* **1:** 1.

Sanner, T. and E. Rivedal. 1985. Tests with the Syrian hamster embryo (SHE) cell transformation assay. *Prog. Mutat. Res.* **5:** 665.

Schulte-Hermann, R., J. Schuppler, I. Timmermann-Trosiener, G. Ohde, W. Bursch, and H. Berger. 1983. The role of growth of normal and preneoplastic cell populations for tumor promotion in rat liver. *Environ. Health Perspect.* **50:** 185.

Seed, J.L. 1982. Mutagenic activity of phthalate esters in bacterial liquid suspension assays. *Environ. Health Perspect.* **45:** 111.

Smith-Oliver, T. and B.E. Butterworth. 1987. Correlation of the carcinogenic potential of di(2-ethylhexyl)phthalate (DEHP) with induced hyperplasia rather than with genotoxic activity. *Mutat. Res.* (in press).

Starr, T.B. 1983. Mechanisms of formaldehyde toxicity and risk evaluation. In *Formaldehyde: Toxicity, epidemiology, mechanisms* (ed. J. Clary et al.), p. 237. Marcel Dekker, New York.

Stenchever, M.A., M.A. Allen, L. Jerominski, and R.V. Petersen. 1976. Effects of bis(2-ethyl hexyl) phthalate on chromosomes of human leukocytes and human fetal lung cells. *J. Pharm. Sci.* **65:** 1648.

Stott, W.T., R.H. Reitz, A.M. Schumann, and P.G. Watanabe. 1981. Genetic and nongenetic events in neoplasia. *Food Cosmet. Toxicol.* **19:** 567.

Thomas, J.A. and M.J. Thomas. 1984. Biological effects of di(2-ethylhexyl)phthalate and other phthalic acid esters. *CRC Crit. Rev. Toxicol.* **13:** 283.

Tomita, I., Y. Nakamura, N. Aoki, and N. Inui. 1982. Mutagenic/carcinogenic potential of DEHP and MEHP. *Environ. Health Perspect.* **45:** 119.

Ward, J.M., R.A. Griesemer, and E.K. Weisburger. 1979. The mouse liver tumor as an endpoint in carcinogenesis tests. *Toxicol. Appl. Pharmacol.* **51:** 389.

Ward, J.M., M. Ohshima, P. Lynch, and C. Riggs. 1984. Di(2-ethylhexyl)phthalate but not phenobarbital promotes N-nitrosodiethylamine initiated hepatocellular proliferative lesions after short-term exposure in male B6C3F1 mice. *Cancer Lett.* **24:** 49.

Ward, J.M., J.M. Rice, D. Creasia, P. Lynch, and C. Riggs. 1983. Dissimilar patterns of promotion by di(2-ethylhexyl)phthalate and phenobarbital of hepatocellular neoplasia initiated by diethylnitrosamine in B6C3F1 mice. *Carcinogenesis* **4:** 1021.

Ward, J.M., B.A. Diwan, M. Ohshima, H. Hu, H.M. Schuller, and J.M. Rice. 1986. Tumor initiating and promoting activities of di(2-ethylhexyl) phthalate in vivo and in vitro. *Environ. Health Perspect.* **65:** 279.

Warren, J.R., N.P. Lalwani, and J.K. Reddy. 1982. Phthalate esters as peroxisome proliferator carcinogens. *Environ. Health Perspect.* **45:** 35.

Yoshikawa, K., A. Tanaka, T. Yamaha, and H. Kurata. 1983. Mutagenicity study of nine monoalkyl phthalates and a dialkyl phthalate using Salmonella typhimurium and Escherichia coli. *Food Chem. Toxicicol.* **21:** 221.

Yotti, L.P., C.C. Chang, and J.E. Trosko. 1979. Elimination of metabolic cooperation in Chinese hamster cells by a tumor promoter. *Science* **206:** 1089.

Zeiger, E., S. Haworth, K. Mortelmans, and W. Speck. 1985. Mutagenicity testing of di(2-ethylhexyl)phthalate and related compounds in Salmonella. *Environ. Mutagen.* **7:** 213.

Zeiger, E., S. Haworth, W. Speck, and K. Mortelmans. 1982. Phthalate ester testing in the National Toxicology Programs environmental mutagenesis test development program. *Environ. Health Perspect.* **45:** 99.

COMMENTS

COHEN: I'm troubled by the fact that you are essentially finding no initiating activity and no promoting activity in rats, and yet it (DEHP) is a liver tumorigen. There is either something very wrong with the assays or the terminology is virtually useless in these situations.

BUTTERWORTH: It must be remembered that DEHP is a very weak carcinogen in the rat. Perhaps this begins to define the limits of sensitivity of the initiation and promotion assays.

SIVAK: I was sparked a little by the question, If it's not an initiator or not a promoter, what is it? I think that our ideas about initiation and promotion imply that we know what the mechanism is. Instead, these words are really operational and describe what we do to the animals in our experimental systems. The fact that we don't understand the mechanism of each of these kinds of processes does not keep us from understanding what is happening when DEHP gives rise to tumors. I'm not troubled by not being able to pigeonhole DEHP or TCDD as initiators or promoters. The fact remains that they do cause tumors. I think it is going to require studies to look at different kinds of biological events that we haven't fully explored yet, rather than be locked into comfortable and traditional ideas with respect to mechanism.

ROSENKRANZ: I find this chemical, DEHP, to be absolutely fascinating, I just served on a hazard assessment panel for DEHP. We came up with a certainty of close to 100% that it was not genotoxic, and we proposed alternate risk assessments, one of which involved a threshold.

SIVAK: You're still alive? You said "threshold" in a public place!

The Mechanism of Urinary Tract Tumorigenesis of Nitrilotriacetate

ROBERT L. ANDERSON
The Procter & Gamble Company
Miami Valley Laboratories
Cincinnati, Ohio 45247

OVERVIEW

Nitrilotriacetate (NTA) is an amino carboxylate cation sequestering agent with potential to replace phosphorus in laundry detergents. NTA is nongenotoxic, as attested by in vitro and in vivo tests, but ingestion of high dosages of NTA is associated with tumors of the renal tubular cells and transitional epithelial cells of the renal pelvis, ureter, and bladder. The urinary tract tumors are associated with NTA-dosage-dependent changes in zinc and calcium disposition in the target tissues that accompany renal clearance and urinary excretion of systemic NTA. The changes in zinc and calcium disposition depend on NTA attaining defined systemic doses. Thus, the limiting conditions necessary for NTA tumorigenicity show thresholds that must be exceeded before NTA can induce any effect in the urinary tract.

INTRODUCTION

Trisodium NTA (Fig. 1) qualifies as a nongenotoxic carcinogen, since it is negative for genotoxicity in 25 assays; yet chronic ingestion of high dosages of NTA is associated with increased tumor incidence in renal tubule cells (RTC) and transitional epithelial cells (TEC) of the renal pelvis, ureter, and bladder (Anderson et al. 1985).

NTA is not metabolized and it does not accumulate to a greater extent in tissues that develop tumors than in tissues that do not. NTA absorption from the gastrointestinal tract, distribution in the body, and excretion in the urine are all zero-order (Anderson et al. 1985). NTA induces a dose-dependent toxicity in the urinary tract that precedes and accompanies any tumors (Anderson et al. 1985). The only chemical activity displayed by NTA is its ability to alter the disposition of ingested minerals, e.g., increase the urinary excretion of zinc and calcium (Anderson et al. 1985).

Rats have been exposed to NTA chronically, together with three nitrosamines, N-methyl-N'-nitro-N-nitrosoguanidine (MNNG), N-nitroso-N-pentyl-1-pentamine (DPN), and 4-(butylnitrosoamino)-1-butanol (NBBN). The simultaneous exposure did not alter the tumorigenicity of MNNG or DPN, and high doses of NTA markedly decreased the bladder tumor incidence noted with NBBN alone (Anderson et al. 1985).

NTA increased the renal tumor incidence in rats initiated with N-ethyl-N-

Banbury Report 25: Nongenotoxic Mechanisms in Carcinogenesis
© Cold Spring Harbor Laboratory. 0-87969-225-1/87. $1.00 + .00

NTA

$$N (CH_2 COO^-)_3 NA_3^+ \cdot H_2O$$

Figure 1
Structure of nitrilotriacetic acid.

hydroxyethylnitrosamine (EHEN) when it was dosed at a renal toxic level but not when it was dosed at a nontoxic level (Hiasa et al. 1985). We recently demonstrated that prior treatment with an initiating dose of NBBN does not alter the dose-response relationship of NTA for inducing the conditions necessary for urinary tract tumorigenesis (Anderson et al. 1986).

RESULTS

To ascertain whether a specific metal salt or complex of NTA might be responsible for the urinary tract toxicity of NTA, the sodium and potassium salts, as well as the calcium, magnesium, and zinc complexes of NTA were infused intravenously for up to 6 days. The salts and the magnesium and calcium complexes, when infused at 6 mmoles/kg for 6 days, caused less renal damage than ingestion of NTA at a dosage producing 1.5 mmoles/kg systemic NTA for 4 days. In contrast, ZnNTA at 3 mmoles/kg for only 2 days caused death due to renal failure associated with coagulative necrosis. This finding led to a series of studies on how NTA might affect zinc metabolism and the role of zinc in renal tubular cell tumorigenicity. These efforts yielded the following findings:

1. Zinc is a renal toxin without NTA.
2. ZnNTA renal toxicity is dependent on renal accumulation of zinc, but not NTA.
3. Increased systemic zinc increases the renal toxicity of ingested NTA.
4. Excess dietary zinc reduces NTA absorption and renal toxicity.
5. Reduced dietary zinc reduces renal toxicity without altering the systemic load of NTA.
6. Renal clearance of NTA is accomplished by simple filtration.
7. Renal clearance of NTA is accompanied by increased renal reabsorption and urinary excretion of zinc because NTA causes an elevated level of plasma ultrafiltrate zinc (species of m.w. $< 10,000$).
8. Only dosages of NTA that increase urinary zinc cause renal toxicity, including tumorigenicity, even after chronic exposure.
9. The dose-response curve for plasma ultrafiltrate NTA versus plasma ultrafiltrate zinc shows a distinct threshold in that NTA must exceed 15 μM before it can increase ultrafiltrate zinc (Fig. 2).
10. E. D. Thompson of our laboratories has recently shown that zinc is mutagenic in some in vitro assays (E. D. Thompson, unpubl.).

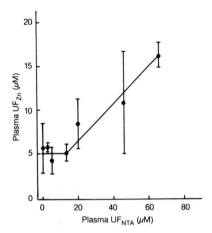

Figure 2

Relationship between plasma ultrafiltrate (species of m.w. < 10,000) NTA concentration and plasma ultrafiltrate zinc concentration. (Reprinted, with permission, from Anderson et al. 1985.)

These results show that renal tubular cell tumorigenesis associated with chronic NTA exposure is dependent on a process that shows a distinct threshold that must be exceeded to induce the limiting conditions required for tumor formation.

The TEC tumors require higher dosages of NTA than the RTC tumors, and tumors in the TEC are associated with NTA-induced changes in calcium disposition in the urinary tract. The role of calcium is established by the following:

1. Only dosages of NTA that increase urinary calcium are associated with TEC tumors.
2. NTA increases urinary calcium only when the urinary concentration of NTA exceeds that of divalent metals ($NTA/M^{++} > 1$) (Fig. 3).
3. These dosages (see item 2) of NTA reduce bladder calcium, but not magnesium, zinc, sodium, or potassium.
4. Infusion of NTA into the bladder causes bladder surface sloughing, ulceration, and increased mitosis (mitotic figures).
5. Infused NTA causes TEC damage only at doses that increase urinary calcium and reduce bladder tissue calcium.
6. Infusion of NTA as the calcium complex prevents TEC toxicity.

These findings demonstrate that NTA, when present in the urine as the uncomplexed ligand, will extract extracellular calcium from the urothelium more rapidly than it can be replaced by diffusion from the plasma. This state causes TEC surface loss, which stimulates TEC division, which can induce TEC tumors when continued for a lifetime.

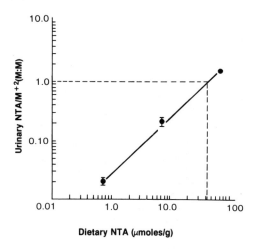

Figure 3

Effect of dietary NTA concentration on the molar ratio of NTA to divalent metals (Ca + Mg + Zn) in the urine.

DISCUSSION

The data reviewed clearly demonstrate that the urinary tract tumors noted in rats after chronic ingestion of high dosages of NTA result from changes in the distribution of divalent metals in the urinary tract that accompany the renal clearance of systemic NTA. RTC tumors result from the chronic toxicity associated with increased zinc resorption that occurs when the ingestion of NTA exceeds the dose (100 μmoles/kg) that induces a plasma filtrate NTA concentration of 15 μM or greater. The TEC tumors result from a chronic mitotic stimulus brought about when uncomplexed NTA in the urine removes extracellular calcium from the urothelium faster than it can be replaced by diffusion from the circulation. This occurs only when NTA intake is greater than 3500 μmoles/kg. Promotion studies indicate that the thresholds demonstrated for NTA acting in naive animals are applicable to animals given an initiating dose of carcinogen.

NTA has been used in laundry detergents in Canada for many years, and in the area of use, the drinking water mean NTA concentration is 2.82 μg/liter (Malaiyandi et al. 1979). Figure 4 depicts the systemic dose of NTA attained as a function of ingested dose and indicates the human exposure level compared to the dosages required to increase zinc delivery to the RTC and to extract calcium from the TEC. This comparison clearly negates the concept that low dosages of NTA could cause urinary tract damage in humans.

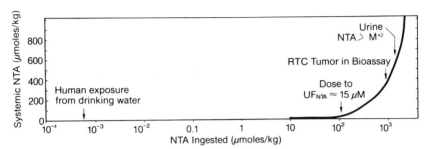

Figure 4

Relationship between the systemic dose of NTA and the ingested dose. The human exposure level and the dosages required to increase zinc delivery to the RTC and to extract calcium from the TEC are indicated.

REFERENCES

Anderson, R.L., W.E. Bishop, and R.L. Campbell. 1985. A review of the environmental and mammalian toxicology of nitrilotriacetic acid. *CRC Crit. Rev. Toxicol.* **15**: 1.

Anderson, R.L., R.L. Kanerva, F.R. Lefever, and W.R. Francis. 1986. Effect of N-nitro-n-butyl-(4-hydroxybutyl)amine exposure on the changes in mineral disposition caused by trisodium nitrilotriacetate. *Food Chem. Toxicol.* **24**: 229.

Hiasa, Y., Y. Kitahori, N. Konishi, and T. Shimoyama. 1985. Dose-related effect of trisodium nitrilotriacetate monohydrate on renal tumorigenesis initiated with N-ethyl-N-hydroxyethyl-nitrosamine. *Carcinogenesis* **6**: 907.

Malaiyandi, M., D.T. Williams, and R. O'Grady. 1979. A national survey of nitrilotriacetic acid in Canadian drinking water. *Environ. Sci. Technol.* **13**: 59.

COMMENTS

TRUMP: I suggest that the vacuoles are arising from the same mechanism as inulin, sucrose, mannitol, and NTA, all filterable and nonmetabolizing.

ANDERSON: Absolutely. We have looked at those vacuoles using both light and electron microscopes, and under no conditions do we see anything different. But, if you continue the NTA exposure, the tissue will rapidly go into a hyperplasia.

TRUMP: You don't think the zinc stays behind?

ANDERSON: Yes. The zinc stays back and the NTA goes out in the urine, very definitely.

TRUMP: That's the same way lead and cadmium seem to enter.

ANDERSON: Well, there is absolutely no reason to suspect that zinc is handled any differently by the kidney than cadmium.

TRUMP: Are you saying that it may be different in the presence of NTA than it is normally?

ANDERSON: Yes. I think the difference is that normally the filterable pool of any of these metals is very small. If you look at renal clearance of excess zinc given intravenously, it will enter the kidney mostly from the blood side. That pool is very rapidly washed out of the kidney. If it's entering from the tubular side, as we are doing with ZnNTA, then it is retained much more tenaciously.

TRUMP: You see, I am suggesting that it's just like cadmium metallothionien. The metallothionien carries the cadmium into the phagolysosome.

ANDERSON: Yes.

TRUMP: The protein in the cadmium then starts working.

ANDERSON: Yes.

BARRETT: You stated that there were two genotoxicity studies that were positive at high doses. Are those reproducible studies? What dose ranges were used, and how do the doses compare to the doses in your in vivo studies?

ANDERSON: One was the V79 cell rescue. The dosage was very high. There was more NTA than there is total divalent metals.

BARRETT: But the NTA dose would have to be very high to get tumors in vivo as well.

ANDERSON: No! The blood levels attained are micromolar. When you're talking the same concentration as the sum of the divalent cations in the medium, you're talking millimolar. As I said, 15 μM NTA is the blood level when we start seeing effects in feeding studies. There are orders of magnitude of difference between the dose that produces an effect in vivo and the level required to exceed the divalent cation level in a serum-containing medium.

BARRETT: So, is it your conclusion then that the mutagenicity of zinc plays a role in the carcinogenesis?

ANDERSON: I will leave that to the mutagenicity people. I don't think it is necessary. My own feeling is there is plenty of toxicity, and I happen to subscribe to the concept of the toxicity being adequate.

BARRETT: I am sure that the zinc mutagenicity is going to depend on the mitogenic stimulus as well. So, it may be improper to call it a nongenotoxic carcinogen if it is working through a genetic mechanism; it is clearly a threshold compound.

ANDERSON: It, itself, is not mutagenic. It is not DNA reactive. The fact that it can deliver zinc does not make it a mutagen to me.

Session 6:
Cell Culture Models

Modulation of Transformed Focus Formation in Cultures of C3H/10T1/2 Cells

CRAIG J. BOREIKO
Department of Genetic Toxicology
Chemical Industry Institute of Toxicology
Research Triangle Park, North Carolina 27709

OVERVIEW

The measured frequency with which chemically induced transformation of C3H/10T1/2 mouse embryo cells occurs can be modulated by "nongenotoxic" variables such as the number of cells present in a culture dish during carcinogen treatment or the subsequent exposure of carcinogen-treated cells to tumor promoters. Observations such as these have suggested that oncogenic transformation may be a multistep process involving high-frequency, potentially nongenotoxic, changes within individual cells. Others have suggested that variations in transformation frequency are the product of complex cell:cell interactions in which nontransformed cells influence the phenotypic expression of malignancy in transformed cells. Recent studies suggest that modulation of focus formation in cultures of C3H/10T1/2 cells may in fact be the product of several discrete processes, not all of which need to be relevant to in vivo carcinogenesis.

INTRODUCTION

Efforts to detect and study human carcinogens have spurred the development of in vitro cell transformation systems that have potential sensitivity to diverse aspects of the multistage carcinogenic process (Heidelberger et al. 1983). Although these systems can be imprecise and difficult to maintain, their use may permit the detection and study of carcinogenic agents and/or processes that do not elicit responses in most short-term tests for genotoxicity. The C3H/10T1/2 cell transformation system (Reznikoff et al. 1973a,b) has emerged as one of the cell transformation systems more commonly used for such purposes.

The C3H/10T1/2 cell transformation system uses a cell line of mouse embryo fibroblasts (Reznikoff et al. 1973b) with firm density-dependent controls over cell division. As a result, C3H/10T1/2 cells inoculated into a cell culture dish will grow to form an even monolayer of cells and then cease cell division. Cells transformed by exposure to a carcinogen exhibit altered growth controls and continue to proliferate at confluence to form foci of multilayered, actively growing, transformed cells. By the time of termination of this 6-week assay, these foci can be easily distinguished from the background monolayer of quiescent nontransformed cells. Three different focus morphologies can be observed at this stage, and they have been designated types I, II, and III by Reznikoff et al. (1973a). Cells from type II and type III foci, but not type I foci, usually grow to form fibrosarcomas when injected into a syngeneic or nude mouse.

The work of numerous laboratories (Heidelberger et al. 1983; Kennedy 1984; Boreiko 1985a) has established that the C3H/10T1/2 cell transformation system responds in an appropriate fashion to a number of known carcinogens. Furthermore, the process of transformation in these cells can be made to proceed through discrete steps of initiation and promotion analogous to that observed in mouse skin or rat liver (Mondal et al. 1976; Kennedy 1984; Boreiko 1985a). For example, tumor promoters that have only weak transforming activity in C3H/10T1/2 cell cultures will provide marked enhancement of focus formation in cultures previously exposed to an initiating agent. The mechanism for this enhancement is usually presumed to be the result of nongenotoxic events.

The nongenotoxic variable of cell density can also be an important determinant of focus formation. Studies by a number of investigators (Haber et al. 1977; Fernandez et al. 1980; Kennedy and Little 1984) have demonstrated that there need not be a linear relationship between the number of cells treated with a carcinogen and the number of transformed foci that subsequently develop. Typically, the frequency of transformation will increase as cell density is lowered until, at very low cell density, exceptionally high frequencies of transformation result. For example, Huband et al. (1985) (Fig. 1A) recently observed that treatment with a 1 μg/ml solution of 3-methylcholanthrene (MCA) could produce frequencies as high as 3×10^{-2} or as low as 5×10^{-4} per cell surviving treatment. Thus, the transformation frequency produced by a 1 μg/ml solution of MCA could be modulated by simply altering the number of cells present in a cell-culture dish. This cell-density effect complicates both the quantitation and the interpretation of C3H/10T1/2 transformation results.

Observations of cell-density effects upon focus formation have provided the experimental basis for multistep models of transformation (Fernandez et al. 1980; Kennedy and Little 1984). Complex mechanistic models have been developed in which the majority of cells present in a culture dish are "activated" by carcinogen treatment. Focus formation is postulated to be the result of a second, low-frequency spontaneous alteration in an activated cell. Promotion could be considered the reverse of this process, providing an activating function to complement previous carcinogen-induced changes.

Others have suggested that interactions between nontransformed cells and transformed cells are responsible for variations of frequency with cell density (Mordan et al. 1983) and are related to the promotion process (Trosko and Chang 1984). Given that nontransformed cells can inhibit the growth of transformed cells

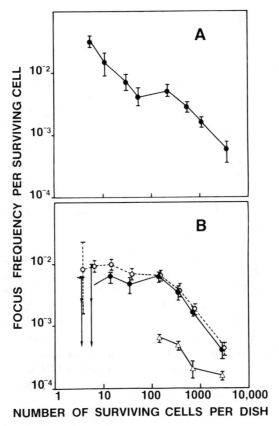

Figure 1
Effect of cell density on focus formation in (A) MCA-treated cultures and (B) MNNG-treated cultures. MNNG data included are for treatment with MNNG alone (△) and for enhancement of MNNG transformation by TPA (○). MNNG + TPA data for which TPA "backgrounds" have been subtracted are also presented (●). Low-cell-density MNNG treatment groups were executed at cell densities identical to the MNNG + TPA low-density data. However, significant levels of focus formation were not observed. (Reprinted, with permission, from Huband et al. 1985.)

(Bertram 1979), increasing the number of nontransformed cells present in a culture could decrease the efficiency with which a transformed cell is able to develop into a focus. Modulation of focus formation by tumor promoters might have a similar mechanistic basis, since inhibition of focus formation by nontransformed cells may be mediated by intercellular communication, a process by which cells in contact would be able to exchange growth-regulating substances through gap junctions. C3H/10T1/2 cell transformation could be enhanced if tumor promoters were to block these suppressive cell:cell interactions.

RESULTS AND DISCUSSION

Interpretation of the mechanistic significance of cell-density-dependent alterations in transformation frequency has been complicated by recent findings on the role of carcinogen residues in the transformation process (Huband et al. 1985). Treatment of C3H/10T1/2 cultures with 1.0 μg/ml MCA for 24 hours was found to result in the deposition of a persistent carcinogen residue upon the dish surface. Reconstruction studies further suggested that most of the transformed foci produced by MCA in low-density cultures were the result of residue-induced events after the supposed termination of MCA treatment. If focus production is the result of a multigeneration exposure to low concentrations of carcinogen, then calculations of transformation frequency based on the number of cells present at the start of treatment will overestimate the actual transformation frequency. Since the length of time a residue persists could be a function of metabolism, exaggeration of transformation frequency by this treatment artifact might be greatest in low-density cultures.

Huband et al. (1985) further observed that transformation frequencies produced by treatment with 0.5 μg/ml of the alkylating agent N-methyl-N'nitro-N-nitrosoguanidine (MNNG) and promotion by 400 nM 12-O-tetradecanoylphorbol-13-acetate (TPA) also varied with cell density (Fig. 1B). However, whereas transformation frequencies rose in very low density MCA-treated cultures, transformation frequencies in low-density MNNG + TPA-treated cultures were relatively constant and averaged 6×10^{-3} per cell surviving treatment. This response plateau is of interest, since it suggests that initiation by MNNG, which is labile and unable to persist as a residue, in low-density cultures is the result of a direct, MNNG-induced event. The declines in transformation frequency in high-density cultures could have resulted from the inhibitory effects of nontransformed cells upon the growth of transformed cells. Transformation by MCA could similarly be produced by a direct carcinogen-induced event, whose quantitation is complicated by residues at low cell density and phenotypic suppression at high cell density.

Participation of carcinogen residues in MCA-induced transformation permits interpretation of cell-density effects as being the product of cell:cell interactions. However, this does not preclude the existence of multistage cellular mechanisms in the transformation process. Unusual density effects have been observed in cultures treated with X-rays (Kennedy 1984; Kennedy and Little 1984), a process in which residue formation is unlikely. Furthermore, involvement of a carcinogen residue in transformation could be consistent with multistage models for transformation. For example, the rodent carcinogen 2,3,7,8-tetrachlorodibenzo-p–dioxin (TCDD) is a potent promoter of C3H/10T1/2 transformation (Abernethy et al. 1985a). The biological activity of TCDD is presumed to result from binding to receptor proteins under the control of the Ah locus. Given that MCA binds to similar receptors, extended exposure of the cells to an MCA residue could provide an ''activating'' influence similar to that postulated in multistage transformation models.

Promotion of C3H/10T1/2 cell transformation by TCDD highlights the ability of nongenotoxic tumor promoters to enhance the focus formation process. The transformation of C3H/10T1/2 cells can be enhanced by numerous compounds known or suspected to possess tumor-promoting activity in vivo (Boreiko 1985a). As shown in Figure 1, the application of a promoter such as TPA to a C3H/10T1/2 culture can dramatically enhance the formation of foci in dishes treated with MNNG. Enhancement of C3H/10T1/2 cell transformation by tumor promoters mirrors many of the operational characteristics of in vivo promotion (Boreiko 1985a) and suggests that the C3H/10T1/2 system may have applications for the detection and study of tumor promoters.

Recent studies with dioxins (Abernethy et al. 1985a,b) established that the potent rodent carcinogen TCDD lacks significant initiating or transforming activity in the C3H/10T1/2 cell transformation system. When examined for its ability to promote transformation, TCDD was found to exert activity at concentrations as low as 4 pM. Subsequent studies established that carcinogenic hexachloro- isomers of dioxin were also potent promoters of transformation and that the equivocal carcinogen 2,7-dichlorodibenzo-p-dioxin exhibited only weak activity at high concentrations. These observations are consistent with the suggestion that the carcinogenicity of dioxin isomers is mediated in large part by tumor-promoting potential. Moreover, the observation of a good correlation between promoting activity in cell culture and in vivo carcinogenicity suggests that the C3H/10T1/2 system may provide an in vitro screen suited for the preliminary evaluation of dioxin isomers of unknown carcinogenic potential.

The mechanism by which promoters enhance focus formation in C3H/10T1/2 cultures is still a matter of speculation. However, a recent study of the BALB/c-3T3 cell transformation system (a focus-formation assay similar to the C3H/10T1/2 system) has demonstrated interesting correlations between the ability of promoters to inhibit intercellular communication, as measured as dye-coupling between cells following microinjection of Lucifer Yellow dye, and their ability to enhance focus formation (Enomoto and Yamasaki 1985; Yamasaki and Enomoto 1985). Promotion in the BALB/c system can thus be linked to the ability of promoters to relieve the suppressive effects exerted on the growth of transformed cells by contact with nontransformed cells. The "initiated" BALB/c-3T3 cell may thus be a phenotypically suppressed transformed cell.

Further support for the importance of intercellular communication in focus formation is provided by the observation that susceptibility of different BALB/c-3T3 clones to transformation correlates with the extent of intercellular communication at confluence (Yamasaki et al. 1985). The subclone most susceptible to transformation was that which exhibited little interaction between the cells within monolayers. Furthermore, BALB/c foci with tumorigenic potential (type III) did not interact with nontransformed cells but exhibited competence for interaction with transformed cells (Enomoto and Yamasaki 1984). Type I foci, which are considered to lack tumorigenic potential, exhibited extensive dye-coupling with nontransformed cells.

The promotion of C3H/10T1/2 cell transformation could also entail inhibition of intercellular communication. However, a number of observations suggest that the "initiated" C3H/10T1/2 cell is not simply a phenotypically suppressed transformed cell (Boreiko 1985b). For example, high cell density inhibits focus formation by MNNG + TPA in a fashion identical to that for MCA (Fig. 1). Furthermore, the low levels of focus production in high-density cultures treated with just MNNG remains insignificant as cell density is reduced. If TPA just facilitates the growth of transformed cells, then focus production in low-density cultures exposed to just MNNG should rise and approach that produced in MNNG + TPA-treated cultures. Moreover, preliminary data (Boreiko 1985b) indicate that expression of a transformed morphology in dishes treated with MNNG + TPA is often dependent on the continued presence of TPA. Withdrawal of TPA from cell-culture medium will cause the rapid "regression" of foci.

The findings of microinjection studies of C3H/10T1/2 cells (Boreiko et al. 1987) indicate that alterations in intercellular communication accompany C3H/10T1/2 focus formation but that the tight correlations observed in the BALB/c system are not directly applicable to the C3H/10T1/2 system. For example, although C3H/10T1/2 cells are susceptible to transformation, extensive intercellular communication occurs within monolayers at confluence. Focus formation is characterized by a lack of dye-coupling between nontransformed and transformed cells. However, this inhibition is more generalized and extends to dye-coupling between transformed cells as well. This generalized inhibition of dye-coupling was evident in both tumorigenic (type II and III) and nontumorigenic (type I) focus types. Finally, the presence of either TPA or TCDD did not alter dye-coupling between nontransformed cells within a confluent monolayer. These studies indicate that alterations in intercellular communication consistently accompany, and are of possible importance to, C3H/10T1/2 cell transformation. However, the process of promotion in the C3H/10T1/2 system does not correlate with the induction of a simple generalized inhibition of intercellular communication. Effects that specifically influence the interaction of nontransformed and transformed cells are, of course, still possible.

CONCLUSIONS

The transformation of C3H/10T1/2 cells can be modulated by a variety of nongenotoxic variables. Some of these are of questionable relevance to in vivo carcinogenesis. For example, cell-density-dependent alterations in focus formation in low-cell-density cultures treated with MCA may result from the action of carcinogen residues bound to the surface of cell-culture dishes. However, although binding to dish surfaces may be of little direct relevance to human exposure situations, the biological effects of residues could be mediated by processes akin to promotion by substances such as TCDD. Indeed, the carcinogenic potential of dioxin isomers correlates with their ability to promote the transformation of C3H/10T1/2 cells.

The mechanism by which high cell density and tumor promoters modulate focus formation is not understood. Inhibition of focus formation by high cell density may be related to the suppressive effects of nontransformed cells on the growth of transformed cells. The consistent observation of disruptions in intercellular communication during focus formation supports this simple selective model but does not rule out more complex multistage mechanisms for transformation. Promotion in the C3H/10T1/2 cell transformation does not appear to entail simple selection for the growth of preexisting transformed cells and is not accompanied by the generalized promoter-induced alterations in intercellular communication observed in the BALB/c-3T3 cell transformation system. The action of tumor promoters upon C3H/10T1/2 cells may thus entail the induction of alterations within individual cells or specifically alter the interaction of transformed cells with nontransformed cells.

REFERENCES

Abernethy, D.J., W.F. Greenlee, J.C. Huband, and C.J. Boreiko. 1985a. 2,3,7,8-Tetrachlorodibenzo-p-dioxin (TCDD) promotes the transformation of C3H/10T1/2 cells. *Carcinogenesis* **6:** 651.

Abernethy, D.J., J.C. Huband, and C.J. Boreiko. 1985b. Effect of polychlorinated dibenzo-p-dioxins upon C3H/10T1/2 cell transformation. *Proc. Am. Assoc. Cancer Res.* **26:** 130.

Bertram, J.S. 1979. Modulation of cellular interactions between C3H/10T1/2 cells and their transformed counterparts by phosphodiesterase inhibitors. *Cancer Res.* **39:** 3502.

Boreiko, C.J. 1985a. Initiation and promotion in cultures of C3H/10T1/2 mouse embryo fibroblasts. *Carcinog. Compr. Surv.* **8:** 329.

Boreiko, C.J. 1985b. Mechanistic aspects of initiation and promotion in C3H/10T1/2 cells *Carcinog. Compr. Surv.* **9:** 153.

Boreiko, C.J., D.J. Abernethy, and D.B. Stedman. 1987. Alterations of intercellular communication associated with the transformation of C3H/10T1/2 cells. *Carcinogenesis* **8:** 321.

Enomoto, T. and H. Yamasaki. 1984. Lack of intercellular communication between chemically transformed and surrounding nontransformed BALB/c-3T3 cells. *Cancer Res.* **44:** 5200.

———. 1985. Phorbol ester-mediated inhibition of intercellular communication in BALB/c-3T3 cells: Relationship to enhancement of cell transformation. *Cancer Res.* **45:** 2681.

Fernandez, A., S. Mondal, and C. Heidelberger. 1980. Probabilistic view of the transformation of cultured C3H/10T1/2 mouse embryo fibroblasts by 3-methylcholanthrene. *Proc. Natl. Acad. Sci. U.S.A.* **77:** 7272.

Haber, D.A., D.A. Fox, W.S. Dynan, and W.G. Thilly. 1977. Cell density dependence of focus formation in the C3H/10T1/2 cell transformation assay. *Cancer Res.* **37:** 1664.

Heidelberger, C., A.E. Freeman, R.J. Pienta, A. Sivak, J.S. Bertram, B.C. Casto, V.C. Dunkel, M.W. Francis, T. Kakunaga, J.B. Little, and L.M. Schechtman. 1983. Cell transformation by chemical agents: A review and analysis of the literature. *Mutat. Res.* **114:** 283.

Huband, J.C., D.J. Abernethy, and C.J. Boreiko. 1985. Potential role of treatment artifact in the effect of cell density upon frequencies of C3H/10T1/2 cell transformation. *Cancer Res.* **45:** 6314.

Kennedy, A.R. 1984. Promotion and other interactions between agents in the induction of transformation in vitro in fibroblasts. In *Mechanisms of tumor promotion: Tumor promotion and carcinogenesis in vitro* (ed. T.J. Slaga), vol. 3, p. 13. CRC Press, Boca Raton, Florida.

Kennedy, A.R. and J. B. Little. 1984. Evidence that a second event in X–ray induced transformation in vitro occurs during cellular proliferation. *Radiat. Res.* **99:** 228.

Mondal, S., D.W. Brankow, and C. Heidelberger. 1976. Two-stage chemical oncogenesis in cultures of C3H/10T1/2 cells. *Cancer Res.* **36:** 2254.

Mordan, L.J., J.E. Martner, and J.S. Bertram. 1983. Quantitative neoplastic transformation of C3H/10T1/2 fibroblasts: Dependence upon the size of the initiated cell colony at confluence. *Cancer Res.* **43:** 4062.

Reznikoff, C.A., J.S. Bertram, D.W. Brankow, and C. Heidelberger. 1973a. Quantitative and qualitative studies of chemical transformation of clones C3H mouse embryo cells sensitive to postconfluence inhibition of cell division. *Cancer Res.* **33:** 3239.

Reznikoff, C.A., D.W. Brankow, and C. Heidelberger. 1973b. Establishment and characterization of a cloned line of C3H mouse embryo cells sensitive to postconfluence inhibition of cell division. *Cancer Res.* **33:** 3231.

Trosko, J.E. and C. Chang. 1984. Role of intercellular communication in tumor promotion. In *Mechanisms of tumor promotion: Cellular responses to tumor promoters* (ed. T.J. Slaga), vol. 4, p. 119. CRC Press, Boca Raton, Florida.

Yamasaki, H. and T. Enomoto. 1985. Role of intercellular communication in Balb/c-3T3 cell transformation. *Carcinog. Compr. Surv.* **9:** 179.

Yamasaki, H., T. Enomoto, Y. Shiba, Y. Kanno, and T. Kakunaga. 1985. Intercellular communication capacity as a possible determinant of transformation sensitivity of BALB/c-3T3 clonal cells. *Cancer Res.* **45:** 637.

COMMENTS

DIAMOND: When you reverse and are removing TPA, what happens to the communication?

BOREIKO: Our results on this are preliminary and have been variable. Some of the foci start communicating with the monolayers; some of them do not. There is very little consistency in the way that this goes. Communication could be involved in the reversion process, but we are not really certain at this point.

YAMASAKI: Did you test many serum batches to see whether transformation frequency can be affected? I think there are some data which suggests that serum batches are playing a role.

BOREIKO: The studies that I was discussing were conducted over the course of one year. We used three different serum lots; so we are not talking about an effect that is necessarily unique to one serum lot. But the serum lots that we used were prescreened for use in promotion studies.

SCRIBNER: We have played a lot with the C3H system promotion, and finally two summers ago, we gave up in disgust after spending an entire summer screening for serum lots that work. We went through 20 different lots. Have you solved that problem in anything but a pragmatic way, and, if you have, what comments do you have about what factors are involved in the serum?

BOREIKO: That is the major problem with the TPA promotion system. We have yet to find a way to get around that. We do a lot of work with the system and can afford to keep screening serum lots. With the proper quality control, the promotion system can be kept going. The question is, Can you allocate sufficient personnel to use it as a routine research tool and keep it going? If you cannot make that commitment, then we advise that it is not the system to be used. Promotion by the dioxins may not be quite as serum-specific. If you don't mind elevated backgrounds, I think you can use the system in a fairly routine fashion for a study of dioxin isomers. The sera that work for transformation by MCA usually work for dioxin promotion.

SCRIBNER: What percentage of your lots work?

BOREIKO: About 90% for MCA, that is, without TPA. With TPA it is the other way around; it is about 10%.

CERUTTI: We have also given up in disgust. Especially for the study of biochemical reactions, the serum lot becomes so critical that results become questionable.

SCRIBNER: When it works, it works beautifully. We have gotten some very nice data. It is just an effort to keep it going.

BARRETT: Have you looked at how soon after MNNG treatment you have to give your TCDD? The reason that I ask is that Dr. Tanaka, working with Paul Nettesheim and myself, has recently shown that he gets a marked enhancement of transformation of rat tracheal epithelial cells by TCDD following MNNG treatment. But in his experiments, he observed that he has to give TCDD fairly soon after MNNG treatment. If he waits until later, he loses the effect; so it is more like a comutagenic or cocarcinogenic effect.

BOREIKO: We figure that whatever TCDD is doing, it probably is receptor-mediated.

BARRETT: Our effect is also receptor-mediated.

BOREIKO: We did our initial studies with addition of TCDD on day 5 and got results that were similar to those that we obtained when we added TCDD on day 1. We now routinely add dioxins on day 1 simply because the receptor-mediated events probably require 48 to 72 hours and we want to ensure effective exposure during logarithmic growth.

BARRETT: You can wait until day 5 and still see an effect?

BOREIKO: Yes.

SWENBERG: Craig, the reversibility of transformed foci when you took away the promoter was very interesting. Have you tried to put the promoter back on any of these cultures and did the foci come back? Do you have remodeling?

BOREIKO: You can clone the foci and put them into mass culture. If you put TPA on them, and they will look transformed. If you take the TPA off, they will revert. Thus far, we have not succeeded in cloning them to homogeneity.

The Role of Cell-to-Cell Communication in Tumor Promotion

HIROSHI YAMASAKI
International Agency for Research on Cancer
69372 Lyon Cedex 08, France

OVERVIEW

Cancer can be regarded as a rebellion in an orderly cellular society. Cancer cells neglect their neighbors and grow autonomously over surrounding normal cells. Since intercellular communication plays an important role in maintaining an orderly society, it must be disturbed during the process of carcinogenesis. Evidence is being accumulated to suggest that blockage of intercellular communication is important in the promotion process of carcinogenesis. Using in vitro cell transformation as a model system, we have obtained several lines of evidence to support this hypothesis. We are investigating whether inhibition of junctional intercellular communication is an appropriate endpoint for a short-term test to detect tumor-promoting activity.

INTRODUCTION

Intercellular communication is considered to play an important role in maintaining and controlling cell growth, cell differentiation, and homeostasis. Since this control system is absent from cancer cells, it has been proposed that disturbed intercellular communication is involved in carcinogenesis. Of the various forms of intercellular communication, junctional communication is considered to be the most important for controlling the mechanisms of cell growth (Loewenstein 1979). Previous studies compared the junctional communication capacity of normal and transformed cells, and the results suggested that only some cancerous cells lose this function (Weinstein et al. 1976; Loewenstein 1979). However, these studies cannot demonstrate whether or how control of junctional communication is involved in carcinogenesis, since the comparison cells were already transformed.

Tumor-promoting phorbol esters are the first cancer-associated compounds that have been shown to inhibit junctional communication in various cell populations, as measured by metabolic cooperation (Murray and Fitzgerald 1979; Yotti et al. 1979), electrical coupling (Enomoto et al. 1981), and by a dye-transfer method (Friedman and Steinberg 1982; Enomoto et al. 1984). Moreover, treatment of cultured cells or mouse skin with phorbol esters results in a decrease in gap junctions (Finbow et al. 1983; Kalimi and Sirsat 1984). It has therefore been proposed that blockage of junctional communication is involved in the promotional phase of carcinogenesis

Banbury Report 25: Nongenotoxic Mechanisms in Carcinogenesis
© Cold Spring Harbor Laboratory. 0-87969-225-1/87. $1.00 + .00

(Trosko et al. 1982; Yamasaki et al. 1984). This hypothesis has been widely accepted, since it fits well with the fact that clonal expansion of initiated cells over surrounding normal cells is essential to promotion. If an initiated cell is isolated from surrounding normal cells, it can undergo altered gene expression and expand clonally, ignoring its neighboring normal cells. Another line of evidence to support this hypothesis is that partial hepatectomy and skin wounding, which are promoting stimuli for liver carcinogenesis (Pound and McGuine 1978) and skin tumors (Clark-Lewis and Murray 1978), respectively, also decrease gap junctions (Loewenstein and Penn 1967; Meyer et al. 1981).

We have used cell transformation as a model system to study the role and mechanisms of inhibition of junctional communication during carcinogenesis. We chose the dye-transfer assay for measuring junctional communication. Unlike other methods such as the metabolic cooperation assay and the electrical coupling assay, it allows study of junctional communication between cells cultured under any conditions and reflects their physiological status.

RESULTS

Inhibition of Junctional Communication between Cultured Cells by Tumor-promoting Phorbol Esters

The methods for measuring junctional communication between cultured cells can be divided roughly into three groups: (1) metabolic cooperation, (2) electrical coupling, and (3) dye transfer. Tumor-promoting agents were first shown to inhibit junctional communication between cultured cells using the metabolic cooperation assay (Murray and Fitzgerald 1979; Yotti et al. 1979). Since this assay measures only the transfer of molecules from one cell to another through gap junctions, we felt it necessary to demonstrate that ion transfer is also blocked by tumor-promoting agents. Since electrical coupling measures ion transfer between cells, presumably through gap junctions, if it is inhibited by phorbol esters, these compounds must block the passage of any physiological factor. Using cultured human amniotic membrane epithelial cells (FL cells), we demonstrated, in collaboration with Y. Kanno's laboratory, that TPA can inhibit the formation and maintenance of electrical coupling between cells (Enomoto et al. 1981; Yamasaki et al. 1983) and reduce junctional communication between BALB/c-3T3 cells (Yamasaki et al. 1985).

This rather laborious electrophysiological method is, however, not optimal for studying the mechanisms by which junctional communication is inhibited by phorbol esters and how this inhibition is involved in carcinogenesis. Metabolic cooperation is also not a suitable assay in this case, since it requires the preparation of mutants and coculture of two types of cells in one petri dish, whereas for cell transformation, one cell type must be cultured for a long time. The dye-transfer assay was found to be the most suitable. This method involves microinjection of a tracer dye into individual cells and observation of the spread of the dye into neighboring cells. Using Lucifer Yellow CH, which does not diffuse through cell membranes (Stewart 1978), the presence of fluorescent cells around microinjected cells indicates passage of the dye through junctions. As shown in Figure 1, with this microinjected dye transfer assay we can show that phorbol ester tumor-promoting agents inhibit junctional communication between cultured cells.

12-O-Tetradecanoylphorbol 13-acetate (TPA) may not totally destroy junctional materials, since de novo protein synthesis is not required for recovery of communication after TPA inhibition (Yamasaki et al. 1983; Enomoto et al. 1984). As for many other effects of TPA, activation of protein kinase C (Nishizuka 1984) appears to be involved in TPA-mediated inhibition of intercellular communication, since a presumptive functional analog of phorbol esters, diacylglycerol, also inhibits communication (Enomoto and Yamasaki 1985a; Gainer and Murray 1985).

Inhibition of Junctional Communication and Enhancement of Transformation of BALB/c-3T3 Cells

Morphological cell transformation of BALB/c-3T3 cells induced by 3-methylcholanthrene can be enhanced by tumor-promoting phorbol esters. In order to establish whether there is a correlation between inhibition of junctional communication and enhancement of cell transformation by phorbol esters, we studied these two phenomena in the same cell line. Addition of phorbol esters induces rapid inhibition of junctional communication from which, however, there is a rapid recovery, due probably to down-regulation of phorbol ester receptors, i.e., protein kinase C. However, continuous addition of phorbol esters twice weekly reactivates the inhibition of intercellular communication when the cells grow to confluence and continues throughout the transformation assay. A good dose-response relationship was seen between TPA inhibition of junctional communication at cell confluence and TPA enhancement of cell transformation. Phorbol-12,13-didecanoate was an even more potent inhibitor of junctional communication and more potent in enhancing cell transformation (Enomoto and Yamasaki 1985b). These results suggest that inhibition of junctional communication may be involved in the enhancement of cell transformation by phorbol esters.

These results are not consistent with those obtained with another cell transformation system, namely, C3H/10T1/2 cells, as reported by Boreiko's group (Dorman et al. 1983). They found that TPA produced a refractory state after a short period of culture and that this inhibition of junctional communication was not involved in the enhancement of cell transformation in this system. However, the difference in the results may be due to the fact that they used the metabolic cooperation assay to measure junctional communication.

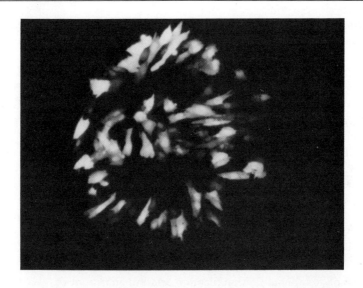

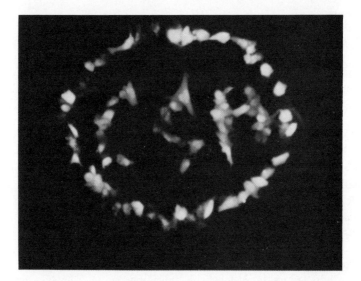

Figure 1

Inhibition of dye-transfer between cultured cells by TPA. Both panels show fluorescent micrographs of Chinese hamster V79 cells injected with Lucifer Yellow CH so that the dye-injected cells form the mark of "CSH." (*Top*) Dye injected to control culture cells; (*bottom*) dye was injected after cells were treated with TPA. Because of the inhibition of the junctional communication (dye-transfer), CSH is visualized only in the lower panel. Microinjection was carried out under Olympus Injectoscope Type IMT2-SYF, coupled with Eppendorf automatic microinjector 5242.

A BALB/c-3T3 Cell Variant That Appears To Be Intrinsically Promotion-proficient

A few subclones of BALB/c-3T3 cell variants that differ in their susceptibility to chemical induction of cell transformation have been isolated and characterized by Kakunaga (Kakunaga et al. 1982). Having found, however, that they were very similar in their ability to respond to initiating agents, Kakunaga suggested that they differ only in the late stage (promotion) of cell transformation. We began a collaborative study to investigate his suggestion.

These cell variants responded similarly to exogenously added phorbol esters. We therefore considered that they must differ in expressing certain promotion-related phenotypes, one of which is blocked intercellular communication. We cultured two variant cell lines, one transformation-susceptible (clone A31-1-13) and one transformation-resistant (clone A31-1-8), for 4 weeks and measured junctional communication capacity. That of the transformation-resistant line was constant over the incubation time, but that of the transformation-susceptible line was reduced markedly when the cells reached confluence (Yamasaki et al. 1985). Thus, at confluence, transformation-susceptible cells can express a TPA-like effect, i.e., blockage of intercellular communication; and initiated cells triggered by chemicals can be transformed easily.

We do not know the mechanism by which cell-transformation-susceptible cell lines lose their capacity for junctional communication at confluence. We have found recently that such cells keep accumulating fibronectin even after confluence, whereas transformation-resistant cell lines do not.

Expression of Morphological Cell Transformation and Inhibition of Intercellular Communication in Syrian Hamster Embryo Cells

Another group of genetic variants in terms of TPA susceptibility was also used to correlate enhancement of cell transformation and blockage of intercellular communication by TPA. Of three cell variants of Syrian hamster embryo cells, isolated by Rivedal and Sanner, only a TPA-sensitive line was also sensitive to TPA-mediated inhibition of junctional communication (Rivedal et al. 1985).

Although these results suggest that there is a good correlation between TPA-enhanced cell transformation and blockage of intercellular communication, the transformation assay with Syrian hamster embryo cells is quite different from that with BALB/c-3T3 cells. The endpoint in the latter is in situ production of transformed foci, whereas that in the Syrian hamster embryo cell system is transformation of colonies and TPA can alter the morphology of all cells in a given colony in a very short time. The effect of TPA in Syrian hamster embryo cell transformation is thus more on expression of transformed morphology, whereas that in BALB/c-3T3 cells is on the process of cell transformation.

Selective Communication between Transformed and Nontransformed Cells

Since promotion involves the clonal expansion of initiated cells over surrounding normal cells, clonally expanded, initiated cells must form a population of cells that differ from normal cells. We have tested this idea by studying the intercellular communication capacity of transformed and nontransformed BALB/c-3T3 cells. When the cells are transformed by 3-methylcholanthrene, the communication capacity among transformed foci is similar to that of normal cells, but there is no communication between transformed cells and surrounding nontransformed cells.

Recently, we have succeeded in transforming BALB/c-3T3 cells by transfection with the EJ Ha-*ras1* oncogene. We have proved that EJ *ras* oncogene is integrated and expressed in transformed cells by means of Southern and Western blot analysis. The same results were obtained: although junctional communication among transformed foci is similar to that in nontransformed cells, there is no communication between oncogene-transformed and surrounding normal cells (Fig. 2).

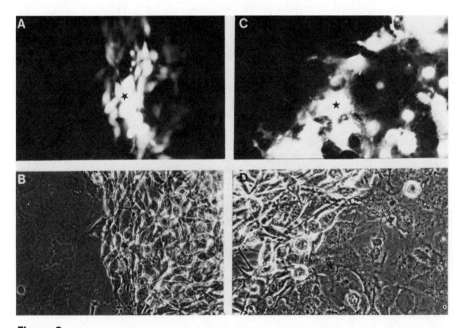

Figure 2
Selective communication between oncogene-transformed and surrounding nontransformed BALB/c-3T3 cells. BALB/c-3T3 cells were transfected with EJ Ha-*ras1* DNA by calcium phosphate coprecipitation method. (*A,B*) Lucifer Yellow CH was microinjected into a single cell in a transformed focus; (*C,D*) dye was injected into a single cell of nontransformed monolayer part; (★) cells into which the dye was injected.

Furthermore, in spontaneously transformed BALB/c-3T3 cells, seen occasionally, junctional communication is absent between normal and transformed cells.

The obvious logical extension of this finding is to investigate the communication pattern in an epithelial cell transformation system. However, it is difficult to induce epithelial cell transformation in situ, and it was necessary to undertake a reconstruction experiment. When we cocultured transformed and nontransformed rat liver epithelial cells, there was again no communication between transformed and nontransformed cells, indicating that selective communication between normal and transformed cells is a universal phenomenon.

Inhibition of Junctional Communication as a Possible Endpoint to Assay Tumor-promoting Activity of Chemicals

On the basis of our finding that inhibition of junctional communication is involved in tumor promotion, we investigated its use as a short-term screening test for tumor-promoting agents. Trosko's group has studied this aspect, with quite convincing results (Trosko et al. 1982). Our results are summarized in Table 1. Several different types of tumor-promoting agents, such as DDT, butylated hydroxyanisole, phenobarbital, and lindane, inhibited junctional communication; however, other known tumor-promoting agents, including anthralin, benzoyl peroxide, and certain bile acids, did not.

DISCUSSION

Using cell culture systems, we have obtained several lines of evidence that blocked intercellular communication is important in the promotion process of carcinogenesis. This is compatible with the idea that initiated cells can expand clonally because they have no communication with surrounding normal cells. Since we have used junctional communication as the measure of intercellular communication, we consider that the blockage of junctional communication per se is important for tumor promotion; however, our results might equally indicate that it is blockage of cell-cell recognition that is important for the isolation of initiated cells. In other words, it may be that in the promotion process, recognition between initiated and surrounding normal cells is blocked and they cannot form gap junctions. We consider, however, that blockage of intercellular communication itself is also important for tumor promotion. If there is junctional communication between normal and initiated cells, there will be an exchange of factors by which normal cells could neutralize the initiated cells. This is analogous to the finding of Stanbridge's group that when nontumorigenic and tumorigenic cells are hybridized, the normal cell phenotype is dominant over the tumorigenic phenotype (Stanbridge et al. 1982), suggesting that normal cells can produce factors that can neutralize the tumorigenicity.

Table 1
The Ability of Various Reported and Suspected Tumor-promoting Agents to Inhibit Junctional Intercellular Communication in Cultured Mammalian Cells

Chemical	Tumor-promoting activity	Inhibition of intercellular communication in V79 cells		Inhibition of junctional communication measured in other cell types and/or by other metabolic cooperation (MC) systems
		Lucifer Yellow CH transfer[a]	metabolic cooperation assay[b]	
TPA	mouse, skin	+	+	+ in mouse epidermal cells/mouse fibroblasts MC assay + in human fibroblasts MC assay + in human fibroblasts/V79 MC assay
p,p'-DDT	rat, liver	+	+	+ in human fibroblast MC assay + in primary rat hepatocytes/rat liver epithelial cells MC assay
Phenobarbital	rat, liver	+	+, −[c]	+ in primary rat hepatocytes/rat liver epithelial cells MC assay
Lindane	not tested[d]	+	+	
BHA	rat, urinary bladder	+	not tested	
BHT	rat, urinary bladder	−	+	
Sodium deoxycholic acid	rat, colon	−	+, −[c]	
Lithocholic acid	rat, colon	−	+	
Benzoyl peroxide	mouse, skin	−	+, −[c]	+ in human keratinocytes MC assay
Anthralin	mouse, skin	−	+, −[c]	

[a]Chinese hamster V79 cells were cultured in the presence or absence of several doses of test chemicals for 24–72 hr, before the dye-transfer was assayed. When the extent of dye-transfer was dose-dependently inhibited at noncytotoxic levels (measured by cloning efficiency assay), we scored the chemical as + (Zeilmaker and Yamasaki, 1986).
[b]Reported in published papers.
[c]Both positive and negative results were reported.
[d]Carcinogenic in mouse liver.

Our trial using the inhibition of junctional communication as an endpoint to detect tumor-promoting activity of various chemicals was rather successful; both phorbol-ester-type and other tumor-promoting agents were positive. We believe that the dye-transfer assay has several advantages over the metabolic cooperation assay used by Trosko's group and others (Trosko et al. 1982). Because of the known tissue specificity of tumor-promoting agents, we plan to use different cell types for further trials of this new short-term test. Since there is no validated short-term test for detecting the tumor-promoting activity of chemicals, and in view of the importance of such chemicals as health hazards, we consider that the junctional communication assay should be further exploited for this purpose.

CONCLUSION

The following results from our laboratory suggest a correlation between blocked junctional communication and tumor promotion: (1) Tumor-promoting agents block junctional communication; (2) there is a good relationship between phorbol-ester-mediated enhancement of cell transformation and inhibition of junctional communication; (3) a cell variant with high susceptibility to chemically induced transformation loses its intrinsic junctional communication ability at confluence; and (4) oncogene-transformed or chemically transformed cells do not communicate with surrounding normal cells. Blockage of junctional communication may thus be used as an endpoint in a short-term test to detect the tumor-promoting activity of chemicals.

ACKNOWLEDGMENTS

This work was partly supported by National Cancer Institute grant R01-CA-40534-01. I thank my collaborators T. Enomoto, Y. Kanno, M. Mesnil, M. Hollstein, T. Kakunaga, E. Rivedal, T. Sanner, M. Zeilmaker, A.M. Aguelon-Pegouries, and F. Katoh, who contributed to this research project; Dr. L. Tomatis and Dr. R. Montesano for their continuous kind encouragement during the course of the study; Ms. C. Fuchez for secretarial aid; and Ms. E. Heseltine for editing the manuscript.

REFERENCES

Clark-Lewis, I. and A.W. Murray. 1978. Tumor promotion and the induction of epidermal ornithine decarboxylase activity in mechanically stimulated mouse skin. *Cancer Res.* **38:** 494.

Dorman, B.H., B.E. Butterworth, and C.J. Boreiko. 1983. Role of intercellular communication in the promotion of C3H10T1/2 cell transformation. *Carcinogenesis* **4:** 1109.

Enomoto, T. and H. Yamasaki. 1985a. Rapid inhibition of intercellular communication between BALB/c-3T3 cells by diacylglycerol, a possible endogenous functional analogue of phorbol esters. *Cancer Res.* **45:** 3706.

―――. 1985b. Phorbol ester-mediated inhibition of intercellular communication in BALB/ c-3T3 cells: Relationship to enhancement of cell transformation. *Cancer Res.* **45:** 2681.

Enomoto, T., N. Martel, Y. Kanno, and H. Yamasaki. 1984. Inhibition of cell communication between BALB/c-3T3 cells by tumor promoters and protection by cAMP. *J. Cell. Physiol.* **121:** 323.

Enomoto, T., Y. Sasaki, Y. Shiba, Y. Kanno, and H. Yamasaki. 1981. Tumor promoters cause a rapid and reversible inhibition of the formation and maintenance of electrical cell coupling in culture. *Proc. Natl. Acad. Sci. U.S.A.* **78:** 5628.

Finbow, M.E., J. Shuttleworth, A.E. Hamilton, and J.D. Pitts. 1983. Analysis of vertebrate gap junction protein. *EMBO J.* **2:** 1479.

Friedman, E.A. and M. Steinberg. 1982. Disrupted communication between late-stage premalignant human colon epithelial cells by 12-*O*-tetradecanoylphorbol-13-acetate. *Cancer Res.* **42:** 5096.

Gainer, H.S.H. and A.W. Murray. 1985. Diacylglycerol inhibits gap junctional communication in cultured epidermal cells. Evidence for a role of protein kinase C. *Biochem. Biophys. Res. Commun.* **126:** 1109.

Kakunaga, T., H. Hamada, J. Leavith, J.D. Crow, T. Hirakawa, and K.Y. Lo. 1982. Evidence for both mutational and nonmutational process in chemically induced cell transformation. In *Mechanisms of chemical carcinogenesis* (ed. C.C. Harris and P.A. Cerutti), p. 517. Alan R. Liss, New York.

Kalimi, G.H. and S.M. Sirsat. 1984. Phorbol esters tumor promoter affects the mouse epidermal gap junctions. *Cancer Lett.* **22:** 343.

Loewenstein, W.R. 1979. Junctional intercellular communication and the control of growth. *Biochim. Biophys. Acta* **560:** 1.

Loewenstein, W.R. and R.D. Penn. 1967. Intercellular communication and tissue growth II. Tissue regeneration. *J. Cell Biol.* **33:** 235.

Meyer, D.J., S.B. Yancey, and J.P. Revel. 1981. Intercellular communication in normal and regenerating rat liver: A quantitative analysis. *J. Cell Biol.* **91:** 505.

Murray, A.W. and D.J. Fitzgerald. 1979. Tumor promoters inhibit metabolic cooperation in cocultures of epidermal and 3T3 cells. *Biochem. Biophys. Res. Commun.* **91:** 395.

Nishizuka, Y. 1984. The role of protein kinase C in cell surface signals transduction and tumor promotion. *Nature* **308:** 693.

Pound, A.W. and L.I. McGuine. 1978. Repeated partial hepatectomy as a promoting stimulus for carcinogenic response of liver to nitrosamines in rats. *Br. J. Cancer* **37:** 585.

Rivedal, E., T. Sanner, T. Enomoto, and H. Yamasaki. 1985. Inhibition of intercellular communication and enhancement of morphological transformation of Syrian hamster embryo cells by TPA. Use of TPA-sensitive and TPA-resistant cell lines. *Carcinogenesis* **6:** 899.

Stanbridge, E.J., C.J. Der, C.J. Doersen, R.Y. Nishimi, D.M. Peehl, B.E. Weissman, and J.E. Wilkinson. 1982. Human cell hybrids: Analysis of transformation and tumorigenicity. *Science* **215:** 252.

Stewart, W.W. 1978. Functional connections between cells as revealed by dye-coupling with a highly fluorescent naphthalimide tracer. *Cell* **14:** 741.

Trosko, J.E., L.P. Yotti, S.T. Warren, G. Tsushimoto, and C.C. Chang. 1982. Inhibition of cell-cell communication by tumor promoters. *Carcinog. Compr. Surv.* **7:** 565.

Weinstein, R.S., F.B. Merk, and J. Alroy. 1976. The structure and function of intercellular junctions in cancer. *Adv. Cancer Res.* **23:** 23.

Yamasaki, H., T. Enomoto, and N. Martel. 1984. Intercellular communication, cell differentiation and tumour promotion. *IARC Sci. Publ.* **56:** 217.

Yamasaki, H., T. Enomoto, N. Martel, Y. Shiba, and Y. Kanno. 1983. Tumor promoter-mediated reversible inhibition of cell-cell communication (electrical coupling). *Exp. Cell Res.* **146:** 297.

Yamasaki, H., T. Enomoto, Y. Shiba, Y. Kanno, and T. Kakunaga. 1985. Intercellular communication capacity as a possible determinant of transformation sensitivity of BALB/c-3T3 clonal cells. *Cancer Res.* **45:** 637.

Yotti, L.P., C.C. Chang, and J.E. Trosko. 1979. Elimination of metabolic cooperation in Chinese hamster cells by a tumor promoter. *Science* **206:** 1089.

Zeilmaker, M.J. and H. Yamasaki. 1986. Inhibition of junctional intercellular communication as a possible short-term test to detect tumor-promoting agents: Results with nine chemicals tested by dye transfer assay in Chinese hamster V79 cells. *Cancer Res.* **46:** 6180.

COMMENTS

CERUTTI: Could you envision that a morphological change upon transformation causes the inhibition of cell communication; that is, is it a final result rather than the cause of transformation?

YAMASAKI: Most of the cell-cell communication studies by Lowenstein and others have been done with already transformed or tumorigenic cells. It has been claimed that tumorigenic cells do not communicate. But, in our study we used agents that are involved in carcinogenesis. We also used Balb/c-3T3 cell variants in which we have not added TPA and we don't see any morphological change at confluency, yet we can show junctional communication inhibition and enhancement of transformation. Of course, it is not really direct, but these studies suggest that communication inhibition may be involved in the process, rather than the result of cell transformation.

TRUMP: How many studies from your group or Trosko's group or any other group have tried to look at the question of gap junction mechanisms; do they correlate with altered gap junctions or not? Has that ever been tested critically, that is, whether the number of gap junctions or the conformation of the subunits of gap junctions correlates with the decreased communication?

YAMASAKI: There were several studies, one in vivo and two in vitro studies, which showed that TPA painting on mouse skin or TPA treatment of cultured cells results in reduced number of gap-junctions. But our studies show that, if you inhibit gap junction communication by TPA and you remove TPA from culture medium, you don't need any protein synthesis to see resumption of the junctional communication. From this we are speculating that gap junctions are dispersed into pieces by TPA and can be reassembled upon TPA removal.

TRUMP: Does phenobarbital do that to gap junctions in vivo; does hepatectomy during regeneration of liver?

YAMASAKI: Yes.

TRUMP: What about phenobarbital-TCDD? Different gap junctions in vivo?

YAMASAKI: Yes. It was reported at the Japanese Cancer Society meeting; feeding phenobarbital to the rat reduced gap junctions 60% in the liver.

DI GIOVANNI: When you showed some of the other compounds and promoters, like anthralin and benzoyl peroxide, were they ambiguous even in the metabolic cooperation assay?

YAMASAKI: No. Benzoyl peroxide was reported to be positive in two different metabolic cooperation systems, one in Chinese hamster V79 cells and another with human epidermal keratimocytes.

DI GIOVANNI: What about anthralin?

YAMASAKI: Anthralin was reported to be positive in the Chinese hamster V79 metabolic cooperation assay from two laboratories, but another laboratory reported to be negative.

DI GIOVANNI: In one of your tables, it appeared that ambiguous results were obtained with benzoyl peroxide and anthralin.

YAMASAKI: When the results from different laboratories were equivocal for one compound, I marked plus/minus in my table.

BUTTERWORTH: What is the correlation with your dye-transfer assay compared to that of the metabolic cooperation assay of Jim Trosco?

YAMASAKI: There is no complete agreement with his data; but I don't believe that Chinese hamster V79 cells can pick up all tumor promoters. I think we have to go to different cell types, and with the microinjection assay we can do that.

BUTTERWORTH: We know that there is organ-to-organ specificity for promotion. Have you considered doing your studies in primary cultures of kidney or liver?

YAMASAKI: That is possible. We can do that.

BUTTERWORTH: Could you do it in the whole organ?

YAMASAKI: Yes, it is possible, even in vivo. It is possible if you combine the dye-transfer assay with the electrical coupling just to measure membrane potential so that you know your injecting capillary is inside the cell. After injection of the dye, you slice the tissue and you examine the spread of dye. This has been done in rat liver.

BUTTERWORTH: That could be very important given the phenomenon of tissue specificity. You could possibly move into the human situation where you could use discarded surgical material.

YAMASAKI: Yes.

Genetic and Epigenetic Mechanisms of Presumed Nongenotoxic Carcinogens

J. CARL BARRETT,* MITSUO OSHIMURA,* NORIHO TANAKA,* AND TAKEKI TSUTSUI†
*Environmental Carcinogenesis Group
Laboratory of Pulmonary Pathobiology
National Institute of Environmental Health Sciences
Research Triangle Park, North Carolina 27709
†Nippon Dental University Tokyo
Tokyo, 102 Japan

OVERVIEW

Several chemicals (e.g., diethylstilbestrol and asbestos) that are not active in most genotoxicity assays are active in inducing morphological transformation of Syrian hamster embryo (SHE) cells in culture. The mechanism of action of these chemicals has been studied in detail. Diethylstilbestrol (DES) induces cell transformation by two possible mechanisms. One apparently does not involve direct DNA damage, but rather a depolymerization of microtubules resulting in aneuploidy due to chromosome nondisjunction. Considerable evidence exists to support a role for aneuploidy in DES-induced cell transformation. The second mechanism by which DES may operate requires exogenous metabolic activation. Under these conditions, DES is metabolized to DNA-reactive and mutagenic metabolites, and an enhancement of transformation is observed. Asbestos and other mineral fibers also induce cell transformation. The ability of mineral fibers to induce cell transformation depends on fiber dimension. Long, thin fibers are most active in the transformation assay; this is similar to the findings on mesothelioma induction in vivo. Asbestos fibers are phagocytized by the cells and accumulate intracellularly around the perinuclear region. The fibers interfere with chromosome segregation during mitosis, resulting in anaphase abnormalities and chromosomal mutations. Cells transformed by asbestos have a nonrandom gain of chromosome 11, a fact that supports the hypothesis that a chromosome mutation is causative in the induction of transformation. These findings indicate that genetic mechanisms (chromosome mutations) are important in the activity of these carcinogens. Since these chemicals may operate also by epigenetic mechanisms, an interplay of genetic and epigenetic changes is probably important in chemical carcinogenesis.

INTRODUCTION

Cell transformation assays have proved to be useful models for studying the genetic and epigenetic mechanisms of chemical carcinogens (Barrett and Fletcher 1987).

Banbury Report 25: Nongenotoxic Mechanisms in Carcinogenesis
© Cold Spring Harbor Laboratory. 0-87969-225-1/87. $1.00 + .00

One of the interesting features of these systems is that certain chemicals, which are often negative in gene mutation assays in bacteria or mammalian cells, are positive in cell transformation assays (Table 1).

One of the difficulties in understanding the role of mutagenesis in carcinogenesis is that different target cells are generally used to measure each endpoint. With cell transformation assays, one can directly compare the ability of a chemical to induce neoplastic transformation and somatic mutation or any other measure of "genotoxicity." This approach allows a more direct determination of the role of genetic events in carcinogenesis. An understanding of epigenetic mechanisms in carcinogenesis requires a knowledge of the role of genetic events in carcinogen-induced tumors.

In this paper, we review our results on the mechanism of induction of heritable cell transformation by certain carcinogens, presumed by some investigators to be "nongenotoxic." In several cases, we have concluded that the mechanism of action for these chemicals in inducing cell transformation, and hence possibly carcinogenesis in vivo, involves genetic mechanisms.

RESULTS

General Description of SHE Cell Transformation Assay

The cell transformation system used in our studies was established initially by Berwald and Sachs (1965) and further characterized in several other laboratories (DiPaolo et al. 1971; Barrett and Ts'o 1978; Pienta 1980; Tu et al. 1986). The basis for the assay is the induction of morphologically transformed colonies of SHE cells, which are observed generally 7–8 days after carcinogen treatment. This assay is quantitative and can be used to study dose-response relationships, although several technical difficulties still persist with the assay (Barrett et al. 1985a).

Table 1
Chemicals That Induce Cell Transformation but Are Reported as Nonmutagenic

Amitrole
Arsenicals[a]
Asbestos[a]
5-Azacytidine[a]
Benzene
Colcemid[a]
Diethylstilbestrol[a]
17β-Estradiol[a]
Ethionine[a]
Sodium bisulfite
Vincristine sulfate[a]

[a]Gene mutation and cell transformation measured concomitantly in the same cells.

As shown in Table 1, several chemicals detected in this assay are generally not positive in short-term tests for mutagens. Furthermore, certain chemicals can induce transformation of these cells in the absence of any detectable mutations at two genetic loci, indicating that this assay can detect chemicals that act by mechanisms other than gene mutations (Barrett et al. 1985b).

The morphologically transformed colonies represent the first step in a progressive, multistep process leading to neoplastic conversion of these cells (Barrett and Ts'o 1978). Additional changes are needed for the cells to become tumorigenic; therefore, an understanding of the mechanism of a chemical in this first step does not preclude other mechanisms (genetic or epigenetic) in the overall carcinogenic response elicited by the chemical.

Diethylstilbestrol

The first chemical shown to induce cell transformation in the absence of detectable induction of gene mutations was the human carcinogen DES (Barrett et al. 1981). We have observed that although a natural estrogen, 17β-estradiol, is similar to DES in its transforming activity, transforming activity and estrogenic activity do not correlate for a number of DES-related compounds (McLachlan et al. 1982). Furthermore, SHE cells have no detectable estrogen receptors and are not stimulated to grow by estrogens. On the basis of these observations, the estrogenic activity of these chemicals does not appear to be involved in their transforming ability (McLachlan et al. 1982). The carcinogenicity of these hormones in vivo can also be dissociated from estrogenic activity (Liehr 1983; Purdy 1984; Li et al. 1985).

In an attempt to understand DES-induced cell transformation, we examined the ability of DES to induce a variety of genetic changes in the SHE cells. We have shown that treatment of SHE cells with DES alone induces cell transformation without causing gene mutations, unscheduled DNA synthesis, sister chromatid exchanges, or structural chromosome aberrations (Tsutsui et al. 1983, 1984b; Barrett et al. 1985b). Thus, DES can induce cell transformation in the absence of detectable DNA damage. However, under these conditions, DES does induce a genetic change (aneuploidy). DES binds with microtubules and disrupts tubulin assembly (Sato et al. 1984; Sharp and Parry 1985; Tucker and Barrett 1986). Treatment of cells in mitosis with doses as low as 10 nM DES results in aneuploidy induction via nondisjunction (Tsutsui et al. 1983). Several lines of evidence, summarized in Table 2, support the hypothesis that aneuploidy is involved in DES-induced cell transformation (Barrett et al. 1985b).

DES is metabolized by SHE cells to Z,Z-dienestrol via a peroxidase-mediated pathway (Degen et al. 1982, 1983). This metabolism may be important in cell transformation (McLachlan et al. 1982). However, since no DNA damage is detected under the conditions that result in cell transformation, these metabolites are either not DNA-reactive or not produced at sufficient levels in SHE cells alone to

Table 2
Lines of Evidence for a Role of DES-induced Nondisjunction in Cell Transformation

1. DES induces significant levels of loss or gain of one or two chromosomes at nontoxic doses.

2. DES induces aneuploidy and cell transformation with parallel dose-response curves.

3. Aneuploidy induction correlates with the ability to induce cell transformation by DES-related compounds.

4. Cell-cycle specificity of aneuploidy induction and cell transformation by DES indicates that G_2/M phase is most sensitive.

5. Neoplastic cell lines induced by DES are near-diploid.

6. DES disrupts microtubule organization in cells providing a biochemical mechanism for induction of anaphase abnormalities and nondisjunction.

induce detectable DNA damage. Treatment of SHE cells with DES in the presence of an exogenous metabolic activation system consisting of rat liver postmitochondrial supernatant changes the pattern of DES metabolism quantitatively and qualitatively (Tsutsui et al. 1984b). Furthermore, this enhanced metabolism of DES results in DNA damage (Tsutsui et al. 1984b), mutagenicity, and enhanced cell transformation (Tsutsui et al. 1986). These results indicate that two pathways may exist for the induction of cell transformation by DES. One apparently does not involve direct DNA damage, and the other, which requires rat liver postmitochondrial supernatant-mediated exogenous metabolic activation, is associated with DNA damage and mutagenicity (Fig. 1).

In vivo DES is also metabolized and a number of metabolites have been identified, some of which may be electrophilic and possibly capable of inducing DNA damage (Metzler and McLachlan 1981). No specific DES-DNA adduct has been identified; however, adduct formation in hamster kidney cells during DES-induced renal carcinogenesis was recently observed (Liehr et al. 1985). Further studies are needed to determine if the metabolites that are active in inducing mutation and transformation in vitro are also involved in the carcinogenicity of DES in vivo.

Asbestos and Mineral Fibers

Asbestos and other mineral fibers are carcinogenic in humans and animals (Wagner et al. 1974). Although asbestos may have cocarcinogenic or tumor-promoting activity (Mossman et al. 1983), it is also active as a complete carcinogen (Wagner et al. 1974; Barrett 1987a). In terms of induction of mesotheliomas in rats following intrapleural injection, the physical rather than the chemical nature of the fibers is related to the carcinogenic potential of diverse mineral dusts. For example long (>8 μm) and thin (<0.25 μm) fibers are more active in

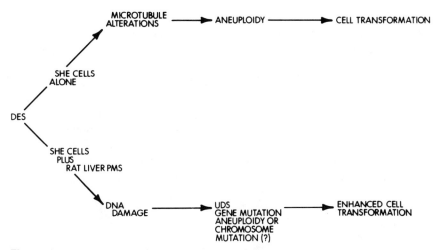

Figure 1
Two possible genetic mechanisms for DES-induced cell transformation and carcinogenicity.

mesothelioma induction in rats than short, thick fibers, regardless of the chemical nature of the fibers. Little is known, however, about the cellular and molecular mechanisms of asbestos carcinogenicity.

Since asbestos and other mineral dusts were known to have toxic and chromosome-damaging effects on cells in culture, we were interested in whether these substances induce cell transformation (Hesterberg and Barrett 1984). We observed that chrysotile and crocidolite asbestos induced morphological and neoplastic transformation of SHE cells which was indistinguishable from the cell transformation induced by other carcinogens such as benzo[a]pyrene. However, asbestos failed to induce gene mutations at specific genetic loci in these cells (Oshimura et al. 1984). The mineral fibers were active in inducing chromosome damage and numerical and structural aberrations. As in the induction of mesotheliomas in vivo, cell transformation by mineral fibers depended on fiber size (Hesterberg and Barrett 1984). Transforming activity of the fibers was destroyed when the fibers were shortened to less than 1 μm in length. The chromosome damage induced by the fibers was likewise dependent on fiber length (Oshimura et al. 1984).

Asbestos induces aneuploidy in the treated cells, causing losses and gains of individual chromosomes. We have proposed a mechanism for this type of genetic change (Hesterberg and Barrett 1985). Asbestos fibers are taken up by the cells by endocytosis within 24 hours after treatment; the intracellular fibers accumulate around the perinuclear region of the cells 24–48 hours after exposure. When the cells undergo mitosis, the physical presence of the fibers results in interference with chromosome segregation. Analysis of anaphases in cells exposed to chrysotile reveals a large increase in the number of cells with anaphase abnormalities (Fig. 2), including lagging chromosomes, bridges, and sticky chromosomes. Asbestos fibers are observed in the mitotic cells and appear, in some cases, to interact directly with the chromosomes. From these studies, we propose that the physical interaction of the asbestos fibers with the chromosomes or structural proteins of the spindle apparatus causes missegregation of chromosomes during mitosis, resulting in aneuploidy. These findings provide a mechanism, at the chromosomal level, by which asbestos and other mineral fibers might induce cell transformation and cancer (Hesterberg and Barrett 1985). This hypothesis is supported by the finding of a nonrandom trisomy of chromosome 11 in asbestos-transformed cells (Oshimura et al. 1986).

Amitrole

Amitrole, a widely used herbicide, is an animal carcinogen and an inducer of cell transformation (IARC 1974; Tsutsui et al. 1984a). However, it is inactive as a mutagen in bacterial test systems (IARC 1974). Thus, it has been suggested that amitrole is a nonmutagenic carcinogen. Over the dose range that induced morphological transformation of SHE cells in culture, amitrole induced gene mutations at the Na^+/K^+ ATPase and hypoxanthine phosphoribosyl transferase loci measured concomitantly in the same cells (Tsutsui et al. 1984a). These findings indicate that amitrole may act via a mutational mechanism and contrast with the negative results

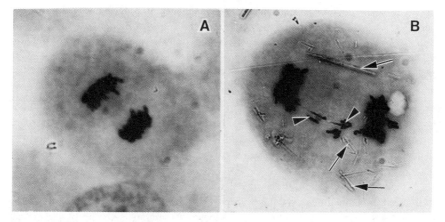

Figure 2
A normal (A) and an abnormal (B) anaphase from asbestos-treated SHE cells. Note the asbestos fibers (arrows), some of which appear to be associated with displaced chromosomes (arrowheads) in the abnormal anaphase.

observed with bacterial mutation assays. Although a variety of mechanisms may account for differences in bacterial versus mammalian cell mutagenesis, the most likely explanation is the necessity for metabolism of amitrole for its activity. SHE cells are able to metabolize a variety of chemical carcinogens to active mutagens and transforming intermediates (Barrett et al. 1985a). Recently, Kraus et al. (1986) have shown that amitrole is metabolized to mutagenic intermediates by peroxidases, including prostaglandin synthetase, which is found in high levels in SHE cells, and lactoperoxidase, a model for thyroid peroxidase. Since the thyroid is the target organ for this carcinogen, these findings suggest that organ-specific metabolism is important in amitrole carcinogenicity.

Chemicals That Fail to Transform SHE Cells

As shown in Table 1, a number of putative nongenotoxic chemicals induce transformation of SHE cells. However, it is important to note the chemicals that are inactive in this assay. Many routinely employed noncarcinogens, such as benzo[e]pyrene, are inactive (Pienta 1980). More importantly, structural analogs of some of the compounds listed on Table 1 are inactive (McLachlan et al. 1982; Hesterberg and Barrett 1984). In addition, other carcinogens proposed as nongenotoxic are inactive in this assay, including phenobarbital (Barrett and Lamb 1985), 2,3,7,8-tetrachlorodibenzo-*p*-dioxin (N. Tanaka and J.C. Barrett, unpubl.), and 12-*O*-tetradecanoyl-phorbol-13-acetate (Pienta 1980; J.C. Barrett, unpubl.).

DISCUSSION

The somatic mutation theory of carcinogenesis remains the main tenet for explaining the carcinogenic activity of chemicals (Barrett 1987a). Some chemicals, however, fail to elicit positive responses in in vitro assays for genetic toxicity. Several possible mechanisms or explanations for these putative nonmutagenic carcinogens can be proposed (Table 3).

A problem that exists in most in vitro assays is the necessity for exogenous metabolic activation, and the lack of a positive response in a mutation assay may relate to this requirement. Even though considerable advances have been made in this area in the last several years, chemicals with unusual metabolic activation pathways will undoubtedly be discovered. Amitrole and DES are possible examples of this problem.

Many genotoxicity assays measure only the activity of a chemical to induce point mutations or induce DNA damage. However, chemicals can also induce genetic changes at the chromosomal level without inducing gene mutations or directly damaging DNA (Oshimura and Barrett 1986; Barrett 1987a) and therefore would be negative in some genotoxicity assays.

Table 3
Possible Mechanisms or Explanations for Putative Nonmutagenic Carcinogens

1. Unusual metabolic activation is required for activity in mutational assays (examples: amitrole and DES).

2. Mutagenic activity of chemical is limited to chromosomal level, i.e., structural or numerical chromosome changes (examples: benzene, arsenicals, DES, and asbestos).

3. Chemicals are inhibitors of DNA methylation (examples: 5-azacytidine and ethionine).

4. Chemicals act as tumor promoters (examples: phenobarbital, 2,3,7,8-tetrachlorodibenzo-*p*-dioxin, hormones, and asbestos).

Certain exceptions to the correlation between carcinogenesis and mutagenicity, including benzene, arsenic, DES, and asbestos, may relate to the ability of certain chemicals to act specifically as chromosome mutagens (i.e., clastogens and/or aneuploidogens). We have already discussed the data that support the conclusion that DES and asbestos are chromosome mutagens. Benzene, a known human carcinogen, has been reported negative in most gene mutation assays, but some positive results have been presented (IARC 1982; Ashby et al. 1985). However, clear evidence exists that cytogenetic effects are induced by benzene (IARC 1982), indicating that it is primarily an inducer of chromosome damage, and this is likely its major mechanism of action. Similarly, arsenic and arsenical compounds are known human carcinogens that are inactive or weak gene mutagens but very potent clastogens (IARC 1982). Sodium arsenite and sodium arsenate induce morphological transformation of SHE cells in culture (Lee et al. 1985). Under these conditions, gene mutations at two genetic loci cannot be detected, but chromosome aberrations are significantly increased, with a similar dose-response curve for induction of cell transformation. Thus, it is likely that these are other examples of carcinogens that are primarily chromosome mutagens.

Methylation of DNA at the 5 position of cytosine is important in the regulation of gene expression and is one possible epigenetic mechanism for the heritable change in cancer cells. Chemicals such as 5-azacytidine and ethionine may effect DNA methylation through an interaction with the DNA methylase enzyme. It has also been suggested that DNA-alkylating agents may heritably alter DNA methylation patterns (Jones 1987). This provides an epigenetic mechanism for heritable alterations in expression of genes involved in carcinogenesis.

Other epigenetic mechanisms for carcinogens can be proposed (Barrett 1987b). A number of these may involve the tumor-promoting activity of the carcinogenic chemical, as discussed elsewhere in this volume. It is imperative, however, to remember that genetic and epigenetic mechanisms for a chemical are not mutually exclusive. Many of the chemicals shown to have genetic activity also display epigenetic properties undoubtedly important in their carcinogenic or tumor-

POSSIBLE MECHANISMS FOR
DIETHYLSTILBESTROL-INDUCED CARCINOGENICITY

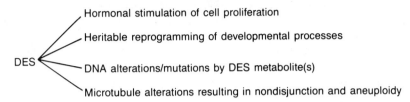

DES

Hormonal stimulation of cell proliferation

Heritable reprogramming of developmental processes

DNA alterations/mutations by DES metabolite(s)

Microtubule alterations resulting in nondisjunction and aneuploidy

Figure 3
Possible genetic and epigenetic mechanisms for DES-induced carcinogenicity.

promoting activity. The thyroid hormone disturbances caused by amitrole (IARC 1974) and the target organ mutagenicity of this chemical are both potential mechanisms that possibly play dual roles in the carcinogenicity of this chemical.

A good example of a carcinogen that possibly operates by a multitude of mechanisms—genetic and epigenetic—is DES. DES can induce genetic changes by two mechanisms, one involving DNA damage and the other involving microtubule malfunction resulting in aneuploidy (Tsutsui et al. 1986). In addition, this chemical is a tumor promoter probably due to its estrogenic properties, and furthermore it can induce heritable, epigenetic changes in developmental processes (Barrett 1987a). All of these mechanisms may be important in DES-induced carcinogenicity (Fig. 3).

CONCLUSION

Certain carcinogens presumed to be nongenotoxic induce morphological and neoplastic transformation of SHE cells in culture (e.g., DES and asbestos). Examination of the mechanism of action of these chemicals revealed that a genetic mechanism, often a chromosomal mutation, is involved. These chemicals also have epigenetic properties that may relate to their tumor-promoting activity. Carcinogenesis is a multistep, multigenic, and multicausal process. As such, both epigenetic and genetic factors are probably important (Barrett 1987b). These mechanisms are not mutually exclusive; rather, they probably work in conjunction during carcinogen-induced neoplastic progression.

REFERENCES

Ashby, J., F. de Serres, M. Draper, M. Ishidate, B. Margolin, B. Matter, and M. Shelby, eds. 1985. Evaluation of short-term tests for carcinogens. In *Report of the international program on chemical safety collaborative study on in vitro assays.* Elsevier/North-Holland, Amsterdam, Netherlands.

Barrett, J.C., ed. 1987a. Relationship between mutagenesis and carcinogenesis. In *Mechanisms of environmental carcinogenesis. Genetic and epigenetic mechanisms of carcinogenesis*, vol. 1. CRC Press, Boca Raton, Florida.

————. 1987b. Genetic and epigenetic mechanism of carcinogenesis. In *Mechanisms of environmental carcinogenesis. Role of genetic and epigenetic changes*, vol. 1. CRC Press, Boca Raton, Florida.

Barrett, J.C. and W.F. Fletcher. 1987. Cellular and molecular mechanisms of multistep neoplastic transformation of cells in culture. In *Mechanisms of environmental carcinogenesis. Multistep models of carcinogenesis* (ed. J.C. Barrett), vol. 2. CRC Press, Boca Raton, Florida. (In press.)

Barrett, J.C. and P.W. Lamb. 1985. Tests with the Syrian hamster embryo cell transformation assay. *Prog. Mutat. Res.* **5:** 623.

Barrett, J.C. and P.O.P. Ts'o. 1978. Evidence for the progressive nature of neoplastic transformation *in vitro*. *Proc. Natl. Acad. Sci.* **75:** 3761.

Barrett, J.C., T.W. Hesterberg, and D.G. Thomassen. 1985a. Use of cell transformation systems for carcinogenicity testing and mechanistic studies of carcinogenesis. *Pharmacol. Rev.* **36:** 53S.

Barrett, J.C., A. Wong, and J.A. McLachlan. 1981. Diethylstilbestrol induces neoplastic transformation without measurable gene mutation at two loci. *Science* **212:** 1402.

Barrett, J.C., T.W. Hesterberg, M. Oshimura, and T. Tsutsui. 1985b. Role of chemically induced mutagenic events in neoplastic transformation of Syrian hamster embryo cells. *Carcinog. Compr. Surv.* **9:** 123.

Berwald, Y. and L. Sachs. 1965. *In vitro* transformation of normal cells to tumor cells by carcinogenic hydrocarbons. *J. Natl. Cancer Inst.* **35:** 641.

Degen, G.H., T.E. Eling, and J.A. McLachlan. 1982. Oxidative metabolism of diethylstilbestrol by prostaglandin synthetase. *Cancer Res.* **42:** 919.

Degen, G.H., A. Wong, T.E. Eling, J.C. Barrett, and J.A. McLachlan. 1983. Involvement of prostaglandin synthetase in the peroxidative metabolism of diethylstilbestrol in Syrian hamster embryo fibroblast cell cultures. *Cancer Res.* **43:** 992.

DiPaolo, J.A., J. Donovan, and R.L. Nelson. 1971. Transformation of hamster cells *in vitro* by polycyclic hydrocarbons without cytotoxicity. *Proc. Natl. Acad. Sci.* **68:** 2958.

Hesterberg, T.W. and J.C. Barrett. 1984. Dependence of asbestos- and mineral dust-induced transformation of mammalian cells in culture on fiber dimension. *Cancer Res.* **44:** 2170.

————. 1985. Induction by asbestos fibers of anaphase abnormalities: Mechanism for aneuploidy induction and possibly carcinogenesis. *Carcinogenesis* **6:** 473.

International Agency for Research on Cancer (IARC). 1974. *Monographs on the evaluation of carcinogenic risk of chemicals to man: Some anti-thyroid and related substances, nitrofurans and industrial chemicals,* vol. 7, p. 31.

————. 1982. *Monograph of the evaluation of the carcinogenic risk of chemicals to humans* (suppl.), vol. 4, p. 50. IARC.

Jones, P. 1987. Role of DNA methylation in regulating gene expression, differentiation and carcinogenesis. In *Mechanisms of environmental carcinogenesis. Role of genetic and epigenetic changes* (ed. J.C. Barrett), vol. 1. CRC Press, Boca Raton, Florida. (In press.)

Kraus, R.S., D.L. Daston, W.J. Caspary, and T.E. Eling. 1986. Peroxidase mediated metabolic activation of the thyroid carcinogen amitrole. *Proc. Am. Assoc. Cancer Res.* **27:** 112.

Lee, T.C., M. Oshimura, and J.C. Barrett. 1985. Comparison of arsenic-induced cell transformation, cytotoxicity, mutation, and chromosome effects in Syrian hamster embryo cells in culture. *Carcinogenesis* **6:** 1421.

Li, S.A., J.K. Klicka, and J.J. Li. 1985. Estrogen 2- and 4-hydroxylase activity, catechol estrogen formation, and implication for estrogen carcinogenesis in the hamster kidney. *Cancer Res.* **45:** 181.

Liehr, J.G. 1983. Modulation of estrogen-induced carcinogenesis by chemical modifications. *Arch. Toxicol.* **56:** 119.

Liehr, J.G., K. Randerath, and E. Randerath. 1985. Target organ-specific covalent DNA damage preceding diethylstilbestrol-induced carcinogenesis. *Carcinogenesis* **6:** 1067.

McLachlan, J.A., A. Wong, G.H. Degen, and J.C. Barrett. 1982. Morphological and neoplastic transformation of Syrian hamster embryo cells by diethylstilbestrol and its analogs. *Cancer Res.* **42:** 3040.

Metzler, M. and J.A. McLachlan. 1981. The metabolism of diethylstilbestrol. *CRC Crit. Rev. Biochem.* **10:** 171.

Mossman, B.T., W.G. Light, and E.T. Wei. 1983. Asbestos: Mechanisms of toxicity and carcinogenicity in the respiratory tract. *Annu. Rev. Pharmacol. Toxicol.* **23:** 595.

Oshimura, M. and J.C. Barrett. 1986. Chemically induced aneuploidy in mammalian cells: Mechanisms and biological significance in cancer. *Environ. Mutagen.* **8:** 129.

Oshimura, M., T.W. Hesterberg, and J.C. Barrett. 1986. An early, nonrandom karyotypic change in immortal Syrian hamster cell lines transformed by asbestos: Trisomy of chromosome 11. *Cancer Genet. Cytogenet.* **22:** 225.

Oshimura, M., T.W. Hesterberg, T. Tsutsui, and J.C. Barrett. 1984. Correlation of asbestos-induced cytogenetic effects with cell transformation of Syrian hamster embryo cells in culture. *Cancer Res.* **44:** 5017.

Pienta, R.J. 1980. Transformation of Syrian hamster embryo cells by diverse chemicals and correlation with their reported carcinogenic and mutagenic activities. *Chem. Mutagens* **6:** 175.

Purdy, R.H. 1984. Carcinogenic potential of estrogen in some mammalian model systems. *Prog. Cancer Res. Ther.* **31:** 401.

Sato, Y., T. Murai, M. Tsumuraya, H. Saito, and M. Kodama. 1984. Disruptive effects of diethylstilbestrol in microtubules. *Gann* **75:** 1046.

Sharp, D.C. and J.M. Parry. 1985. Diethylstilbestrol: The binding and effects of diethylstilbestrol upon the polymerization of purified microtubule protein *in vitro*. *Carcinogenesis* **6:** 865.

Tsutsui, T., H. Maizumi, and J.C. Barrett. 1984a. Amitrole-induced cell transformation and gene mutations in Syrian hamster embryo cells in culture. *Mutat. Res.* **140:** 205.

Tsutsui, T., H. Maizumi, J.A. McLachlan, and J.C. Barrett. 1983. Aneuploidy induction and cell transformation by diethylstilbestrol: A possible chromosome mechanism in carcinogenesis. *Cancer Res.* **43:** 3814.

Tsutsui, T., N. Suzuki, H. Maizumi, J.A. McLachlan, and J.C. Barrett. 1986. Alteration in diethylstilbestrol-induced mutagenicity and cell transformation by exogenous metabolic activation. *Carcinogenesis* **7**: 1415.

Tsutsui, T., G.H. Degen, D. Schiffman, A. Wong, H. Maizumi, J.A. McLachlan, and J.C. Barrett. 1984b. Dependence of exogenous metabolic activation for induction of unscheduled DNA synthesis in Syrian hamster embryo cells by diethylstilbestrol and related compounds. *Cancer Res.* **44**: 184.

Tu, A., W. Hallowell, S. Pallotta, A. Sivak, R.A. Lubet, R.D. Curren, M.D. Avery, C. Jones, B.A. Sedita, E. Huberman, R. Tennant, J. Spalding, and R.E. Koury. 1986. An interlaboratory comparison of transformation in Syrian hamster embryo cells with model and coded chemicals. *Environ. Mutagen.* **8**: 77.

Tucker, R.W. and J.C. Barrett. 1986. Decreased numbers of spindle and cytoplasmic microtubules in hamster embryo cells treated with a carcinogen, diethylstilbestrol. *Cancer Res.* **46**: 2088.

Wagner, J.C., G. Berry, J.W. Skidmore, and V. Timbrell. 1974. The effects of the inhalation of asbestos in rats. *Br. J. Cancer* **29**: 252.

COMMENTS

COHEN: You mentioned the effects of DES, without the liver microsomes having an effect, that may not be due to metabolic activation. But, as you said, SHE cells have high levels of prostaglandin synthetase. DES is readily oxidized by that enzyme. Do you have any evidence for or against that enzyme's role in the effect of DES?

BARRETT: We have shown that DES is metabolized by the SHE cells to primarily (exclusively, to our ability to detect it) Z,Z-dienestrol, which is mediated by prostaglandin synthetase. There is a correlation between the ability of certain DES-related compounds to be metabolized and their ability to transform the cells. That is suggestive evidence that, indeed, metabolism might be playing a role. But, we have been unable to add either inhibitors or enhancers of metabolic activation and show an appropriate effect on a transformation, with perhaps the exception of the rat liver microsomes, where we see a large quantitative increase in that one metabolite; there are qualitative changes in metabolic activation also. So, it is still unclear to us whether with liver microsomes the transformation is going through other metabolites or whether we are just getting more of the essential metabolites that are there in the absence of the rat liver microsomes but in insufficient amounts.

ROE: In your final slide, you identified DES as a specific chromosomal mutagen. Have you got comparable data for 17β-estradiol?

BARRETT: What we know is that it induces transformation and induces nondisjunction. Aneuploidy, of course, is a consequence of the nondisjunction; so, yes, we have evidence that it is a chromosomal mutagen.

ROE: So, you have found nothing that distinguishes DES from 17β-estradiol?

BARRETT: In these measurements, yes. Their doses are slightly different. DES is effective at slightly lower doses.

ROE: When you say dose, do you mean concentration?

BARRETT: Yes.

PITOT: Ten micrograms per milliliter is a fairly high concentration of estrogen.

BARRETT: Right. We can see it at much lower doses. That's at the peak. The dose-response curves are interesting in that they are much shallower than benzo[a]pyrene. They are linear, but the slope is less than 1. Whereas with benzo[a]pyrene it is 1, with DES it's 0.3. We still see effects at very low doses of DES, 1 ng/ml, for instance. The effects go up very slowly with dose. That is true for the effects of aneuploidy induction as well as transformation.

PITOT: It is possible that the SHE system is peculiar. Is there evidence that these compounds induce aneuploidy in the same way in vivo, in mammals for example?

BARRETT: There is evidence that the early preneoplastic lesions of the cervix following exposure to estrogens and DES are aneuploid, but it's not clear whether that is a cause or an effect. But it is really very difficult to measure, of course, aneuploidy induction in vivo.

PITOT: Is DES or other estrogens positive in the in vivo bone marrow micronucleus test?

BARRETT: In bone marrow there is some evidence, although conflicting, that it induces cytogenetic effects in vivo.

MAGEE: Could you remind me what the animal carcinogenicity data are for DES?

BARRETT: DES is carcinogenic in the newborn mice, causing tumors very similar to what is seen in humans if the mice are treated during the right gestational period. It is also carcinogenic to the hamster kidney, and there carcinogenicity does not correlate with estrogenicity, even though the tumors that are induced are estrogen-dependent. Thus, an epigenetic effect plays a role in the carcinogenicity of the hamster kidney, but that isn't sufficient because there are estrogenic compounds that are not carcinogenic. Recently, Kurt Randerath has actually identified adducts formed in the hamster kidney following DES exposure which are not observed in nontarget tissues. That would be consistent with a mutagenic event. Also, if you modify metabolism with α-naphthoflavone, you can make DES carcinogenic to the hamster liver.

PITOT: Estrogen is a good promoting agent in the liver.

BARRETT: That's right. The studies I mentioned were examples of estrogens as complete carcinogens. There are a number of examples, on the other hand, where estrogen can act as a classical promoter; that is, in the liver as well as in the vagina, it has been shown that after treatment with an initiator, estrogens are promoters in the classical sense. Thus, it can work as an epigenetic carcinogen. I think this is not at all mutually exclusive with it acting as a mutagenic carcinogen. Quite the contrary, when a compound has multiple mechanisms of action, there is all the more reason to consider it to be a good carcinogen.

ROE: Personally, I do not automatically regard natural chemicals as safe. Nevertheless, does it not worry you a bit that something like a natural hormone, such as 17β-estradiol, gives a positive result, which you are prepared to accept as evidence of chromosomal mutagenicity? You said, in answer to my earlier question, that this is so. Does it not make you suspicious that your test system isn't giving you useful information, when you have a natural hormone which is normally present in blood and normally endogenously produced in the body and which ends up being classified as a mutagen? Doesn't that worry you?

BARRETT: No. There is evidence that it is a mutagen in vivo. It's very difficult to demonstrate conclusively mutagenicity in vivo, but it's certainly possible that it's causing similar effects.

ROE: I give up! I thought that common sense counted for something!

Genotoxic Oxidant Tumor Promoters

PETER A. CERUTTI
Department of Carcinogenesis
Swiss Institute for Experimental Cancer Research
Lausanne, Switzerland

INTRODUCTION

Researchers usually agree that DNA damage and the resulting sequence changes (i.e., "genotoxicity") play a role in early steps in carcinogenesis. Support for this contention derives from the observations that there exists a good correlation between mutagenic and carcinogenic potencies of a majority of xenobiotic initiators and that point mutations, gene rearrangements, and gene amplification can result in the activation of certain oncogenes (Bishop et al. 1984). In contrast, it is often felt that later events, in particular tumor promotion, occur by epigenetic mechanisms (Hecker et al. 1982). Indeed, many tumor promoters are not inducing DNA damage in the usual test systems, and the benign mouse skin papillomas induced by two-step (initiation-promotion) protocols are usually devoid of any gross cytogenetic abnormalities. Genetic instability, which is reflected in multiple chromosomal aberrations, is characteristic for the progression stage in which benign tumors become more aggressive, invade surrounding tissues, and may metastasize.

The paradigm that tumor promoters such as 12-O-tetradecanoylphorbol-13-acetate (TPA) act exclusively by "nongenotoxic" mechanisms has been seriously questioned over the last few years (Emerit and Cerutti 1981; Cerutti et al. 1983; Cerutti 1985). For example, TPA induces abundant chromosomal aberrations in mouse epidermal cells treated in culture (Dzarlieva-Petrusevska and Fusenig 1985) and in situ in mouse skin (N. Fusenig, pers. comm.). Further support for the suspicion that TPA may cause chromosomal changes in mouse skin derives from the observation that it induces irreversible, hereditary changes (Fürstenberger et al. 1983; Cerutti 1985). Bona fide oxidant promoters (e.g., benzoylperoxide, organic hydroperoxides, superoxide, autooxidized anthralin [DiGiovanni, this volume] induce DNA strand breakage with high efficiency.

Indirect effects of promoters are not always detectable in simple cell-culture systems. In many instances, promoters may cause chromosomal damage in target cells via the intermediacy of clastogenic materials released from the surrounding tissue (Emerit and Cerutti 1982, 1983; Cerutti et al. 1983). In particular, inflammatory phagocytes can play a role. Indeed, the infiltration of polymorphonuclear leukocytes, and later of macrophages, has been adjudged to be necessary (but not sufficient) for mouse skin promotion (Slaga et al. 1981a; Lewis and Adams 1985), and in a recent comparative study with genetically different mouse strains, a striking relationship could be observed between promotability by phorbol esters and the extent of promoter-induced inflammation (DiGiovanni et al. 1986). Inflammation is likely to participate in lung carcinogenesis by tobacco smoke and mineral fibers, in certain forms of breast cancer, in malignancies at the site of chronic osteomyelitic infections, in certain rheumatoid inflammatory diseases with increased cancer incidence, etc. Upon stimulation by xenobiotics or certain endogenous promoters, phagocytes react with an oxidative burst, i.e., the production of short-lived forms of active oxygen (Volkman 1984), the release of metastable diffusible clastogenic factor (CF) (Emerit and Cerutti 1982, 1983), and a host of paracrine mediators including prostaglandins, thromboxanes, leukotrienes, complement components, lytic enzymes, tumor necrosis factor, and monokines (Volkman 1984). Whereas active oxygen has the capability to cause chromosomal damage in initiated cells in the immediate vicinity (Goldstein et al. 1980; Dutton and Bowden 1985; Lewis and Adams 1985), CF can exert long-range effects and appear in the blood serum (Emerit 1982; Emerit and Cerutti 1982, 1983; Emerit et al. 1982). The formation of CF is not restricted to phagocytic cells. Even noninitiated epithelial-cells and mesenchymal cells have the potential to release clastogenic components following exposure to oxidants (Cerutti 1986).

It follows that tumor promotion must be considered a tissue phenomenon to which initiated and noninitiated epithelial cells, surrounding fibroblasts, inflammatory leukocytes, etc., contribute. In many cases, promoters interact with the initiated cell itself; in others, they mostly disturb short- and long-range cellular interactions. Multiple cellular and molecular mechanisms contribute to the end result, and their relative importance depends on the promoters and the tissue. Some mechanisms may be obligatory; others may merely facilitate the process. Major mechanisms are (1) modulation of the expression of growth- and differentiation-related genes, which may result from the direct interaction of the promoter with the target cell or from the action of paracrine or clastogenic mediators that originate from non-target cells; and (2) selective toxicity to the noninitiated surrounding tissue by the promoter itself or by clastogenic mediators from non-target cells, in particular inflammatory leukocytes. In view of the complexity of the situation, it is reasonable to conclude that both genotoxic and nongenotoxic mechanisms are likely to contribute to tumor promotion and that their relative importance depends on the promoter and the particular tissue. For oxidant promoters, which are emphasized in this paper, there is ample evidence that they induce DNA damage. Although this does not necessarily imply that this damage plays a crucial role for their promotional activity, it should be noted that DNA breaks per se, when induced by liposome-encapsulated DNase I, sufficed to transform Syrian hamster embryo cells (Zajac-Kaye and Ts'o 1984).

PROMOTER-INDUCED PROOXIDANT STATES AND BONA FIDE OXIDANT PROMOTERS

The participation of prooxidant states (i.e., increased stationary concentrations of intracellular active oxygen) in carcinogenesis is well documented (Cerutti 1985).

There are numerous mechanisms by which xenobiotics can induce prooxidant states either by causing the overproduction of active oxygen or by inhibiting its elimination. Regardless of the mechanism of formation, prooxidant states appear to exert a promotional and/or progressional effect on initiated target cells, whereas antioxidants are anticarcinogenic in many systems (Kozumbo and Cerutti 1986). In the simplest case, the initiated tissue is directly exposed to exogenous active oxygen, organic peroxides, and radicals. For initiated mouse skin, the following peroxides were found to possess promotional activity: peroxyacetic acid, chlorobenzoic acid, benzoylperoxide, decanoylperoxide, cumenehydroperoxide, p-nitrobenzoic acid, and H_2O_2 (Slaga et al. 1981b, 1983); for cultured mouse epidermal cells JB6 (clone 41), the list additionally includes IO_4^- and superoxide ion O_2^- (Nakamura et al. 1985). Recent results from O'Connell et al. (this volume) indicate that benzoylperoxide also acts as a potent progressor, stimulating the conversion of benign mouse skin papilloma to carcinoma. Oxidants also exert promotional and/or cocarcinogenic effects in lung tumorigenesis. For example, exposure of DMBA-treated rats to hyperbaric oxygen (Heston and Pratt 1959) or ozone (Hussein et al. 1985) increased the tumor yield. Even the normal air that we breathe may not be completely inert because molecular oxygen is always contaminated with minute traces of active oxygen.

The mechanism of action of oxidants in carcinogenesis is unknown. Presumably, it differs substantially from that of the most intensively studied phorbol ester promoters, which act on the signal transduction pathway of polypeptide hormones and growth factors (Berridge and Irvine 1984; Nishizuka 1984). Oxidant promoters are expected to cause ubiquitous damage to the cellular constituents. Lipids are particularly sensitive to oxidation, and the destruction of the structural and functional integrity of the plasma membrane could play a role in the inhibition of cell-cell communication by oxidant promoters (Slaga et al. 1981b). Support for this notion derives from the mouse epidermal cell JB6 system. Srinivas and collaborators demonstrated that exposure to oxidants (Srinivas and Colburn 1984) or TPA (Srinivas et al. 1982) leads to the rapid disappearance of the surface ganglioside GT_1 in the promotable clone 41, but not in the promotion-resistant clone 30 (Srinivas and Colburn 1984). It is also conceivable that oxidants affect growth factors and growth factor receptors and disturb the auto- and paracrine homeostasis of the tissue. Candidates that may be particularly sensitive are TGF-β and protein kinase C (the phorbol ester receptor), which contain cysteine-rich domains.

Oxidants set in motion a cascade of secondary reactions that could play a role in carcinogenesis. Like several polypeptide growth factors, they activate membrane phospholipase A_2 (and C?). Whereas growth factors release the lipase from its inhibition by lipocortin (Wallner et al. 1986), oxidants may stimulate the enzyme because the oxidation of surface components results in the disturbance of the native conformation of the plasma membrane (Yasuda and Fujika 1977). In both cases, large amounts of free arachidonic acid become available to the metabolic enzymes.

Furthermore, oxidants at low concentrations activate cyclooxygenase (Hemler et al. 1979) and lipoxygenase, which are the key enzymes of the arachidonic acid cascade. The hydroperoxy-arachidonic acid metabolites prostaglandin G_2, 15-hydroperoxy-prostaglandin E_2, and hydroperoxy-5,8,11,13-icosatetraenoic acid (HPETES) are formed as metastable intermediates on the pathways to prostaglandins, thromboxanes, and leukotrienes. They have the potential to further activate cyclooxygenase and lipoxygenase in a feedback loop. This intricately tuned "trigger-amplification" system (Lands 1984) results in the overproduction of hydroperoxy-arachidonic acid derivatives that possess clastogenic activity (see below). As a model for lung carcinogenesis, we have compared the stimulation of the arachidonic acid cascade by superoxide (produced extracellularly with xanthine/xanthine-oxidase) and TPA in human epithelioid lung tumor cells A549. Both agents strongly stimulated the cyclooxygenase pathway, resulting in the formation of prostaglandins E_2 and $F_2\alpha$ and of a mixture of as yet unidentified metabolites that may contain prostaglandins A_2 and B_1. Free arachidonic acid increased only moderately, and there was no evidence for the overproduction of lipoxygenase products (I. Zbinden et al., unpubl.). This is in contrast to human TPA-stimulated monocytes, which secreted increased amounts of prostaglandins, thromboxane, HHT, and HETES (hydroxy-arachidonic acids) and a large amount of free arachidonic acid (Cerutti 1985; Kozumbo et al. 1987). Superoxide, H_2O_2, and *tert*-butylhydroperoxide also stimulated prostaglandin synthesis in pig aorta endothelial cells (Ager and Gordon 1984) and lung fibroblasts (Taylor et al. 1983). It should be noted that the overproduction of prostaglandins E_2 and $F_2\alpha$ has been adjudged to be necessary for the induction and maintenance of hyperproliferation in TPA-treated mouse skin (Fürstenberger et al. 1984).

CLASTOGENIC ACTION OF ARACHIDONIC ACID HYDROPEROXIDES

As mentioned above, the biosynthesis of stable arachidonic acid metabolites proceeds via the intermediacy of hydroperoxy- derivatives. These intermediates are metastable in aqueous solutions (half-life times range from a few minutes to an hour). In contrast to active oxygen species, they possess a sufficient radius of action in the tissue to reach cells that are remote from the site of their generation. Indeed, under certain conditions, hydroperoxy-fatty acids can be detected in the blood serum. We had shown previously that TPA stimulated human monocytes to release a diffusible, low-molecular-weight CF (Emerit and Cerutti 1983) that contains, among other metabolites, sizable amounts of 5,11 and 15-hydroperoxy-arachidonic acid (5,11- and 15-HPETE) (Cerutti 1985; Kozumbo et al. 1987). We therefore measured the capacity of synthetic HPETES to induce DNA single-strand breaks in mouse embryo fibroblasts C3H/10T1/2. Using the alkaline elution and alkaline unwinding assay, we found that HPETES induced DNA breaks regardless of the position of the hydroperoxy- group. Figure 1 shows the dose-response curves for

DNA breakage by 15-HPETE and aerobic γ-rays as measured by alkaline elution. From the comparison with γ-rays, we estimate that 15-HPETE induces breaks with an efficiency of $0.75 \pm 0.1 \times 10^{10}$ dalton^{-1} μM^{-1} (15-min treatment at 37° C). Higher efficiency was observed at doses below 10 μM (Ochi and Cerutti 1987).

Insight into the breakage mechanism was obtained in experiments with chelators of iron and calcium. Desferrioxamine, an extracellular chelator of Fe^{+++}, inhibited 15-HPETE-induced breakage by approximately 40%. It appears likely that alkoxy radicals are formed from HPETE in Fe^{++}-catalyzed reactions. Alkoxy radicals are lipophilic and expected to penetrate readily the plasma membrane. Alternatively, desferrioxamine-inhibitable DNA breakage by HPETE might be due to cooxygenation reactions (Marnett and Reed 1979; Dix and Marnett 1983; Reed et al. 1984). Peroxy- radicals can serve as the ultimate oxygen donors in peroxidase-catalyzed reactions. The observation that extracellular CuZn-superoxide dismutase and catalase had no effect on HPETE-induced DNA breakage is compatible with the above mechanisms (Ochi and Cerutti 1987). An additional 40% of the HPETE-induced DNA breakage was inhibited by the extra- and intracellular Ca^{++} chelators EGTA and Quin 2. The following observations suggest that Ca^{++}-dependent DNA breakage might be due to the activation of a Ca^{++} (Mg^{++})-dependent endonuclease (Yoshihara et al. 1975). We have recently found that HPETE mobilizes mitochondrial Ca^{++} with particular efficiency. This

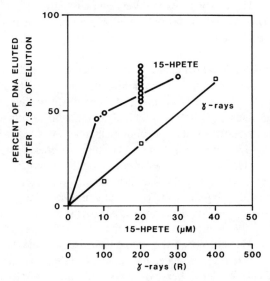

Figure 1

Dose-response curves for the formation of DNA strand breaks (alkali-labile sites) by 15-HPETE and aerobic α-rays in mouse embryo fibroblasts C3H/10T1/2 as determined by alkaline elution.

reaction entails a decrease in mitochondrial glutathione, an increase in nicotinamide-adenine-dinucleotide (NAD), and the stimulation of NAD hydrolysis. ADP-ribosylation of the Ca^{++}/proton antiport and/or the inactivation of a Ca^{++}ATPase then results in the release of mitochondrial Ca^{++} (C. Richter et al., unpubl.). A consecutive increase in cytosolic and nuclear Ca^{++} may result in the activation of certain lysosomal and nuclear enzymes (Smith et al. 1985). It is expected that prostaglandin-hydroperoxides (e.g., 15-hydroperoxy-prostaglandin E_2 and prostaglandin G_2) and organic hydroperoxides with promotional activity may act in a similar fashion.

Our results with HPETES are particularly relevant to the role of inflammation in tumor promotion (see Introduction). It may be interesting to note that stable prostaglandin-endoperoxide analogs (U-46619 and U-44069) possessed promotional activity on mouse skin (Lupulescu 1984) and HPETES induced ornithine decarboxylase in rat colonic mucosa (Bull et al. 1984).

INDUCTION OF POLY-ADP-RIBOSYLATION OF CHROMOSOMAL PROTEINS BY OXIDANT PROMOTERS

The posttranslational phosphorylation of proteins plays a central role in the mechanism of action of polypeptide growth factors, hormones, and phorbol-ester-type promoters. Although certain physiological substrates have been identified for the protein kinases participating in these reactions, the pathways that ultimately result in the modulation of gene expression remain obscure. The phosphorylation of topoisomerase II by protein kinase C could play a role (Sahyoun et al. 1986).

We have proposed a working hypothesis involving poly-ADP-ribosylation in the mechanism of action of oxidant promoters (Cerutti 1985). The following characteristics of poly-ADP-ribose make it an attractive candidate: (1) Poly-ADP-ribosylation is a nuclear reaction that modifies chromosomal proteins (Althaus et al. 1985). (2) Poly-ADP-ribose is synthesized from NAD residues by the action of ADP-ribose transferase. (3) Exposure of cells to oxidants results in a diminution of the cellular reducing power and a concomitant increase in NAD, which serves as the substrate for the ADP-ribose transferase. (4) The transferase is stimulated by DNA containing strand breaks. As discussed above, oxidant promoters cause DNA breaks and probably other types of DNA and chromosomal damage.

We have tested this hypothesis in promotable mouse epidermal cells JB6, clone 41. For these cells, several oxidants such as benzoylperoxide, IO_4^-, and MnO_4^- have been shown to possess promotional activity. We have recently found that the exposure of clone 41, but not of the promoter-resistant clone 30, to a single burst of extracellular superoxide (produced by xanthine/xanthine-oxidase) had a moderate promotional effect. A single burst of superoxide also efficiently induced DNA strand breakage and poly-ADP-ribosylation of nuclear proteins in these cells. In the context of our mechanistic studies of Ca^{++} mobilization and DNA breakage by

HPETE (see above), it was of particular interest that the Ca^{++} chelator Quin 2 completely suppressed the stimulation of poly-ADP-ribosylation by superoxide but not by the alkylating agent N-methyl-N'-nitro-N-nitrosoguanidine (D. Mühlematter and P. Cerutti, unpubl.). The latter observation suggests that the inhibition by Quin 2 was not due to the inactivation of ADP-ribosyl transferase, which is known to require CA^{++} for full activity. At present, we do not know which chromosomal proteins serve as poly-ADP-ribose acceptors following treatment with oxidant promoters. We had shown previously that TPA induces poly-ADP-ribosylation of nuclear proteins in mouse embryo fibroblasts C3H/10T1/2 in a reaction that was inhibitable by CuZn superoxide dismutase and catalase (Singh et al. 1985a). Acceptor proteins in C3H/10T1/2 cells were the core histones H2B, A24, and H3d (Singh and Cerutti 1985) and numerous medium- and high-molecular-weight nonhistone proteins. The major acceptor was ADP-ribose transferase itself and its proteolytic fragments of 20–25, 45, and 72–95 kD (Singh et al. 1985b). It should be noted that TPA-induced poly-ADP-ribosylation, in contrast to bona fide oxidant promoters, was not accompanied by any detectable DNA strand breakage (Singh et al. 1985a).

ACKNOWLEDGMENTS

This work was supported by the Swiss National Science Foundation and the Swiss Association of Cigarette Manufacturers.

REFERENCES

Ager, A. and J. Gordon. 1984. Differential effects of hydrogen peroxide on indices of endothelial cell function. *J. Exp. Med.* **159:** 592.

Althaus, F., H. Hilz, and S. Shall, eds. 1985. *ADP-ribosylation Proteins.* Springer Verlag, New York.

Berridge, M. and R. Irvine. 1984. Inositol triphosphate, a novel second messenger in cellular single transduction. *Nature* **312:** 315.

Bishop, M., J. Rowley, and M. Greaves, eds. 1984. *Genes and cancer.* A.R. Liss, New York.

Bull, A., N. Nigro, W. Golembieski, J. Crissman, and L. Marnett. 1984. In vivo stimulation of DNA-synthesis and induction of ornithine decarboxylase in rat colon by fatty acid hydroperoxides, autoxidation products unsaturated fatty acids. *Cancer Res.* **44:** 4924.

Cerutti, P. 1985. Prooxidant states and tumor promotion. *Science* **227:** 375.

———. 1986. Oxidant tumor promoters. In *Growth factors, tumor promoters and cancer genes* (ed. N. Colburn et al.). A.R. Liss, New York. (In press.)

Cerutti, P., I. Emerit, and P. Amstad. 1983. Membrane mediated chromosomal damage. In *Genes and proteins in oncogenesis* (ed. I.B. Weinstein and H.J. Vogel), p. 55. Academic Press, New York.

DiGiovanni, J., K. Chenicek, and M.W. Ewing. 1986. Skin tumor promotion susceptibility in inbred mouse strains. *J. Cell. Biochem. Suppl.* **10C:** 163 (Abstr. L189).

Dix, T. and L. Marnett. 1983. Metabolism of polycyclic aromatic hydrocarbon derivatives to ultimate carcinogens during lipid peroxidation. *Science* **221**: 77.

Dutton, D. and G. Bowden. 1985. Indirect induction of a clastogenic effect in epidermal cells by a tumor promoter. *Carcinogenesis* **6**: 1279.

Dzarlieva-Petrusevska R. and N. Fusenig. 1985. Tumor promoter 12-0-tetradecanoylphorbol-13-acetate (TPA) induced chromosome aberrations in mouse keratinocyte cells lines: A possible genetic mechanism of tumor promotion. *Carcinogenesis* **6**: 1447.

Emerit, I. 1982. Chromosome breakage factors: Origin and possible significance *Prog. Mutat. Res.* **4**: 61.

Emerit, I. and P. Cerutti. 1981. Tumor promoter phorbol-12-myristate-13-acetate induces chromosomal damage via indirect action. *Nature* **293**: 144.

————. 1982. Tumor promoter phorbol-12-myristate-13-acetate induces a clastogenic factor in human lymphocytes. *Proc. Natl. Acad. Sci. U.S.A.* **79**: 7509.

————. 1983. Clastogenic action of tumor promoter phorbol-12-myristate-13-acetate in mixed human leukocyte cultures. *Carcinogenesis* **4**: 1313.

Emerit, I., P. Jalbert, and P. Cerutti. 1982. Chromosome breakage factor in the plasma of two Bloom Syndrome patients. *Hum. Genet.* **61**: 68.

Fürstenberger, G., B. Sorg, and F. Marks. 1983. Tumor promotion by phorbolesters in skin: Evidence for a memory effect. *Science* **220**: 89.

Fürstenberger, G., M. Gross, and F. Marks. 1984. Involvement of prostaglandins in the process of skin tumor promotion. In *Icosanoids and cancer* (ed. H. Thaler-Dao et al.), p. 91. Raven Press, New York.

Goldstein, B., G. Witz, M. Amoruso, D. Stone, and W. Troll. 1980. Retinoid inhibition of superoxide amion radical production by human PMN stimulated by tumor promoters. *Biochem. Biophys. Res. Commun.* **97**: 883.

Hecker, E., N. Fusenig, W. Kunz, F. Marks, and H. Thielmann, eds. 1982. *Carcinog. Compr. Surv.* **7**.

Hemler, M., H. Cook, and W. Lands. 1979. Prostaglandin biosynthesis can be triggered by lipid peroxides. *Arch. Biochem. Biophys.* **193**: 340.

Heston, W. and A. Pratt. 1959. Effect of concentration of oxygen on occurrence of pulmonary tumors in strain A mice. *J. Natl. Cancer Inst.* **22**: 707.

Hussein, M., M. Mustafa, Q. Ghani, and R. Bhataagar. 1985. Stimulation of poly (ADP-ribose) synthetase activity in the lungs of mice exposed to a low level of ozone. *Arch. Biochem. Biophys.* **241**: 477.

Kozumbo, W. and P. Cerutti. 1986. Antioxidants as antitumor promoters. In *Mechanisms of antimutagenesis and anticarcinogenesis* (ed. A. Hollaender et al.), p. 491. Plenum Press, New York.

Kozumbo, W., D. Mühlematter, A. Jörg, I. Emerit, and P. Cerutti. 1987. Phorbol ester-induced formation of clastogenic factor from human monocytes. *Carcinogenesis* **8**: 521.

Lands, W. 1984. Biological consequences of fatty acid oxygenase mechanisms. *Prostaglandins Leukotrienes Med.* **13**: 35.

Lewis, J. and O. Adams. 1985. Induction of 5,6-ring saturated thymine bases in NIH-3T3 cells by phorbol ester-stimulated macrophages: Role of reactive oxygen intermediates. *Cancer Res.* **45**: 1270.

Lupulescu, A. 1984. Tumorigenic potential of endoperoxide analogs. *Experientia* **40:** 209.

Marnett, L. and G. Reed. 1979. Peroxidatic oxidation of benzo(a)pyrene and prostaglandin synthesis. *Biochemistry* **18:** 2923.

Nakamura, Y., N. Colburn, and T. Gindhart. 1985. Role of reactive oxygen in tumor promotion: Implication of superoxide anion in promotion of neoplastic transformation in JB6 cells by TPA. *Carcinogenesis* **6:** 229.

Nishizuka, Y. 1984. The role of protein Kinase C in cell surface signal transduction and tumor production. *Nature* **308:** 693.

Ochi, T. and P. Cerutti. 1987. Clastogenic action of hydroperoxy-5,8,11,-13-icosatetraenoic acids on the mouse embryo fibroblasts C3H/10T1/2. *Proc. Natl. Acad. Sci.* **84:** 990.

Reed, G., E. Brooks, and T.E. Eling. 1984. Phenylbutazone-dependent epoxidation of 7,8-dihydroxy-7,8-dihydrobenzo(a)pyrene. *J. Biol. Chem.* **259:** 5591.

Sahyoun, N., M. Wolf, J. Besterman, T.S. Hsieh, M. Sander, H. LeVine III, K.J. Chang, and P. Cuatrecasas. 1986. Protein Kinase C phosphorylates topoisomerase. II. Topoisomerase activation and its possible role in phorbol ester-induced differentiation of HL-60 cells. *Proc. Natl. Acad. Sci. U.S.A.* **83:** 1603.

Singh, N. and P. Cerutti. 1985. Poly ADP-ribosylation of histones in tumor promoter phorbol-12-myristate-13-acetate treated mouse embryo fibroblasts C3H101/2. *Biochem. Biophys. Res. Commun.* **132:** 811.

Singh, N., G. Poirier, and P. Cerutti. 1985a. Tumor promoter phorbol-12-myristate-13-acetate induces poly ADP-ribosylation in fibroblasts. *Eur. Mol. Biol. Organ. J.* **4:** 1491.

Singh, N., Y. Leduc, G. Poirier, and P. Cerutti. 1985b. Non-histone chromosomal protein acceptors for poly ADP-ribose in phorbol-12-myristate-13-acetate treated mouse embryo fibroblasts (C3H10T1/2) *Carcinogenesis* **6:** 1459.

Slaga, T., V. Solanki, and M. Logani. 1983. Studies on the mechanism of action of antitumor promoting agents: Suggestive evidence for the involvement of free radicals in promotion. In *Radioprotectors and anticarcinogens* (ed. O. Nygaard and M. Simic), p. 471. Academic Press, New York.

Slaga, T., S. Fisher, C. Weeks, and A. Klein-Szanto. 1981a. Cellular and biochemical mechanisms of mouse skin tumor promoters. In *Reviews in biochemical toxicology* (ed. E. Hodgson et al.), vol. II. Elsevier/North-Holland, New York.

Slaga, T., A. Klein-Szanto, L. Triplett, L. Jotti, and J. Trosko. 1981b. Skin tumor-promoting activity of benzoylperoxide a widely used free-radical generator. *Science* **213:** 1023.

Smith, M., C. Evans, H. Thor, and S. Orrenius. 1985. Quinone-induced oxidative injury to cells and tissues. In *Oxidative stress* (ed. H. Sies), p. 91. Academic Press, New York.

Srinivas, L. and N. Colburn. 1984. Preferential oxidation of cell surface sialic acid by periodate leads to promotion of transformation in JB6 cells. *Carcinogenesis* **5:** 515.

Srinivas, L., T. Gindhart, and N. Colburn. 1982. Tumor promoter resistant cells lack trisialoganglioside response. *Proc. Natl. Acad. Sci. U.S.A.* **79:** 4988.

Taylor, L., M. Menconi, and P. Polgar. 1983. The participation of hydroperoxides and oxygen radicals in the control of prostaglandin synthesis. *J. Biol. Chem.* **258:** 6855.

Volkman, A., ed. 1984. *Mononuclear phagocyte biology.* Marcel Dekker, New York.

Wallner, B., R. Mattaliano, C. Hession, R. Cate, R. Tizard, L. Sinclair, C. Foeller, E. Pingchang Chow, J. Browning, K. Ramachandran, and R. Pepinsky. 1986. Cloning and expression of human lipocortin, a phospholipase A_2 inhibitor with potential anti-inflammatory activity. *Nature* **320**: 77.

Yasuda, M. and T. Fujika. 1977. Phospholipase activation by membrane oxidation. *J. Pharmacol.* **27**: 429.

Yoshihara, Y., L. Tanigawa, L. Burzio, and S. Koide. 1975. Evidence for adenosine diphosphate ribosylation of Ca^{2+} Mg^2-dependent endonuclease. *Proc. Natl. Acad. Sci. U.S.A.* **72**: 289.

Zajac-Kaye, M. and P. Ts'o. 1984. DNase I encapsulated in liposomes can induce neoplastic transformation of syrian hamster embryo cells in culture. *Cell* **39**: 427.

COMMENTS

COHEN: Although there is an inflammatory reaction with TPA and many of the skin promoters, in most other tissues where you have promotion, inflammation doesn't play a role—certainly not in the bladder; I don't know about the liver and the kidney.

CERUTTI: You really don't observe inflammation in bladder tumorigenesis?

COHEN: You don't see an inflammatory reaction, certainly not an influx of poly's or macrophages.

CERUTTI: I think that inflammation can contribute to transformation. For instance, there exists a very good correlation between inflammatory infiltration and promotability with TPA of different mouse strains. I just heard convincing data from Dr. DiGiovanni. Another example is lung carcinogenesis, where carcinomas often arise at bronchial bifurcations. That is also where the highest degree of inflammation occurs. There are other examples. In osteomyelitis, sarcomas are induced at increased frequencies, probably because of the chronic inflammatory process. There is Crohn's disease, chronic ileocolitis where tumorigenesis is apparently related to inflammation. In summary, there are many examples supporting a role of inflammation in carcinogenesis, but I do not think it is a prerequisite.

YAMASAKI: Is the poly-ADP-ribosylation induction transient with TPA?

CERUTTI: With TPA, we found that an in vitro cell-culture system it reached a maximum within about 3 hours and then decreased.

YAMASAKI: JB6 cell transformation is an irreversible step. How do you reconcile this reversible effect with the reversible effect on ribosylation?

CERUTTI: As I have shown, active oxygen induces DNA strand breaks in JB6. DNA strand breaks can induce the system for poly-ADP-ribosylation, which finally may change gene expression in a transitory fashion, as you indicated. There are two effects. There is the induction of single-strand breaks, which can be related to poly-ADP-ribosylation—they are repaired, of course, rapidly—by being a cofactor for the poly-ADP-synthetase, but that is a transitory effect.

BARRETT: I'm somewhat confused about the C3H/10T1/2 results. Weitzman reported that neutrophils activated by TPA were complete transforming agents, and you reported that xanthine/xanthine-oxidase was a promoter only. How do you reconcile that?

CERUTTI: No, it is not a promoter only. The data of Weitzman et al. and ourselves agree very nicely. In our work and theirs, xanthine/xanthine-oxidase is a weak complete carcinogen. Weitzman et al. only studied this effect, whereas we emphasized promotion.

Session 7:
Regulatory Considerations

Some Implications and Limitations of in Vitro Genetic Toxicity Data in Regulatory Decisions

RAYMOND W. TENNANT
Cellular and Genetic Toxicology Branch
National Toxicology Program
National Institute of Environmental Health Sciences
Research Triangle Park, North Carolina 27709

INTRODUCTION

The principal sources of results that are currently used to identify potential carcinogens are studies conducted in rodents. The National Toxicology Program (NTP) uses two rodent species, generally B6C3F$_1$ hybrid strain mice and Fischer 344 (F344) inbred strain rats, in studies that are conducted in accord with established toxicological principles (NTP Report 1984; Huff et al. 1986). Among these principles is the requirement that animals be exposed to high enough concentrations of a chemical for a duration sufficient to detect a response in the relatively limited numbers of animals used (50 animals of each sex/species at each concentration). In other words, the ability to detect a potential low frequency of tumor induction is limited by the numbers of animals that can be used due to economic and logistical constraints. Therefore, a chemical is administered at an estimated maximum tolerated dose (MTD) to increase the possibility of observing low-level effects. The responses observed in such studies are evaluated by statistical methods, but observation, experience, and judgment are also used in relating effects to historical incidence rates, overall conduct of the study, etc. (Haseman et al. 1984a, 1985; Huff et al. 1986). These results provide the basis for determining carcinogenic potential of chemicals, but, since animals are exposed for 2 years ($\geq 60\%$ of their life span) to doses that should demonstrate some minimal evidence of toxicity, these results also help to identify substances that show no evidence of carcinogenicity in rodents (Shelby and Stasiewicz 1984). Also, since the studies are conducted according to defined protocols in the same genetically identical strains of rodents, the results are also useful for making comparisons between the effects of diverse and related chemicals (Tennant et al. 1986). However, the chemicals are studied under well-defined protocols, and any inferences regarding mode of action or mechanism of action of a chemical can only be speculative, since rigorous experimentation related to specific properties of individual chemicals is needed to define the latter. Parenthetically, it is probably more meaningful to talk about mode of action rather than mechanism of effect, since the latter is so imprecisely known. Discussions of chemical mechanisms must involve biochemical and molecular biological phenomena. At this time, we do not know the actual mechanism(s) by

Banbury Report 25: Nongenotoxic Mechanisms in Carcinogenesis
© Cold Spring Harbor Laboratory. 0-87969-225-1/87. $1.00 + .00

which any chemical induces neoplasia, although we do know a great deal about the mode of action of many chemicals, such as whether they are toxic, bind to cytosol receptors, form adducts, etc. Therefore, the discussion in this paper is limited to the mode(s) of action of chemicals. For the majority of chemicals recently studied under the aegis of the NTP (Haseman et al. 1984b), there was little information available about the potential mode of action, and any inferences are made retrospectively on the basis of the observed effects of the chemical.

In the early 1970s, efforts were mounted to develop and utilize short-term tests, predominantly in vitro, to identify potential carcinogens. These efforts were based principally on the somatic mutation hypothesis and on the preliminary evidence and speculation that carcinogens are mutagens (Ames et al. 1973). However, as various tests were applied to a greater variety of chemical classes, it became apparent that some of the chemicals identified as carcinogens were not mutagenic. These observations led to efforts to classify carcinogens on the basis of whether they were "genotoxic" or "epigenetic" (Williams 1985). The former term was used to encompass not just mutation, but also other effects of chemicals, such as induction of clastogenic effects (e.g., chromosomal aberrations and sister chromatid exchange [SCE], unscheduled DNA synthesis [UDS], and in vitro neoplastic transformation) that are also indicative of direct interaction with DNA. The term epigenetic was proposed to identify substances that indirectly affected the neoplastic process (this usage does not correspond to the classic genetic meaning). Included in this category were chemicals identified as tumor promoters in any one of a number of systems proposed for measuring tumor promotion (Williams 1983). It must be recognized, however, that these conditional definitions are valid only to the extent that the substances have been tested.

The interpretation was extended further to imply that genotoxic chemicals would all act by direct effects on the cell genome and would demonstrate linear, nonthreshold effects. The epigenetic carcinogens were proposed to act indirectly and therefore implicitly demonstrate some threshold of effect. Genetic toxicity thus became the basis for defining the probable mode(s) of action of carcinogens and was proposed as a basis for regulatory decisions (Weisburger and Williams 1981). It was not possible to adequately evaluate this hypothesis, since the data required to do so were inadequate or unavailable (Perrera 1984). Major problems with the data base were (1) the absence of results generated without potential bias, i.e., genetic toxicity data generated on a number of substances prior to knowing the tumorigenicity results; and (2) inadequate numbers of noncarcinogenic chemicals studied under similar conditions.

To address these and other issues, the NTP initiated development, validation, and evaluation of short-term (in vitro and in vivo) test systems. The principles underlying this program were (1) to develop experimental protocols with demonstrated intra- and interlaboratory reproducibility of results, and (2) to evaluate the results of chemicals tested under code (i.e., the identity of the chemical is unknown to the laboratory conducting the test). Among the short-term assays being evaluated in this project were the *Salmonella* and mouse lymphoma (L5178Y) cell mutagenesis systems, and the induction of chromosome aberrations and SCE in Chinese hamster ovary (CHO) cells. Details of the protocols used and specific test results have been reported previously (Haworth et al. 1983; Galloway et al. 1985; Myhr et al. 1985), and preliminary interpretations of results have been discussed (Shelby and Stasiewicz 1984; Zeiger and Tennant 1986). In addition, an extensive evaluation of these and other in vitro and in vivo short-term genetic toxicity assays is currently in progress and is based on 73 chemicals tested for carcinogenicity in two rodent species. The results discussed in this paper are likewise preliminary and represent hypothetical inferences that must be critically evaluated.

RESULTS

One preliminary but very important observation is that, in contrast to reports that a large proportion of carcinogens are mutagens (McCann et al. 1975; Sugimura et al. 1976; Purchase et al. 1978), the NTP data base revealed an overall concordance of 50–60%. That is, a significantly greater number of chemicals than predicted by other investigators demonstrated some evidence of tumorigenicity but did not show evidence for mutagenicity in *Salmonella* (Zeiger and Tennant 1986). Conversely, a high percentage (78%) of chemicals that were mutagenic in *Salmonella* did demonstrate tumorigenicity. That is, the number of mutagens among all of the carcinogens was rather low, but if the chemical was identified as a mutagen, there was a high probability that it was carcinogenic (Zeiger 1987). *Salmonella* mutagenicity is therefore an effective and efficient means of demonstrating potential genetic toxicity, and a positive response carries a high likelihood, but not a certainty, of tumorigenicity. However, a negative response in *Salmonella* is not very informative. Since the focus of this volume is on substances that are nongenotoxic, the following discussion is limited to such chemicals studied by the NTP.

Twenty-four chemicals from the NTP data base that show little or no overall evidence of genetic toxicity are listed in Table 1. These chemicals have been tested by the NTP for tumorigenicity in both rodent species, and the tumorigenicity sex/species patterns are presented in the table. In addition to being tested for mutagenicity in *Salmonella* and mouse lymphoma cells, the chemicals were also tested for induction of chromosome aberrations or SCE in CHO cells. Where possible, the same lot of a chemical that was used in the rodent carcinogenicity studies was also used in the assays for genetic toxicity. All genetic toxicity tests were conducted with coded chemicals to ensure objectivity. Although several chemicals showed evidence of a positive or equivocal effect in one of the four assay systems, the weight of evidence favors an overall classification of nongenotoxic. Such overall conclusions call for very careful evaluation to ensure that the chemical has been tested adequately (i.e., up to a high concentration that demonstrates some

Table 1
NTP Genetic Toxicity Results for Selected Carcinogens and Noncarcinogens

Chemical name	Bioassay				Genetic toxicity			
	MR	FR	MM	FM	SAL	ML	CA	SCE
Di(2-ethylhexyl)phthalate (DEHP)	+	+	+	+	−	−	−	+
2,3,7,8-Tetrachlorodibenzo-*p*-dioxin	+	+	+	+	−	−	−	−
Polybrominated biphenyl mixture (PBB)	+	+	+	+	−	−	−	−
Benzene	+	+	+	+	−	−	−	?
Cinnamyl anthranilate	+	−	+	+	−	+	−	−
Reserpine	+	−	+	+	−	−	−	−
Di(2-ethylhexyl)adipate	−	−	+	+	−	−	−	?
Benzyl acetate	E	−	+	+	−	+	−	−
Tris(2-ethylhexyl)phosphate	E	−	−	+	−	−	−	−
D & C Red 9	+	E	−	−	+	−	−	−
11-Aminoundecanoic acid	+	−	E	−	−	−	−	+
Melamine	+	−	−	−	−	−	−	?
Butyl benzyl phthalate	I	+	−	−	−	−	−	−
D-mannitol	−	−	−	−	−	−	−	−
Hamamelis water (witch hazel)	−	−	−	−	−	−	−	−
C.I. Acid Red 14	−	−	−	−	−	−	−	−
Caprolactam	−	−	−	−	−	−	−	−
DL-menthol	−	−	−	−	−	−	−	−
Ethoxylated dodecyl alcohol	−	−	−	−	−	−	−	−
FD & C Yellow No. 6	−	−	−	−	−	+	−	?
Bisphenol A	−	−	−	−	−	−	−	?
Titanium dioxide	−	−	−	−	−	−	?	−
Dimethyl terephthalate	−	−	E	−	−	−	−	−
Sodium (2-ethylhexyl)alcohol sulfate	−	−	−	E	−	−	−	−

MR indicates male F344 rat; FR, female F344 rat; MM, male B6C3F$_1$ mouse; FM, female B6C3F$_1$ mouse; SAL, *Salmonella* mutagenesis; ML, mouse lymphoma (L5178Y) cell mutagenesis; CA, chromosome aberration induction in CHO cells; SCE, sister chromatid exchange induction in CHO cells; +, positive result; −, negative result; E, equivocal evidence of carcinogenicity; I, inconclusive study; ?, equivocal genetic toxicity result.

evidence of cellular toxicity) in each of the systems in which no effect was observed. The positive genetic toxicity evaluations shown in this table represent either statistical and/or biologically distinct effects in that particular system. This discordance (i.e., a single positive or equivocal result) with the negative results obtained in the other systems in which the chemicals have been adequately tested does not constitute clear evidence of genetic toxicity of the chemical. For the purposes of our evaluation, equivocal responses in either rodent tumorigenicity assays or genetic toxicity tests are combined with the negative responses.

It is clear that if the genetic toxicity results for these chemicals were available prior to testing the chemicals in rodents for tumorigenicity, it would not have been possible to predict, on this basis alone, the potential carcinogenicity or non-carcinogenicity. On the basis of these in vitro short-term test results alone, it is therefore not possible to distinguish prospectively between these nongenotoxic carcinogens and nongenotoxic noncarcinogens.

The patterns of tumors induced by the various nongenotoxic carcinogens represent some interesting paradoxes. It is first apparent that these chemicals represent diverse structural classes; however, the number of chemicals in the group is not sufficient to determine if there are any consistent chemical class-related properties. The tumor patterns represented by species, sex, tumor type or site, and number of sites induced are all quite diverse. In Table 2, three of the nongenotoxic carcinogens in group A induced neoplastic nodules or hepatocellular carcinomas (DEHP, TCDD, and PBB), but only one (DEHP) induced only neoplasia of the liver. The fourth chemical, benzene, did not induce hepatocarcinogenicity but did induce neoplasia at multiple sites in both sex/species. All of these substances were administered by feed or gavage. Although none of the four substances showed clear evidence of genetic toxicity in vitro, benzene induced micronuclei in hetero- chromatic erythrocytes of exposed mice (Choy et al. 1985) and chromosome aberrations in the bone marrow of exposed rats and mice (Dean 1985). No clear evidence of genetic toxicity in vivo was seen for the other three chemicals.

Table 2, group B presents some interesting contrasts also. The chemicals are structurally diverse and induced diverse patterns of tumors, but no increased incidence of tumors was detected in female rats that were exposed comparably to the other groups. Three of the four chemicals induced liver tumors, but di(2-ethylhexyl)adipate was the only one that induced only liver neoplasia and also the only one of the four that was tumorigenic in only one species.

Groups C and D include nongenotoxic chemicals that show much more restricted tumorigenicity patterns. Only tris(2-ethylhexyl)phosphate induced tumors in both species, and three of the other six chemicals induced tumors only in male rats. Four of the seven chemicals induced liver tumors, alone or in combination with some other tumor/site. Three of the chemicals, dimethyl terephthalate and butyl benzyl phthalate, and sodium (2-ethylhexyl)alcohol sulfate, were judged to be equivocal studies, i.e., they showed a chemically related marginal increase of neoplasms.

DISCUSSION

The idea has been put forward that meaningful distinctions between chemicals, that could be used in regulatory policy, could be made on the basis of in vitro genetic toxicity test results (Weisburger and Williams 1981). The idea is based on the assumption that positive genetic toxicity results carry the implication that the chemical may produce neoplastic change at any dose. Nongenotoxic substances are presumed to act via some epigenetic mechanism and therefore would not carry an equal risk at every dose. The epigenetic effects are proposed to involve tumor promotion, generally requiring continuous prolonged exposure to the chemical.

The first presumption on which this proposal is based, the ability to demonstrate genotoxicity by in vitro tests, is not correct, since some substances that fail to show clear evidence of genetic toxicity in vitro have genotoxic potential that may be

Table 2
Tumorigenicity Patterns for Some Chemicals That Do Not Show In Vitro
Genetic Toxicity

Chemical name	Tumorigenicity		
Group A			
di(2-ethylhexyl)phthalate (DEHP)	MR:	+	liver: hepatocellular carcinoma, neoplastic nodule
	FR:	+	liver: hepatocellular carcinoma
	MM:	+	liver: hepatocellular carcinoma
	FM:	+	liver: hepatocellular carcinoma
2,3,7,8-tetrachlorodibenzo-*p*-dioxin (TCDD)	MR:	+	thyroid gland: follicular cell adenoma
	FR:	+	liver: neoplastic nodule
	MM:	+	liver: hepatocellular carcinoma
	FM:	+	liver: hepatocellular carcinoma thyroid gland: follicular cell adenoma
polybrominated biphenyl mixture (PBB) (Firemaster FF-1)	MR:	+	liver: neoplastic nodule, hepatocellular carcinoma, cholangiocarcinoma
	FR:	+	liver: neoplastic nodule, hepatocellular carcinoma, cholangiocarcinoma
	MM:	+	liver: hepatocellular carcinoma
	FM:	+	liver: hepatocellular carcinoma
benzene	MR:	+	zymbal gland: carcinoma, squamous cell papilloma oral cavity: squamous cell papilloma skin: squamous cell papilloma and carcinoma
	FR:	+	zymbal gland: carcinoma, squamous cell papilloma oral cavity: squamous cell papilloma
	MM:	+	zymbal gland: squamous cell carcinoma lymphatic system: malignant lymphoma lung: alveolar/bronchiolar carcinoma and adenoma harderian gland: adenoma prenupital gland: squamous cell carcinoma
	FM:	+	zymbal gland: squamous cell carcinoma lymphatic system: malignant lymphoma lung: alveolar/bronchiolar carcinoma ovary: granulosa cell tumors and mixed tumors (benign) mammary gland: carcinoma and carcinosarcoma
Group B			
cinnamyl anthranilate:	MR:	+	pancreas: acinar cell adenoma or carcinoma kidney/renal cortex: adenoma or adenocarcinoma
	FR:	−	none
	MM:	+	liver: hepatocellular adenoma
	FM:	+	liver: hepatocellular adenoma and carcinoma
reserpine	MR:	+	adrenal glands: malignant pheochromocytoma or pheochromocytoma
	FR:	−	none
	MM:	+	seminal vesicles: undifferentiated carcinoma
	FM:	+	mammary glands: malignant tumors, all types

Table 2
(Continued)

Chemical name	Tumorigenicity	
Group B (continued)		
di(2-ethylhexyl)adipate	MR: −	none
	FR: −	none
	MM: +	liver: hepatocellular adenoma
	FM: +	liver: hepatocellular carcinoma
benzyl acetate	MR: E	pancreas: acinar cell adenoma
	FR: −	none
	MM: +	liver: hepatocellular adenoma and carcinoma
		stomach: squamous cell papilloma or carcinoma
	FM: +	liver: hepatocellular adenoma and carcinoma
		stomach: squamous cell papilloma or carcinoma
Group C		
tris(2-ethylhexyl)phosphate	MR: E	adrenal gland: pheochromocytoma
	FR: −	none
	MM: −	none
	FM: +	liver: hepatocellular carcinoma
D & C Red 9	MR: +	spleen: sarcoma
		liver: neoplastic nodule
	FR: −	none
	MM: −	none
	FM: −	none
11-aminoundecanoic acid	MR: +	liver: neoplastic nodule
		urinary bladder: transitional cell carcinoma
	FR: −	none
	MM: −	none
	FM: −	none
melamine	MR: +	urinary bladder: transitional cell carcinoma
	FR: −	none
	MM: −	none
	FM: −	none
Group D		
dimethyl terephthalate	MR: −	none
	FR: −	none
	MM: E	lung: alveolar/bronchiolar adenoma or carcinoma
	FM: −	none
butyl benzyl phthalate	MR: I	none
	FR: E	hematopoietic system: mononuclear cell
		leukemia
	MM: −	none
	FM: −	none
sodium (2-ethylhexyl)alcohol sulfate	MR: −	none
	FR: −	none
	MM: −	none
	FM: E	liver: hepatocellular carcinoma and adenoma

For abbreviations and symbols, refer to Table 1.

expressed in the whole animal (e.g., benzene). Second, although the overall data base for in vitro and in vivo genetic toxicity data on carcinogens is still not very large, many carcinogens are not genotoxic (Table 1). Therefore, in a prospective evaluation of chemicals that have not yet been tested for tumorigenicity, the absence of positive in vitro genetic toxicity results carries no clear implications. It is clear that further in vivo characterization is required to provide some confidence that the substance is probably not genotoxic.

The relationship between nongenotoxicity and epigenetic mechanisms, likewise, is uncertain. The category of epigeneticity is so large that it can include substances that may indirectly interact with the cellular genome (e.g., induce chromosome aberrations via interference with the mitotic process) or amplify unexpressed, spontaneous, neoplastically transformed cells. Furthermore, any relationship between epigenetic mechanisms and the phenomena of tumor promotion is even more uncertain due to the lack of a consensus definition of the term and the broad category of effects that can be classified as tumor promotion. The terms tumor promotion and epigenetic mechanism are therefore only empirical designations for chemicals that are thought to induce or enhance the processes of tumorigenesis by one of several different modes of action and/or different mechanisms.

The chemicals listed in Table 2 all have undergone full characterization, i.e., exposure of two sex/species for 104 weeks followed by complete pathologic examination. It is obviously very difficult to make retrospective inferences regarding mode or mechanism of action, even when the genetic toxicity profile is defined. It is particularly difficult to interpret effects as either "complete carcinogenesis" or "promotion," since so few known tumor promoters have been subjected to tests that utilize long-term, high-dose exposure in the absence of initiation. Two chemicals that have shown evidence of tumor promotion in experimental systems, however, were listed in Table 2 (group A). Both TCDD (Pitot et al. 1980) and PBB (Nishizumi 1976) have demonstrated promotional activity in so-called two-stage initiation-promotion systems. The effects of these chemicals in the long-term rodent carcinogenicity studies might be consistent with this mode of action, since both chemicals are associated with increased incidences of hepatocellular neoplasms, which occur as spontaneous tumors in both species. However, there are two other observations of interest related to their effects. The first is that the induced incidence is not proportional to the spontaneous incidence of hepatocellular carcinoma in each of the four sex/species; i.e., male mice show more than ten times the spontaneous incidence of these tumors than, for example, female rats, but they do not show a proportional increase after exposure to TCDD or PBB. Second, both chemicals are associated with the induction of tumors at other sites or of cell types. PBB induces cholangiocarcinomas that occur very rarely as spontaneous tumors (Haseman et al. 1984a), and TCDD induces in male rats and female mice follicular cell adenomas of the thyroid that are not related to the spontaneous incidence of these tumors. Therefore, these presumptive tumor promoters show at least some evidence that they may act through more than one mode of action. Both the diet and endogenous sources of initiation (Totter 1980; Ames 1983) have been proposed to account for spontaneous tumors in rodents. However, the fact that spontaneous tumor patterns are reproducible from generation to generation suggests that they may be influenced by one or more genetic loci in these animals. If tumor promoters act only to selectively enhance the proliferation of spontaneously initiated cells, then the effect is not an epigenetic mode of action. If promoters can act through indirect effects on cells (epigenetically?), then the effects may not be confined only to spontaneously initiated cells and may be seen in noninitiated cells after prolonged exposure. In any case, it is clear that tumor promotion is not synonymous with nongenotoxic and that nongenotoxic is not synonymous with epigenetic; moreover, promotion is not synonymous with epigenetic. It will be possible in the near future to empirically define fairly precisely what is clear evidence of genetic toxicity. The NTP has initiated a project that will provide for in vitro and in vivo characterization of the genetic toxicity of a number of chemicals studied in the rodent carcinogenesis bioassay for tumorigenicity and nontumorigenicity. These studies are being conducted under standardized protocols in more than one laboratory, with chemicals tested under code and evaluated by predetermined criteria. This project will provide a highly objective data base with which to define more clearly parameters of genetic toxicity.

The problem of defining tumor promotion is far more difficult, since it can be measured, observed, or inferred in so many different ways. However, regardless of the means by which promotion may occur, a fundamental property of promotion is the capacity of neoplastic lesions to regress in the absence of the promoter (Pitot, this volume). If this characteristic were used as the basic property of a tumor promoter, it would be possible to prospectively test the assumption by conducting a modified rodent carcinogenicity bioassay that provides for observation of animals following cessation of treatment after an appropriate but limited time of exposure. Comparison of these groups with those treated for the full 104-week period would be a basis for judging the characteristics of chemicals identified as carcinogens. Neoplastic lesions, however, can progress to an autonomous state even after prolonged exposure to tumor promoters (Pitot, this volume), so that duration of exposure is an important factor that has to be considered in relation to the concentration of complete carcinogens that can induce autonomous growth following limited exposure. In some cases, these phenomena may be separated by only the doses required to induce autonomy.

Overall, current regulatory policies do not appear to explicitly utilize the presence or absence of in vitro genetic toxicity results in establishing human exposure limits or use restriction (Food and Drug Administration 1982). However, such results appear to be used implicitly as guidelines for future testing in animals (Flamm and Dunkel 1983; Glocklin 1984; Environmental Protection Agency 1985). Regulatory policy is the product of a process that incorporates public health, economics, and risk-benefit factors. The fundamental aspects of any policy, however, must be built on scientific consensus. It is unrealistic to expect unambiguous policy where we lack a logical scientific framework for utilizing the scientific data. It is clear from other papers in this volume that we lack information in some critical areas in order to achieve concensus on several important aspects of carcinogenesis. Our collective fate, therefore, is one of having to use the limited facts available and to exercise judgment in their application.

ACKNOWLEDGMENTS

The opinions and interpretations expressed in the paper represent those of the author and do not necessarily represent policies of the National Toxicology Program or federal regulatory agencies. I am indebted to my colleagues in the National Institute of Environmental Health Sciences who have provided unpublished results and contributed thoughts and discussions related to this paper. In particular, I thank Drs. Jud Spalding, Barry Margolin, Errol Zeiger, James Huff, and Michael Shelby. I also thank Stan Stasiewicz for help in compiling results.

REFERENCES

Ames, B.N. 1983. Dietary carcinogens and anticarcinogens. *Science* **221:** 1256.
Ames, B.N., W.E. Durston, E. Yamasaki, and F.D. Lee. 1973. Carcinogens are mutagens: A simple test test system combining liver homogenates for activation and bacteria for detection. *Proc. Natl. Acad. Sci. U.S.A.* **70:** 2281.
Choy, W.N., J.T. MacGregor, M.D. Shelby, and R.R. Maronpot. 1985. Induction of micronuclei by benzene in B6C3F$_1$ mice: Retrospective analysis of peripheral blood smears from NTP carcinogenesis bioassay. *Mutat. Res.* **143:** 55.
Dean, B.J. 1985. Recent findings on the genetic toxicology of benzene, toluene, xylenes and phenols. *Mutat. Res.* **154:** 153.
Environmental Protection Agency. 1985. Toxic substances; mesityl oxide; final test rule. *Fed. Regul.* **50:** 51857.
Flamm, W.G. and V.C. Dunkel. 1983. Impact of short-term tests on regulatory action. *Ann. N.Y. Acad. Sci.* **407:** 395.
Food and Drug Administration (FDA). 1982. *Toxicological principles for safety assessment of direct food additives and color additives used in food.* U.S. Bureau of Foods, Washington, D.C.
Galloway, S.M., A. Bloom, M. Resnick, B.H. Margolin, F. Nakamura, P. Archer, and E. Zeiger. 1985. Development of a standard protocol for in vitro cytogenetic testing with CHO cells: Comparison of results for 22 compounds in two laboratories. *Environ. Mutagen.* **7:** 1.
Glocklin, V.C. 1984. Current FDA considerations about the role of mutagenicity studies in drug safety evaluation. In *Critical evaluation of mutagenicity tests.* (ed. R. Bass et al.), p. 527. MMV Medizin Verlag, Munich, Federal Republic of Germany.

Haseman, J.K., J. Huff, and G.A. Boorman. 1984a. Use of historical control data in carcinogenicity studies in rodents. *Toxicol. Pathol.* **12**: 126.

Haseman, J.K., D. Crawford, J.E. Huff, G.A. Boorman, and E.E. McConnell. 1984b. Results from 86 two-year carcinogenicity studies conducted by the National Toxicology Program. *J. Toxicol. Environ. Health* **14**: 621.

Haseman, J.K., J.E. Huff, G.N. Rao, J.E. Arnold, G.A. Boorman, and E.E. McConnell. 1985. Neoplasms observed in untreated and corn oil gavage control groups of F344/N rats and (C57B1/6N X C3H/HeN)F$_1$ mice (B6C3F$_1$). *J. Natl. Cancer Inst.* **75**: 975.

Haworth, S., T. Lawlor, K. Mortlemans, W. Speck, and E. Zeiger. 1983. Salmonella mutagenicity for 250 chemicals. *Environ. Mutagen.* (Suppl. 1)**5**: 3.

Huff, J.E., J.K. Haseman, E.E. McConnell, and J.A. Moore. 1986. The National Toxicology Program, toxicology data evaluation techniques and long-term carcinogenesis studies. In *Safety evaluation of drugs and chemicals* (ed. W.E. Lloyd), p. 411. Hemisphere, Washington, D.C.

McCann, J., E. Choi, E. Yamasaki, and B.N. Ames. 1975. Detection of carcinogens as mutagens in the Salmonella/microsome test: Assay of 300 chemicals. *Proc. Natl. Acad. Sci. U.S.A.* **72**: 5135.

Myhr, B., L. Bowers, and W.C. Caspary. 1985. Assays for the induction of gene mutations at the thymidine kinase locus in L5178Y mouse lymphoma cells in culture. In *Evaluation of short-term tests for carcinogens* (ed. J. Ashby et al.), p. 555. Elsevier Science Publishers, New York.

Nishizumi, M. 1976. Enhancement of diethylnitrosamine hepatocarcinogenesis in rats by exposure to polychlorinated biphenyls or phenobarbitol. *Cancer Lett.* **2**: 11.

Perrera, F.P. 1984. The genotoxic/epigenetic distinction relevance to cancer policy. *Environ. Res.* **34**: 175.

Pitot, H.C., T. Goldsworthy, H.A. Campbell, and A. Poland. 1980. Quantitative evaluation of promotion by 2,3,7,8-tetrachlorodibenzo-p-dioxin of hepatocarcinogenesis from diethylnitrosamines. *Cancer Res.* **40**: 3616.

Purchase, I.F.H., E. Longstaff, J. Ashby, J.A. Styles, D. Anderson, P.A. Leferre, and F.R. Westwood. 1978. An evaluation of six short-term tests for detecting organic chemical carcinogens. *Br. J. Cancer* **37**: 873.

N.T.P. Report. 1984. Report of the NTP Ad Hoc Panel on Chemical Carcinogenesis Testing and Evaluation, Board of Scientific Counselors, National Toxicology Program, U.S. Department of Health and Human Services. U.S. Government Printing Office, Washington, D.C.

Shelby, M.D. and S. Stasiewicz. 1984. Chemicals showing no evidence of carcinogenicity in long-term, two-species rodent studies: The need for short-term test data. *Environ. Mutagen.* **6**: 871.

Sugimura, T., S. Sato, M. Nago, T. Yahagi, T. Matsushima, Y. Seino, M. Takeuchi, and T. Kawachi. 1976. Overlapping of carcinogens and mutagens. In *Fundamentals of cancer prevention* (ed. P.N. Magee et al.), p. 191. University Park Press, Baltimore, Maryland.

Tennant, R.W., S. Stasiewicz, and J.S. Spalding. 1986. Comparison of multiple parameters of rodent carcinogenicity and in vitro genetic toxicity. *Environ. Mutagen.* **8**: 205.

Totter, J.R. 1980. Spontaneous cancer and its possible relationship to oxygen metabolism. *Proc. Natl. Acad. Sci. U.S.A.* **77**: 1763.

Weisburger, J.H. and G.M. Williams. 1981. Carcinogen testing: Current problems and new approaches. *Science* **214:** 401.

Williams, G.M. 1983. Epigenetic effects of liver tumor promoters and implications for health effects. *Environ. Health Perspect.* **50:** 177.

———. 1985. Identification of genotoxic and epigenetic carcinogens in liver culture systems. *Regul. Toxicol. Pharmacol.* **5:** 132.

Zeiger, E. 1987. Carcinogenicity of mutagens: Predictive capability of the *Salmonella* mutagenesis assay for rodent carcinogenicity. *Cancer Res.* **47:** 1287.

Zeiger, E. and R.W. Tennant. 1986. Mutagenesis, clastogenesis and carcinogenesis: Expectations, correlations and relations. In *Genetic toxicology of environmental chemicals,* part B: *Genetic effects and applied mutagenesis* (ed. C. Ramel et al.), vol. 209B, p. 75. A.R. Liss, New York.

COMMENTS

ANDERSON: Ray, since you say no mechanism (of carcinogenesis) has been demonstrated, would you define what is adequate proof of mechanism? I think that is always a tough decision.

TENNANT: We have to establish the equivalent of Koch's postulates. That is, there has to be a systematic and logical construct through which an etiologic relationship between chemical-induced effect and tumor phenotype can be clearly demonstrated. I do not have the magic formula; if I did, I would immediately run back to the laboratory and go to work. It is a very complex problem. The problem of causality in carcinogenesis is literally at the state that I believe infectious diseases were in the latter part of the nineteenth century.

TRUMP: I was wondering about the premise that you mentioned concerning the cholangial carcinomas (in other words, that there is no background and therefore no background initiation) because it seems to me, if you have a compound that forces the targets for some bizarre reason on a particular cell and forces proliferation, you could easily have background initiation and never know it until you get such a compound. The same principle, for example, could apply to the proximal tubule, very low instance in the Fischer rat. We know now of several compounds that target there and may do it in some way. We have had two discussions about that. I was just worried about the premise that because there is no background tumor incidence there is no background initiation.

TENNANT: I can't really answer that. I really only want to raise the possibility that one interpretation is that TCDD has more than one mode of action. Even though there is no demonstrated genotoxicity, there is at least some evidence that it may not be clearly acting only as a tumor promoter in the strict sense that we are thinking of tumor promotion. There are obviously major problems in trying to retrospectively evaluate rodent assay results in terms of the mode of action, either as complete carcinogen, promoter, cocarcinogen, or whatever. It seems to me that there is no solution to this problem but to do additional studies. I don't think we can simply reason to the mode of action. I think that where there are substances that we suspect of having promotional activity, a key feature has to be that we do "stop dosing studies" that tell us whether or not lesions progress or regress in the absence of the chemical. That seems to me to be a fundamental property of promoters, irrespective of what they do in any in vitro system, and that this would have a very important implication for any sort of regulatory action on a chemical.

PITOT: I would take some objection to your point about TCDD because the evidence is overwhelming that its effects are mediated through the receptor. The difference in incidence of different tumors is not surprising, since it is known that promoters have tissue specificity. Thus, to suggest different mechanisms just because different tumors are obtained with different agents, is only one of a number of possible explanations.

TENNANT: That's all I wanted to indicate.

PITOT: But your suggestion is not the most likely possibility. For example, dioxin action occurs primarily through a receptor mechanism.

TENNANT: I agree.

PITOT: I think the evidence is very strong that we have a single mechanism of action for this chemical. We can imagine many possible mechanisms for chemicals. If we continue to do this, we are not going to get anywhere because we will always take the worst possibility. That's the central thinking in the regulatory agencies, that the worst possibility is the one that is considered.

TENNANT: But, on the other hand, I know you would agree that the theories have to be fitted to the facts, and not vice versa. I see this as a logical inconsistency in evaluating TCDD as solely a promoter.

PITOT: From the fact that you get different tumors?

TENNANT: Yes, tumors at a site at which tumors so rarely occur.

ROE: It seems to me that to attempt to match the results of tests for mutagenicity and those of tests for carcinogenicity is an incredibly superficial exercise.

TENNANT: I agree.

ROE: On the carcinogenicity side, a great deal of information which is subject to numerous, often poorly controlled, variables is reduced to a simple all-or-none answer: *Yes* it is a carcinogen or *no* it isn't. Whereas on the genotoxicity side, the results of many tests may be available—some giving negative results and some, positive results. The fact is that if there are positive results both for genotoxicity and carcinogenicity, the mechanisms involved may be quite different. Tumors resulting from nongenotoxic mechanisms may well end up as matched with false positives in tests for genotoxicity.

TENNANT: That's right.

SWENBERG: I would like to bring us back to the last two slides that I showed on the tremendous influence of age of the animal in cancer studies. In comparing the life-span study with the 2-year study, this 25% increase in life span results in anywhere from a twofold increase to a 31-fold increase in spontaneous tumors. Anything you do could modulate this. I think we have to be awfully careful in assuming a genotoxic mechanism when we have those kinds of data. As an example, you said that we don't have any agents for which we know a mechanism. What about the antithyroid agents, where you clearly have TSH chronically stimulating the thyroid gland, and you get thyroid adenomas? That's not genotoxic.

TENNANT: Yes, there is an association, Jim. I don't think that is proof.

SWENBERG: If you supplement T4 during the whole time you are exposing animals to these chemicals, you don't get any tumors.

WILLIAMS: Regarding the cholangiocarcinomas with PBB, I think we have a similar problem. First of all, that is a histological diagnosis which is subject to a lot of disagreement. There are many people who would say that so-called cholangiocarcinomas are merely hepatocellular adenocarcinomas. This debate has been raging for decades. Now, one thing about PBB is that it alters the gene expression in the liver. I see no reason why the pattern of liver tumors cannot differ with an agent that alters gene expression. For example, the closely related compound, polychlorinated biphenyl, will actually induce metaplasia of hepatocytes to pancreatic acimar-like cells. So, I think one has to be very cautious about using the histologic patterns of tumors to infer that the occurrence of a rare tumor means that it stems from ab initio induction of neoplastic conversion in a cell type that is not the source of a spontaneously occurring tumor.

TENNANT: I can't really address that.

BRAND: I would warn against using something like Koch's postulates as a goal to strive for because I think we would be in great trouble, simply because the concept of Koch's postulates is in big trouble, and it always has been. That is because most of the infections we encounter are opportunistic infections caused by members of our normal flora, and the reason we get sick is because our resistance goes down or the susceptibility goes up, something which is possibly very much related to the problems we see in carcinogenicity as well.

TENNANT: I agree. It's a naive analogy, but it's the most scientifically visible, logical construct for etiology that has ever been defined. I just simply say that the field of carcinogenesis is in need of a similar conception. That clearly is going to have to take place at a molecular level in carcinogenesis.

Practical Approaches to Evaluating Nongenotoxic Carcinogens

HARVEY E. SCRIBNER, KAY L. McCARTHY, AND DAVID J. DOOLITTLE*
Toxicology Department, Rohm and Haas Company
Spring House, Pennsylvania 19477

OVERVIEW

Quantitative risk assessment of animal carcinogens to establish acceptable human exposure levels has traditionally been modeled using linear extrapolation. However, if data are available to demonstrate that the response is nonlinear with dose, then the appropriateness of linear extrapolation models is challenged. In practice, the nature of the studies that evaluate the dose-response relationship depends on the type of cellular damage that results from exposure to the chemical.

The in vivo/in vitro UDS S-phase assay in mouse hepatocytes, as validated in our laboratory, provides a simultaneous in vivo assessment of both genotoxicity (unscheduled DNA synthesis [UDS]) and a sensitive indicator of hyperplasia (scheduled DNA synthesis or S phase). We will discuss an example of the use of this assay in developing mode-of-action information to evaluate the significance of mouse liver tumor results obtained using an experimental chemical. The data indicate that the mouse hepatic tumors induced by the experimental chemical are secondary effects resulting from chronic cytotoxicity by a nongenotoxic chemical. Consequently, because the cytotoxic response in the target tissue exhibits nonlinearity with dose, then the use of linear extrapolation models to evaluate risk to humans may be overly stringent.

INTRODUCTION

The potential carcinogenic risk associated with the use of commercial chemicals poses important scientific and regulatory issues. A reasonable approach is to develop the best scientific data for assessing carcinogenic hazard in the belief that accurate, scientifically acceptable risk assessment will ensure the safe use of chemicals, as well as favorable regulatory action.

Quantitative risk assessments based only on adverse oncogenic studies in animals are modeled using linear extrapolation from the effect levels and usually result in extremely low (or zero) acceptable human exposure limits. If, however, data are available to demonstrate that the mode of action of a chemical is compatible with nonlinear response, then higher, less-conservative human exposure limits may be acceptable.

*Present address: Toxicology Research, Bowman Gray Technical Center, R.J. Reynolds Tobacco Company, Winston-Salem, North Carolina 27102.

In practice, the nature of experiments to explore the mode of action of a chemical is determined by the type of cellular damage that results from exposure. If, for example, a chemical is demonstrated to be genotoxic by using a battery of short-term genetic tests, then additional experiments demonstrating a nonlinear relationship between dose-to-target (DNA) and exposure would challenge the appropriateness of using a linear model of risk assessment. This approach has been used to defend the continued use of formaldehyde, whereby the Chemical Industry Institute of Toxicology (CIIT) developed data showing that formaldehyde, even though mutagenic in short-term tests and carcinogenic in animal studies, poses no risk to humans under use conditions (for review, see Starr et al. 1985). It should be noted, however, that although the scientific basis of formaldehyde safety has been generally accepted by the industrial and academic communities, regulatory decisions are still uncertain.

Alternatively, if a chemical is negative in a battery of short-term genetic tests, additional testing in support of a nongenotoxic mode of action could be done (e.g., induction of hyperplasia in the target tissue, or promotion in cells in culture, or in vivo). Unfortunately, data supporting a nongenotoxic mode of action are circumstantial in that there always exists a finite probability that any battery of short-term genetic tests is imperfect and the test chemical might be genotoxic. Nevertheless, in the absence of adverse genotoxic effects, the demonstration of a nonlinear relationship between dose and hyperplasia and/or promotion would question the use of linear extrapolation for risk assessment.

Testing programs are designed on a case-by-case basis, depending on the chemical class and the toxicity data available. Evaluation of the mode of action may be prospective, since information on potential genotoxic and nongenotoxic activity is frequently obtained early in product development; or it may be retrospective, in the case of studies initiated after a finding of adverse carcinogenic effects.

We discuss below the in vivo/in vitro UDS S-phase assay in mouse hepatocytes, as validated in our laboratory, for use as both a prospective tool and a retrospective tool; we also examine a representative approach for demonstrating that an oncogenic dose response may be nonlinear.

RESULTS

Mouse liver tumors are the most common type of tumor observed in chronic rodent bioassays (Ward et al. 1979). Unfortunately, the available batteries of short-term genetic tests used to predict carcinogenicity are generally inadequate for predicting the potential of a chemical to induce this type of tumor. The development of the in vivo/in vitro UDS S-phase assay in rat hepatocytes and other tissues by Butterworth, Mirsalis, and Doolittle (Mirsalis and Butterworth 1980; Mirsalis et al. 1982; Doolittle et al. 1984) has provided a tool for assessing the organ-specific genotoxic potential of chemicals. We have validated the in vivo/in vitro UDS S-phase assay for hepatocarcinogens and hepatotoxins in the CD-1 mouse.

Male CD-1 mice, 50–100 days old, were treated by gavage with dimethyl-nitrosamine (DMN), trichloroethylene (TCE), phenobarbital (PB), 2-acetyl-aminofluorene (2-AAF), 4-acetylaminofluorene (4-AAF), or vehicle control (water or corn oil). At 3, 16, 24, and 48 hours after dosing, hepatocytes were isolated by an in situ perfusion procedure, incubated in the presence of [³H]thymidine, and then fixed. UDS, an indicator of DNA damage and repair, and S phase, an indicator of DNA replication, were assessed by quantitative autoradiography. No mortality or morbidity was observed in this study. The results are shown in Figure 1 (D.J. Doolittle et al., in prep.). DMN at 10 mg/kg induced DNA repair and increased the number of cells in S phase; whereas, at 2 mg/kg, DMN induced DNA repair but did not increase the number of cells in S phase. TCE at 1000 mg/kg, PB at 100 mg/kg, and 4-AAF at 200 mg/kg increased the number of cells in S phase, but all failed to induce DNA damage and repair. 2-AAF (200 mg/kg) did not induce DNA damage or an increase in cells in S phase. The vehicle controls, distilled water or corn oil, did not induce either DNA repair or increase the number of cells in S phase (data not shown).

These results indicate that the assay might be useful for detecting potential mouse liver carcinogens. The induction of DNA repair is obviously a response to hepatic DNA damage. It is unclear, however, whether the induction of S phase represents regenerative hyperplasia in response to hepatotoxicity or is a result of direct mitogenic stimulation of hepatocytes by the chemical. To examine the relationship between hepatic toxicity and the induction of S phase, the level of specific liver enzymes (serum glutamic-oxaloacetic transaminase [SGOT], serum glutamic-pyruvic transaminase [SGPT], alkaline phosphatase [AP], and gamma glutamyl transpeptidase [GGT]) present in mouse serum following chemical exposure was compared to induction of S phase.

Carbon tetrachloride (CCl₄), a nonmutagenic mouse liver carcinogen, was administered to male CD-1 mice as single or multiple doses (D.J. Doolittle et al., in prep.). At various times after treatment, hepatic DNA repair, induction of S phase in hepatic cells, and serum levels of SGOT, SGPT, AP, and GGT were measured. The induction of S phase coincided with the appearance of elevated levels of SGOT and SGPT at 50 and 100 mg/kg of CCl₄ in single-dose studies. A single dose of CCl₄ at 25 mg/kg did not increase S phase or SGOT or SGPT, but when 20 mg/kg was administered for 7 days, the number of cells in S phase, as well as SGOT and SGPT serum levels, increased dramatically. After administration of 20 mg/kg/day for 14 days, the levels of SGOT and SGPT decreased to control values and the percentage of cells in S phase remained elevated, whereas at a dose level of 100 mg/kg/day, the number of cells in S phase and the SGOT and SGPT serum levels remained high throughout the 14-day treatment period. CCl₄ did not induce DNA repair with any dosing regimen and did not affect serum levels of AP or GGT in any experiment.

These data support the hypothesis that S-phase induction in the mouse liver following CCl₄ administration is a regenerative response to hepatotoxicity. These

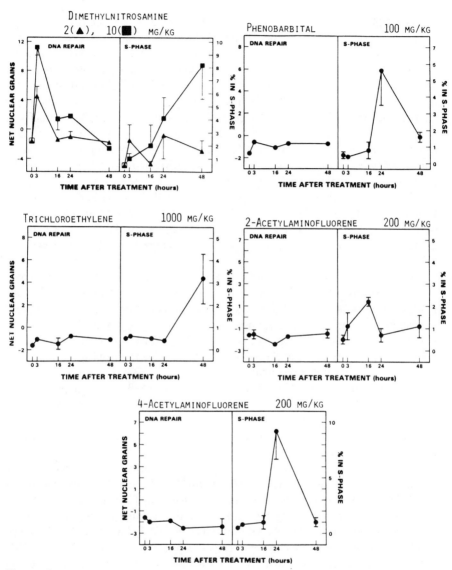

Figure 1

Time course for the induction of DNA repair and DNA replication in the liver of male CD-1 mice following a single oral administration of either 2 mg/kg (▲) or 10 mg/kg (■) of DNN, 1000 mg/kg of TCE, 100 mg/kg PB, 200 mg/kg of 2-AAF, or 200 mg/kg of 4-AAF. Hepatocytes were isolated O, 3, 16, 24, and 48 hr after dosing, incubated in the presence of [³H]thymidine, and subjected to quantitative autoradiography (D.J. Doolittle et al., in prep.). Each point represents the mean ± S.D. obtained from at least three animals; three slides were prepared from each animal. If the error bar is not shown, the standard deviation was within the symbol. For DNA repair (expressed as net nuclear grain count), 50 cells were scored per slide (450 cells/data point); and for DNA replication (expressed as percentage of the total hepatocyte population found in S phase), 1000 cells were scored per slide (9000 cells/data point).

methods have utility to provide information on the mode of action, which may be useful in demonstrating nonlinearity in the dose response, or alternatively, which may assist in dose-level selection for subchronic and chronic studies.

As a practical example of the retrospective use of mode-of-action information, we describe below how we at Rohm and Haas Company have approached evaluating the significance of adverse tumor data obtained in a mouse oncogenic study. The test chemical of interest is a proprietary chemical currently in development.

The experimental chemical has been extensively tested in a comprehensive program to assess potential toxic effects, including subchronic and chronic studies in rats, mice, and dogs; teratogenic studies in rats and rabbits; a multigeneration reproductive study in rats; and a battery of short-term genetic tests (Table 1). The experimental chemical was not oncogenic in the rat (data not shown). In the mouse chronic study, the liver was the primary target organ, exhibiting increased liver weight at necropsy in the mid- and high-dose groups, nonneoplastic histologic changes (megalocytic hepatocytes, sinusoidal cell hyperplasia, necrosis and degeneration of individual hepatocytes, pigment in Kupffer cells, diffuse hepatocytic enlargement and coagulative necrosis), and neoplasms (Table 2).

Two experiments were performed to evaluate the mouse oncogenic result: a 90-day dietary study (including a 30-day recovery period following treatment) in mice at dose levels including the dose levels in the oncogenic study, and an in vivo/in vitro UDS S-phase assay in mice. The experimental design and summary of pertinent results in the 90-day study are shown in Table 3 and Figure 2.

In the 90-day study, gross changes related to treatment were observed in the liver of male mice at 250 ppm after 30 days, and in both sexes at 250 ppm after 90 days, but not in any groups after the recovery period. Treatment-related microscopic changes were limited to the liver (data not shown). Specifically, at 1 month, there was an increased incidence and severity of hepatocellular hypertrophy in the high-dose male mice. After 3 months of treatment, these same histological changes occurred at the high dose in both sexes, with males demonstrating more severe changes than females. Hypertrophy of hepatocytes was primarily localized in the centrilobular regions and was characterized by increased cytoplasmic volume and

Table 1

Experimental Chemical: Short-term Genetic Test Results

Test	Result
Ames test	+/−*
Chinese hamster ovary cells/hypoxanthine-guanine phosphoribosyl transferase	−
Cytogenetic, in vitro (chinese hamster ovary cells)	−
Cytogenetic, in vivo (mouse bone marrow)	−
Cell transformation (C3H/10T1/2)	−

(−) No adverse result; (*) current technical product is negative (not adverse).

Table 2
Experimental Chemical: 88-week Dietary Oncogenicity Study in Mice

	Tumor incidence at the following treatment levels (ppm)				
	0	0	10	50	250
Males					
carcinoma	3	0	4	4	1
adenoma	7	13	4	19	17
hyperplastic nodules	3	1	1	1	1
foci/areas of cellular alteration	0	0	0	0	0
Total	13	14	9	24	19
Females					
carcinoma	0	0	0	3	6
adenoma	3	1	2	3	2
hyperplastic nodules	0	0	0	0	0
foci/areas of cellular alteration	0	0	0	1	1
Total	3	1	2	7	9

For both male and female animals, 80 animals were used for the 0 ppm treatment level and 100 animals were used for the 10, 50, and 250 ppm treatment level.

increased nuclear size. In addition, centrilobular necrosis of individual hepatocytes, pigment within Kupffer cells, and sinusoidal cell hyperplasia were observed in the high-dose mice after 3 months of treatment. Following the 1-month recovery period, the incidence and severity of hepatocellular hypertrophy in the mice treated with the experimental chemical were comparable to those in control animals. A

Table 3
Experimental Chemical: 90-day Dietary Study in CD-1 Mice

Dose levels
  0, 0.4, 2, 10, 50, 250 ppm

Number of animals
  35 mice/sex/group

Treatment regimen
  30 days (10 mice/sex/group)
  90 days (15 mice/sex/group)
  90 days + 30 days recovery (10 mice/sex/group)

Results
  no deaths occurred
  no treatment-related clinical signs
  no effect on body weight
  no effect on feed consumption
  no effect on hepatic mixed function oxidase activity
  increased liver weights after 30 days, high-dose males only
  increased liver weights after 90 days, high-dose males and females
  no increase in liver weights after recovery period (30 days)

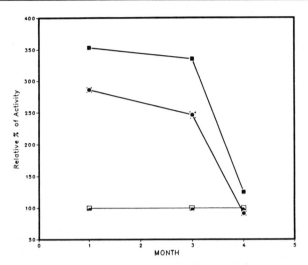

Figure 2

Hepatic peroxisomal β-oxidation activity in male (■) and female (●) CD-1 mice was assayed following administration of an experimental chemical in the diet at 250 ppm for 1 or 3 months, and following a 1-month recovery period after 3 months of treatment. Peroxisomal β-oxidation measured the oxidation of [^{14}C]palmitoyl-CoA to [^{14}C]acetyl-CoA in hepatic post mitochondrial supernatant fractions (1650 g). The data points represent the mean [^{14}C]palmitoyl-CoA oxidase activity determined for five mice relative to the mean activity of the respective control group (□) for each sex. Control peroxisomal β-oxidation activities during the 4-month study ranged from 0.96 to 1.37 and 0.54 to 0.83 μmoles [^{14}C]palmitoyl-CoA oxidized/min/total liver for male and female mice, respectively.

minimal amount of pigment remained in Kupffer cells in scattered centrilobular regions in the high-dose mice after the recovery period.

Hepatic peroxisome proliferation, as measured by [^{14}C]palmitoyl-CoA oxidase activity, was dramatically increased in the high-dose mice after 1 month and after 3 months of treatment, but it decreased to control values after the 1-month recovery (Fig. 2). There was no significant increase in [^{14}C]palmitoyl-CoA oxidase activity in any other treatment group at any time examined.

In the mouse liver UDS S-phase assay, the experimental chemical did not induce DNA repair, but it did induce a slight increase in the number of cells in S phase 48 hours after an acute dose of 500 mg/kg (approximately 40% of the oral LD_{50}; Fig. 3). The doses at which tumors were observed in the mouse oncogenicity study were excessively high, as shown by the clear liver toxicity in the absence of tumors at 10 ppm. The lack of adverse results in a battery of short-term genetic tests, the inability to demonstrate DNA repair (UDS) in the target organ in vivo, and the in vivo induction of hepatic peroxisome proliferation concomitant with liver toxicity support a nongenotoxic mode of action. Moreover, there is a demonstrable nonlinear relationship between dose and hypertrophy and/or necrosis, as shown in the 90-day

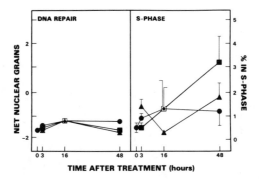

Figure 3

Time course for the induction of DNA repair and DNA replication (S phase) in the liver of male CD-1 mice following a single oral administration of either 0 mg/kg as corn oil vehicle (●) or 125 mg/kg (▲) or 500 mg/kg (■) of an experimental chemical. Hepatocytes were isolated 0, 3, 16, and 48 hr after dosing, incubated in the presence of [³H]thymidine, and subjected to quantitative autoradiography. Each point represents the mean ± s.d. of the mean values obtained from four animals; three slides were prepared per animal. If the error bar is not shown, the standard deviation was within the symbol. For DNA repair, 50 cells were scored per slide (450 cells scored per point), and for DNA replication (expressed as the percentage of the total hepatocyte population found in the S phase) 1000 cells were scored per slide (9000 cells scored per point).

study. The probable consequence of the liver damage is reparative hyperplasia, as evidenced by the increase in cells in S phase following even acute administration. From these results, it is concluded that the increased incidence of hepatic tumors in mice occurred secondarily to toxic effects produced by long-term administration of high doses of the experimental chemical. Expected human exposure to the chemical will be several orders of magnitude too low to result in liver toxicity and will therefore not present a carcinogenic hazard to humans under use conditions.

DISCUSSION

Although the determination of whether a carcinogen is genotoxic or nongenotoxic is important, the practical implication of that information is its relevance to quantitative risk assessment. The results from genotoxicity tests can provide direction for further testing to support the nonlinear extrapolation of risk.

If a chemical is clearly positive (adverse) in a battery of short-term genetic tests, one approach is to evaluate the "delivered dose." This is done by measuring the effective dose-to-target (adducts covalently bound to DNA) and comparing that value to potential exposure. If the results of a scientifically valid battery of short-term genetic tests are negative (not adverse), a number of possible approaches exist to provide data to support (but not prove) a nongenotoxic mode of carcinogenic action. These include in vivo and in vitro promotion assays, classic animal studies with an emphasis on histology of the target tissue, and the use of S-phase induction in the target organ as a sensitive indicator of hyperplasia. Peroxisome proliferation may also be measured as an indicator of potential indirect genetic effects. The data generated must, however, be evaluated within the context of all of the toxicity information available: other toxic effects, hormone balance, and immunological aspects may contribute to or attenuate the potential carcinogenicity of a chemical.

Difficulties arise when the short-term genetic test data are conflicting, i.e., positive results in some tests and negative results in others. It is important to keep in mind that false positives exist in these systems. ("False positive" is used here, in the true sense of the term, to mean that the endpoint measured is not indicative of the phenomena of concern.) False positives are known to occur in the Ames test via phenotypic curing (Ames 1971), in the point mutation *tk* locus assay in mouse lymphoma L5178Y cells as a result of pH effects (Cifone et al. 1984), and in cytogenetic assays in vitro at high concentrations and osmolalities (Galloway et al. 1985). Consequently, appropriate care must be taken in evaluating genotoxicity test results and using them to support a mode-of-action basis for risk assessment.

CONCLUSIONS

In evaluating the carcinogenic potential posed by the commercial use of a chemical, the emphasis should be toward developing data to determine whether the dose-response relationship is linear or nonlinear. Even with genotoxic chemicals, physical, chemical, and biologic factors may attenuate the effective dose-to-target (DNA) such that no hazard exists under use conditions.

Although no definitive methodology exists to demonstrate nongenotoxicity, a number of useful assays have been developed. Nongenotoxic results (e.g., in the in vivo/in vitro UDS S-phase assay) may be used in conjunction with metabolism, pharmacokinetic, and other appropriately designed animal studies to demonstrate nonlinear dose-response relationships, if, in fact, they exist.

If metabolic and biologic thresholds can be demonstrated for toxic effects that precede and are prerequisite to tumor formation, then the use of linear extrapolation models to evaluate risk to humans may be overly stringent.

ACKNOWLEDGMENTS

We express appreciation for the contributions of Mr. Greg Muller, Dr. William T. Lynch, Dr. Barbara Kulwich, Dr. Patricia Goldman, and Dr. Stephen L. Longacre.

REFERENCES

Ames, B.N. 1971. The detection of chemical mutagens with enteric bacteria. In *Chemical mutagens, principles and methods for their detection* (ed. A. Hollaender), p. 267. Plenum Press, New York.

Cifone, M.A., J. Fisher, and B. Myhr. 1984. Evidence for pH effects in the L5178Y Tk +/- mouse lymphoma forward mutation assay. *Environ. Mutagen.* **6:** 423.

Doolittle, D.J., E. Bermudez, P.K. Working, and B.E. Butterworth. 1984. Measurement of genotoxic activity in multiple tissues following inhalation exposure to dimethyl-nitrosamine. *Mutat. Res.* **141:** 123.

Galloway, S.M., C.L. Bean, M.A. Armstrong, D. Deasy, A. Kraynak, and M.O. Bradley. 1985. False positive *in vitro* chromosome aberration tests with non-mutagens at high concentrations and osmolalities. *Environ. Mutagen.* **7 (53):** 48.

Mirsalis, J.C. and B.E. Butterworth. 1980. Detection of unscheduled DNA synthesis in hepatocytes isolated from rats treated with genotoxic agents: An in vivo—in vitro assay for potential carcinogens and mutagens. *Carcinogenesis* **1:** 621.

Mirsalis, J.D., C.K. Tyson, and B.E. Butterworth. 1982. Detection of genotoxic carcinogens in the in vivo—in vitro hepatocyte DNA repair assay. *Environ. Mutagen.* **4:** 553.

Starr, T.B., J.E. Gibson, C.S. Barrow, C.J. Boreika, H.d'A. Heck, R.J. Levine, K.T. Morgan, and J.A. Swenberg. 1985. Estimating human cancer risk from formaldehyde: Critical issues. In *Formaldehyde-analytical chemistry and toxicology* (ed. V. Turaski), publ. no. 210, p. 299. American Chemical Society, Washington, D.C.

Ward, J.M., R.A. Griesemer, and E.K. Weisburger. 1979. The mouse liver tumor as an endpoint in carcinogenesis tests. *Toxicol. Appl. Pharmacol.* **51:** 389.

COMMENTS

WILLIAMS: When you showed the data on your battery of in vitro tests, you described it as being comprehensive. This raises the question that has been touched on only a bit: What is an adequate in vitro battery for genotoxicity?

SCRIBNER: Actually, I said it was a comprehensive program of testing. I didn't mean a comprehensive battery per se. I meant that we have done a lot of animal studies.

WILLIAMS: I'm going to comment on the battery. I would say that today any battery that lacks a system that has intrinsic biotransformation capability is an inadequate battery, because we now know that there are so many aberrations in the biotransformation that occurs in subcellular preparations that it has really become absolutely essential to have a whole-cell system. And, of course, the one that I think is the best is the hepatocyte because of its broad metabolic capability.

SCRIBNER: Certainly, there is no one test that will solve all the problems. I think that you have to look at point mutations, at chromosomal aberrations, and ultimately we would like to look at some aspect of aneuploidy, which we are not set up to do. It is also important to look at the biochemistry and metabolism.

ROSENKRANZ: I would like to say something about short-term tests. There is no single test that is highly predictive; each test has drawbacks. Some are highly sensitive and some are highly specific, but not both. I think that we can use this knowledge to construct batteries of tests, and these really have to reflect the philosophy that we have in testing. We can construct a battery that is highly risk-averse and which will minimize the false classification of carcinogens as noncarcinogens. We can also construct balanced batteries that serve other purposes, such as the inclusion of various endpoints. No one has spoken about the potency of the chemical. We have done a lot of studies and find no correlation between the potency of a chemical in a short-term test and its carcinogenicity, but we find a strong correlation between the carcinogenic potency of a chemical and whether or not it will give a signal in the short-term test. We can even construct a battery that will detect only highly potent carcinogens and a battery that will detect weak as well as strong carcinogens.

SCRIBNER: It amazes me in a sense that people expect these short-term tests to be 100% accurate. There is a lot of biology involved. You're talking about interaction with the DNA, a change in the DNA which may or may not become a mutational event, a mutational event that may or may not lead to a change in the cell, which may or may not lead to a tumor cell. At each stage, a lot of biology is involved. It's no surprise that these tests may not be predictive of carcinogenicity.

BUTTERWORTH: Gary [Williams] suggested that the battery of tests should include an assay system with intrinsic biotransformation capability, such as the hepatocyte UDS assay. In the studies described here, Dr. Scribner did look at UDS in the hepatocytes in the intact animal, where additional factors such as uptake, distribution metabolism, detoxification, and excretion were inherently accounted for. I think this is a good illustration of a chemical where forced cell proliferation may be the primary driving force for the induction of tumors. If one has a test that is not based on a genotoxic mechanism but gets at the true action of the chemical, then you can use that endpoint in choosing a safer substitute.

SCRIBNER: I would also like to talk about ethyl acrylate, which is a monomer. Ethyl acrylate has been tested in a number of chronic studies. By inhalation and by the dermal route, it is negative for tumor induction. But, when you give high doses, 200 mg/kg/day and 100 mg/kg/day, in high concentrations of 4% and 2% respectively, to the rat over the lifetime by gavage, forestomach tumors result. We are examining that in three ways. First, we are doing a lot of metabolism work. We know, in the whole animal, that ethyl acrylate is detoxified in two ways: (1) glutathione conjugation, and we have identified the substituted conjugates; and (2) we know that there is a carboxyesterase that breaks the ethyl acrylate into ethanol and acrylic acid. We are looking at those pathways in the forestomach specifically, and we are comparing the metabolism at different dose levels to the resulting histopathological effects (hyperplasia, irritation). Within 3 or 4 days at 200 mg/kg/day, hyperplasia is obvious. Secondly, we are also doing a 90-day study using the same doses, but in drinking water; so the concentrations are considerably lower. Finally, we plan to examine UDS and S-phase induction in the forestomach. Our approach will be to correlate the histopathological data, the continued hyperplasia (using S phase as an indicator of the hyperplasia), with the metabolism data.

YAMASAKI: We are singling out some chemicals that may work nongenotoxically. But, when we are considering that both nongenotoxic and genotoxic mechanisms are working during multistage carcinogenesis, I don't see how you can really regulate a chemical on the basis of the dose-response relationship of hyperplasia alone.

SCRIBNER: True, the mode of action of many of these chemicals is going to be multifold. One may see genotoxic and nongenotoxic effects at different dose levels, and maybe different effects in different tissues. All we can do is persevere and try to generate as much relevant data as possible. Proving a negative is an impossibility.

WEINSTEIN: There seems to be consensus that there are many variables that influence genotoxicity, so no simple criterion or a single test system can be easily extrapolated. I would think the same would apply to hyperplasia. Why do you think that's so simple? Perhaps the dose-response relationship for hyperplasia varies between species for the same compound. You assume that if an agent induces hyperplasia, but doesn't show genotoxicity, that that's how it works. You believe that if the hyperplasia is only seen at high doses in your animal system, choosing a much lower dose represents a reasonable safety factor for humans. But, do you really know that? What do we know about interspecies differences of dose response? Maybe the human is a hundredfold more sensitive to your agent in terms of hyperplasia.

REITZ: In any rodent studies, we extrapolate from animals to humans. What I think you're asking is can we act on probabilities or do we have to be absolutely certain? If we have to have absolute certainty, then I think we have all agreed that we're in an impossible position. The question is: Are we in a position where we can act on probabilities derived from experimental data?

WEINSTEIN: Do you also know that the hyperplasia you are scoring for is the mechanism by which your chemical works?

SCRIBNER: We will never be 100% certain. We must examine all the biology and make the most probable judgments. I think there are some clear-cut biological changes going on here and I believe it is reasonable to work from those.

Definition of a Human Cancer Hazard

GARY M. WILLIAMS
American Health Foundation
Valhalla, New York 10595

INTRODUCTION

The precise definition of a human chemical carcinogen requires evidence that the chemical has actually caused cancer in humans. Chemicals that have produced cancer in animal bioassays are really only experimental carcinogens. Nevertheless, to protect humans from causation of cancer by chemicals, data from experimental studies must be used to assess whether or not an experimental carcinogen represents a human cancer hazard.

One approach to extrapolation of animal data to assessment of human hazard is to assume that all experimental carcinogens represent hazards. This is, in fact, what most regulatory agencies have done. If this approach were uniformly applied, together with the assumption that any level of exposure represents a risk, the use of many valuable chemicals would be precluded, notably a number of pharmaceuticals that have led to neoplasm development in experimental animals through exaggerated pharmacologic effects produced at the maximally tolerated doses used for bioassay (Williams and Weisburger 1985).

The treatment of all experimental carcinogens as representing identical hazards is predicated largely on the assumptions that all carcinogens act alike and therefore the properties exhibited by some are possessed by all. This belief was fostered by the finding that many carcinogens could be converted to electrophilic reactants and hence were mutagenic or otherwise genotoxic. However, extensive information that has accrued on a broad spectrum of experimental carcinogens now reveals that these properties are not inherent in all carcinogenic chemicals (Williams and Weisburger 1987). Accordingly, chemical carcinogens have been categorized on the basis of whether they undergo chemical reaction with DNA, or, in the absence of evidence for reaction with DNA by the carcinogen or a derivative of it, whether they produce another biologic effect that could be the basis for carcinogenicity (Table 1). The effects of DNA-reactive and epigenetic carcinogens differ both qualitatively and quantitatively (Williams 1985).

QUALITATIVE EFFECTS OF DNA-REACTIVE AND EPIGENETIC CARCINOGENS

DNA-reactive Carcinogens

As a consequence of their ability to react with and alter DNA, carcinogens of the DNA-reactive type display a number of characteristic properties. In general, they

Banbury Report 25: Nongenotoxic Mechanisms in Carcinogenesis
© Cold Spring Harbor Laboratory. 0-87969-225-1/87. $1.00 + .00

Table 1
Classification of Carcinogenic Chemicals

Category and class	Example
DNA-reactive carcinogens	
activation-independent	alkylating agent
activation dependent	polycyclic aromatic hydrocarbon, nitrosamine
inorganic	metal
Epigenetic carcinogens	
promoter	organochlorine pesticides, saccharin
cytotoxic	nitrilotriacetic acid
hormone-modifying	estrogen, amitrole
peroxisome proliferator	clofibrate
immunosuppressor	purine analog
solid state	plastics
Unclassified	
miscellaneous	dioxane

lead to a high incidence of cancer within a short expression time and usually induce cancer in more than one organ and in different species. Other features of their carcinogenicity which indicate their potential hazard are listed in Table 2.

Epigenetic Carcinogens

Generalizations about epigenetic carcinogens must be cautious because they are diverse (Table 1) and operate through several different mechanisms. Nevertheless, typically, they lead to a low or moderate incidence of neoplasms after a lengthy expression time. The neoplasms may be predominantly benign and occur only in specific tissues and in specific species, often those with a significant cryptogenic background of the type of neoplasm whose occurrence was increased by the chemical. The features of the carcinogenicity of epigenetic carcinogens that function as neoplasm promoters are given in Table 3.

Table 2
Features of the Carcinogenic Effects of DNA-reactive Carcinogens

Occasionally active with single exposure
Frequently active at low (i.e., subtoxic) doses
Can have additive or synergistic effects with one another
Can be active transplacentally, and carcinogenicity often increased in neonates
Subcarcinogenic effects can be made manifest by subsequent promoting action
Effects can be enhanced by cocarcinogens
Organotropism shifted by inhibitors of biotransformation

Table 3
Features of the Carcinogenic Effects of Epigenetic Carcinogens of the Promoter Type

Not demonstrated to be active with single exposure
May be active at low dose but require a level of exposure to produce relevant biological effect
Additivity uncertain; can inhibit one another
None active transplacentally
No evidence of enhanced susceptibility of neonates
Shifts in organotropism not reported

QUANTITATIVE EFFECTS OF DNA-REACTIVE AND EPIGENETIC CARCINOGENS

As with the qualitative features of DNA-reactive and epigenetic carcinogens, their quantitative effects differ.

DNA-reactive Carcinogens

In numerous experiments using appropriate quantitative parameters, detailed dose-response relationships have been demonstrated for carcinogens. Most of the carcinogens studied were of the DNA-reactive type. Two effects are usually observed with DNA-reactive carcinogens: with increasing dose (1) the incidence and multiplicity of neoplasms increases, and (2) the expression time required for neoplasm appearance decreases. In most cases, the overall neoplasm yield in any specific organ is proportional to the total dose, but the speed or rate of neoplasm appearance is related to the amount in an individual dose or dose rate (Druckrey 1967; Littlefield and Gaylor 1985). With many DNA-reactive carcinogens, the lower the dose and dose rate, the lower the incidence of specific neoplasms. In the extreme, some DNA-reactive carcinogens, such as 2-acetylaminofluorene, which are potent carcinogens when administered chronically, are not at all active when given as a single large dose (Weisburger 1982). However, in a few instances, such as polycyclic aromatic hydrocarbons injected subcutaneously, the same total dose, when administered as smaller doses over a longer period of time, may actually be more effective than when given as larger, yet fewer individual doses in a shorter period of time (Hueper and Conway 1964).

DNA-reactive carcinogens vary greatly in their potency. For example, among liver carcinogens, to achieve a greater than 50% incidence with lifetime administration requires 1 ppb aflatoxin B_1, 5 ppm diethylnitrosamine, and 1000–5000 ppm safrole. Relatively few studies have been done on the effect of dose rate or even dose response with the weaker DNA-reactive carcinogens. Long et al. (1963) fed safrole in the diet to groups of 50 rats at levels of 100, 500, 1000, and 5000 ppm. Malignant liver cancers were obtained only at the highest dose level, and benign adenomas were obtained at the two highest doses, but not the lower doses. Shimkin et al. (1966) examined the potential of alkylating drugs of diverse structures to induce pulmonary tumors in mice. Strong carcinogens were active over a broad dose range, whereas the weaker ones gave evidence of some carcinogenicity only at the highest, but not at lower, dose levels. From considerations of metabolism, the barriers to electrophiles in reaching critical targets in DNA, protective DNA repair processes, and the like, it seems probable that for every DNA-reactive carcinogen there must be a no-effect threshold. It may be very low for powerful carcinogens, as suggested by the two large-scale studies, one using 2-acetylaminofluorene in mice (Brown and Hoel 1983) and the other using several nitrosamines in rats (Peto et al. 1984), but it seems to be correspondingly higher for weak carcinogens.

These dose-response studies on DNA-reactive carcinogens have provided data from which a number of mathematical models have been proposed (Office of Technology Assessment 1982; Hoel et al. 1983; Krewski et al. 1984). Although some of these have a biological basis (e.g., multistage) and others are tolerance-distribution models (e.g., probit), several can fit a data set equally well and therefore none can be considered superior from this perspective. The assumptions in some of these models, however, are not currently supported by experimental evidence. For example, linearity at low dose is not established. In fact, even for the less complicated process of chemical mutagenesis in vivo, a drop below linearity at low doses has been demonstrated (Russell et al. 1982). Consequently, a sublinear curve probably best fits current data and concepts on carcinogenic effects at low levels of exposure (Hoel et al. 1983). Also, as noted, the absence of a threshold has not been demonstrated for any carcinogen. To the contrary, no-observed-effect-levels (NOELs) have been observed in many studies, particularly with weak carcinogens, although there are always statistical limitations on the certainty of such observations. In addition, all models have been developed from data on DNA-reactive carcinogens, which ignores the observation (discussed below) that thresholds may be quite high with some epigenetic carcinogens of the promoter class. Thus, there is clearly a need for a model with a better biological basis. Unfortunately, the process of carcinogenesis is so complex and multifactorial that this may never be possible.

Relatively little information exists on quantitative effects in humans. In the few situations where human exposures and subsequent carcinogenicity could be quantified, dose-dependent carcinogenic effects have been observed (Williams et al. 1985). The most reliable quantitative data on human cancer resulting from exposure to specific carcinogens come from studies of occupational or therapeutic exposures. In these situations, adequate data for several carcinogens show that human cancer incidence is proportional to dose, often measured by length of employment, since there are virtually no actual data on the prevailing levels of any chemical in the industrial environment, especially in the past when exposures were high enough to lead to cancer. The cancer incidence in workers exposed to benzidine, vinyl chloride, or bis(chloromethyl)ether indicates a general relationship between exposure and disease occurrence. Workers engaged in uranium or asbestos mining exhibit a risk of cancer broadly related to the length of time an individual was engaged in these particular occupations. Likewise, with the drug chlornaphazine, where intake was reasonably well established, the percentage of treated patients that subsequently developed bladder cancer was proportional to the amount of drug administered.

The question of whether there are thresholds in human exposure to DNA-reactive carcinogens is of great contemporary importance in light of the sensitivity of analytic techniques to measure accurately (at the parts-per-billion or even the parts-per-trillion level) the presence of carcinogens in environmental samples. Application of such techniques have shown that humans are intermittently exposed to a wide variety of DNA-reactive carcinogens. A major source is food, which can contain naturally occurring carcinogens such as mycotoxins, carcinogens introduced as environmental contaminants, and carcinogens formed from food constituents. Likewise, drinking water contains many carcinogens at minute levels. Other sources of exposure are intentional cigarette smoking and involuntary inhalation of cigarette smoke and carcinogens in the air as a result of natural events such as forest fires, as well as industrial polution. It is virtually certain that every human is exposed to one or more DNA-reactive carcinogens at some time during life. If no threshold existed for carcinogenesis, it would be expected that every human surviving to old age would develop cancer. This does not happen, and so it is reasonable to conclude that, as with animal studies, there are indeed exposures that do not lead to cancer. This inference is supported by observations that not every worker exposed to DNA-reactive carcinogens in the work place develops cancer, nor does every patient receiving alkylating chemotherapeutic drugs, which are themselves carcinogenic, develop a second cancer.

Epigenetic Carcinogens

For carcinogens that are not DNA-reactive and operate by producing other cellular effects, the carcinogenic effects might be expected to parallel the dose-response relationships for the cellular effect that underlies carcinogenicity. Unfortunately, relatively few dose-response studies have been done with carcinogens of the epigenetic type, and almost none with regard to underlying toxicologic or pharmacologic effects. Data exist for the chelating agent nitrilotriacetic acid, which produces kidney and bladder tumors after exposure to about 75 mmoles/kg diet. This effect diminishes dramatically, in a nonlinear fashion, when the exposure is reduced below 50 mmoles/kg diet (Anderson et al. 1982; Kitahori et al. 1985). The mechanistic explanation is based on the cytotoxicity of high levels of the agent resulting from chelation of divalent cations. In a dose-response study with amitrole in rats (Steinhoff et al. 1983), thyroid tumors were induced at 100 ppm, which perturbed thyroid function, but not at 10 or 1 ppm, which did not affect the thyroid. No tumors occurred in mice or hamsters.

For several types of epigenetic carcinogens, especially promoters, theoretical considerations as well as available data from experimental studies strongly support the concept and existence of NOELs. When the promoting agents DDT, phenobarbital, or butylated hydroxyanisole (BHA) were tested by themselves for carcinogenicity in rats, an effect was evident only at the highest dose levels given in lifetime studies. These observations are supported by tests for promotion, where, after an appropriate genotoxic carcinogen is administered, higher yields of neoplasms are induced in a shorter time. After exposure to the appropriate tissue-specific genotoxic carcinogens, NOELs have been observed in promotion assays for butylated hydroxytoluene (Maeura and Williams 1984) and phenobarbital (Peraino et al. 1977) in liver carcinogenesis.

BHA, a useful food antioxidant, has been reported to induce squamous cell neoplasms in the forestomach of rats and hamsters, but not of mice (Ito et al. 1985). In appropriate tests for genotoxicity, BHA proved negative (Williams 1986), and in animal studies, it exerted a promoting effect in the forestomach (Ito et al. 1985). The dose-response characteristics of promotion were explored by administration of a single gavage dose of the direct-acting gastric carcinogen N-methyl-N'-nitro-N-nitrosoguanidine to male rats, followed 1 week later by feeding of diets containing between 60 and 12,000 ppm BHA for life. Increases in squamous cell forestomach tumors were obtained with concentrations of 12,000 and possibly 6000 ppm, but no enhancing effect was apparent with 3000 ppm and lower doses (Weisburger and Williams 1986; Williams 1986). These results are supported by the finding of increased proliferative lesions with 20,000 ppm BHA, fewer with 5000 ppm, and none with 2500 ppm. Even with 20,000 ppm BHA feeding, there was reversibility after 1–2 weeks of cessation of BHA intake (Altmann et al. 1985; Iverson et al. 1985). Thus, the information available suggests both the existence of a threshold and reversibility, as is typically expected of agents operating through epigenetic mechanisms.

Useful data exist for the quantitative effects of promoting agents in humans. Bile acids are demonstrated promoters for colon cancer. In high-risk populations for colon cancer in the western world, the prevailing concentration of bile acids is about 12 mg/g of feces, stemming from consumption of high-fat, low-fiber diets. In Japan, where fat intake is lower, or in Finland, where cereal fiber intake is high, the risk for colon cancer is low and the concentration of fecal bile acids is about 4 mg/g, only one third of the concentration associated with high risk (Reddy et al. 1980; Wynder et al. 1983). Complex tobacco smoke contains relatively small amounts of genotoxic polycyclic aromatic hydrocarbons, nicotine-derived nitrosamines, and certain heterocyclic amines (Surgeon General Report 1982). The major effect of tobacco stems from the enhancing effect of the acidic fraction of the smoke. It is established that an individual chronically smoking 40 cigarettes per day is at high risk, but with 10 cigarettes per day the risk is much lower, and with 4 cigarettes per day the risk is difficult to evaluate accurately. These observations represent evidence that enhancing factors have steep dose-response curves in humans, as in experimental animals. Cessation of smoking reduces the risk considerably because promotion is removed (Wynder 1983).

Human beings have been exposed to significant levels of a variety of epigenetic carcinogens such as certain of the organochlorine pesticides, phenobarbital, and physiologic levels of estrogens without evidence of cancer causation (Clemmesen et al. 1980; Hayes 1982). Yet, carcinogens that are not DNA-reactive have produced human cancer, such as asbestos through occupational exposure and diethylstilbestrol at high pharmacologic levels. These two chemicals, however, are special cases. Inhaled asbestos fibers remain in the lung; thus, there is lifelong continuing exposure of the tissue, even after inhalation ceases. With high levels of transplacental diethylstilbestrol, there appears to be permanent alteration of genital tissues and imprinting of the endocrine system of the fetus, which is eventually expressed at puberty as a special type of endocrine-related neoplasm, clear cell carcinoma of the vagina. The negative findings with other epigenetic agents suggest that their exposure levels have been below the thresholds for cancer production.

Thus, epigenetic carcinogens, like DNA-reactive carcinogens, act in a dose-dependent fashion, although the dose-response relationships appear to be different. Thresholds have been observed for both types of carcinogens in experimental animals and humans. The thresholds for DNA-reactive carcinogens vary greatly and may be low. Those for nongenotoxic, epigenetic carcinogens, particularly of the promoter class, have been fairly high and are a function of well-established pharmacologic and toxicologic phenomena. These observations indicate that the interpretation of carcinogenic tests to delineate human hazard must incorporate mechanistic considerations (Weisburger 1985).

DEFINITION OF A HUMAN CANCER HAZARD

Given the qualitative and quantitative differences between DNA-reactive and epigenetic carcinogens, it would be expected that the former represent a much greater hazard to humans. Indeed, this is the case; most human carcinogens are of the DNA-reactive type (Table 4). Therefore, based on mechanistic considerations and available data, it seems likely that experimental carcinogens of the DNA-reactive type represent definite human cancer hazards. The finding of biochemical DNA binding or definitive genotoxicity in short-term tests, together with the carcinogenic effects described in the section on qualitative effects, therefore provides the profile for an experimental carcinogen that should be regarded as a definite potential human carcinogenic hazard (Table 5). This constellation of findings is similar to that described by Squire (1981) as carcinogen class I.

The same conclusions cannot be drawn for epigenetic carcinogens. Although several (e.g., diethylstilbestrol) have caused cancer in humans, this usually occurs only under specific conditions of exposure. In the case of hormones, cancer has

Table 4

Genotoxicity of Chemicals Judged to be Carcinogenic to Humans by the International Agency for Research on Cancer

Chemical	Evidence for activity in short-term tests[a]	Assessment[b]
4-Aminobiphenyl	sufficient	D
Arsenic and arsenic compounds	limited	?
Asbestos	inadequate	E
Azathioprine	limited	E
Benzene	limited	E
Benzidine	sufficient	D
N-N-Bis(2-chloroethyl)naphthylamine	limited	D
Bis(chloromethyl)ether	limited	D
Chlorambucil	sufficient	D
Chromium and certain chromium compounds	sufficient	D
Conjugated estrogens	inadequate	E
Cyclophosphamide	sufficient	D
Diethylstilbestrol	inadequate	E
Melphalan	sufficient	D
Mustard gas	sufficient	D
Myleran	sufficient	D
2-Naphthylamine	sufficient	D
Nickel and certain nickel compounds	inadequate	?
Treosulphan	inadequate	?
Vinyl chloride	sufficient	D

[a]Data extracted from International Agency for Research on Cancer (1982).
[b]Categorization by Williams and Weisburger (1987). D indicates DNA-reactive; E, epigenetic; ?, data insufficient.

occurred with dosages that produce perturbations of the endocrine system. Many other epigenetic carcinogens, such as phenobarbital, DDT, saccharin, nitrilotriacetic acid, have not been associated with human cancer despite significant exposures. Therefore, experimental carcinogens of the epigenetic type cannot be assumed to represent human carcinogenic hazards.

EXPOSURE CONTROL

Control of exposure to all types of carcinogens should be done on a case-by-case basis with utilization of all relevant pharmacologic and toxicologic data (Interna-

Table 5

Definition of Human Cancer Hazard

DNA-reactive or genotoxic
Produces a high incidence of malignant neoplasms with a short expression time in experimental animals
Produces cancer in several organs and several experimental species

tional Life Sciences Institute 1984). With regard to DNA-reactive carcinogens, for the few chemicals for which quantitative data from humans could be compared with those from experimental animals, there was for each at least one species whose sensitivity was comparable to that of humans within an order of magnitude (Williams et al. 1985). Therefore, after development of sufficient data (i.e., multispecies dose-response data), it may be possible to set reasonably safe limits of exposure (i.e., virtually safe doses) by using extrapolation procedures. As discussed above, the models for extrapolation from the high doses used in testing to the low exposures that might occur to humans have certain deficiencies. One that does not depend on any mathematical model is the linear interpolation algorithm of Gaylor and Kodell (1980). This may be used to determine a "de minimus" risk, usually taken to be less than a 1 in 10^6 lifetime risk of developing cancer (Cornfield 1977). Although such procedures are presently used out of necessity, they do not incorporate critical factors that characterize the human situation, such as multiple exposures, concurrent action of cocarcinogens, enhancement by promoters, and conditions of possible enhanced sensitivity. For these reasons, the objective for DNA-reactive carcinogens should be zero exposure where this is technologically feasible.

For epigenetic carcinogens, safety assessment should be based on the recognition that an antecedent biologic or toxic effect underlies their carcinogenicity. Thus, attention should be focused on delineating NOELs for such effects in multispecies testing. Control can then follow standard food safety practices (Office of Technology Assessment 1979) that have been demonstrated to provide adequate protection against noncancer toxicity from foodborne chemicals. Briefly, an acceptable daily intake (ADI) is calculated from the NOEL by dividing by a safety factor that is determined by the adequacy of the quantitative data. Specific applications have been discussed for di(2-ethylhexyl)phthalate (Turnbull and Rodricks 1985) and BHA (Williams 1986), whose limited carcinogenic effects were described above.

CONCLUSIONS

The immense progress in the understanding of the mechanisms of carcinogenesis has led to the recognition that there are different types of carcinogens. These differ both qualitatively and quantitatively in ways that suggest that different procedures for risk management are indicated. There will always be uncertainty regarding the risk of cancer from environmental exposures because of the complexities of the carcinogenic process and of the human situation; the goal of research is to minimize the uncertainty.

ACKNOWLEDGMENT

During preparation of this paper, the author received support from grant CA-17613 from the National Cancer Institute.

REFERENCES

Altmann, H.J., P.W. Webster, G. Mathiaschk, W. Grunow, and C.A. van der Heijden. 1985. Induction of early lesions in the forestomach of rats by 3-tert-butyl-4-hydroxyanisole (BHA). *Food Chem. Toxicol.* **8**: 723.

Anderson, R.L., C.L. Alden, and J.A. Merski. 1982. The effects of nitrilotriacetate on cation disposition and urinary tract toxicity. *Food Chem. Toxicol.* **20**: 105.

Brown, K.G. and D.G. Hoel. 1983. Modeling time-to-tumor data: Analysis of the ED_{01} study. *Fundam. Appl. Toxicol.* **3**: 458.

Clemmesen, J., D.M. Conning, D. Henschler, and F. Oesch, eds. 1980. Quantitative aspects of risk assessment in chemical carcinogenesis. *Arch. Toxicol.* (Suppl.) **3**: 1.

Cornfield, J. 1977. Carcinogenic risk assessment. *Science* **198**: 693.

Druckrey, H. 1967. Quantitative aspects in chemical carcinogenesis. *Union Int. Contre Cancer Monogr. Ser.* **7**: 60.

Gaylor, D.W. and R.L. Kodell. 1980. Linear interpolation algorithm for low dose risk assessment of toxic substances. *J. Environ. Pathol. Toxicol.* **4**: 305.

Hayes, W.J., Jr. 1982. *Pesticides studied in man.* Williams and Wilkins, Baltimore, Maryland.

Hoel, D.G., N.L. Kaplan, and M.W. Anderson. 1983. Implication of nonlinear kinetics on risk estimation in carcinogenesis. *Science* **219**: 1032.

Hueper, W.C. and W.D. Conway. 1964. *Chemical carcinogenesis and cancers.* Charles Thomas Publishers, Springfield, Illinois.

International Agency for Research on Cancer (IARC). 1982. *Monographs on the evaluation of the carcinogenic risk of chemicals to humans: Chemicals, industrial processes and industries associated with cancer in humans,* suppl. 4. International Agency for Research on Cancer, Lyon, France.

International Life Sciences Institute. 1984. Interpretation and extrapolation of chemical and biological carcinogenicity data to establish human safety standards. In *Current issues in toxicology* (ed. H.C. Grice), p. 1. Springer-Verlag, New York.

Ito, N., S. Fukushima, and T. Hiroyuki. 1985. Carcinogenicity and modification of the carcinogenetic response by BHA, BHT and other antioxidants. *CRC Crit. Rev. Toxicol.* **15**: 109.

Iverson, F., E. Lok, E. Nera, K. Karpinski, and D.B. Clayson. 1985. A 13-week feeding study of butylated hydroxyanisole: The subsequent regression of the induced lesions in male Fischer 344 rat forestomach epithelium. *Toxicology* **35**: 1.

Kitahori, Y., N. Konishi, T. Shimoyama, and Y. Hiasa. 1985. Dose-dependent promoting effect of trisodium nitrilotriacetate monohydrate on urinary bladder carcinogenesis in Wistar rats pretreated with N-butyl-N-(4-hydroxylbutly) nitrosamine. *Jpn. J. Cancer Res. (Gann)* **76**: 818.

Krewski, D., C. Brown, and D. Murdoch. 1984. Determining "safe" levels of exposure: Safety factors or mathematical models? *Fundam. Appl. Toxicol.* **4**: S383.

Littlefield, N.A. and D.W. Gaylor. 1985. Influence of total dose and dose rate in carcinogenicity studies. *J. Toxicol. Environ. Health* **15**: 545.

Long, E.L, A.A. Nelson, O.G. Fitzhugh, and W.H. Hansen. 1963. Liver tumors produced in rats by feeding safrole. *Arch. Pathol.* **75**: 595.

Maeura, Y. and G.M. Williams. 1984. Enhancing effect of butylated hydroxytoluene on the development of liver altered foci and neoplasms induced by N-2-fluorenylacetamide in rats. *Food Chem. Toxicol.* **22:** 191.

Office of Technology Assessment. 1979. *Environmental contaminants in food.* U.S. Government Printing Office, Washington, D.C.

————. 1982. *Cancer risk: Assessing and reducing the dangers in our society.* U.S. Government Printing Office, Washington, D.C.

Peraino, C., R.J.M. Fry, E. Staffeld, and J.P. Christopher. 1977. Enhancing effects of phenobarbitone and butylated hydroxytoluene on 2-acetylaminofluorene-induced hepatic tumorigenesis in the rat. *Food Cosmet. Toxicol.* **15:** 93.

Peto, R., R. Gray, P. Brantom, and P. Grasso. 1984. Nitrosamine carcinogenesis in 5120 rodents: Chronic administration of sixteen different concentrations of NDEA, NDMA, NPYR and NPIP in the water of 4440 inbred rats, with parallel studies on NDEA alone of the effect of the age of starting (3,6, or 20 weeks) and of the species (rats, mice or hamsters). *Int. Agency Res. Cancer Sci. Publ.* **57:** 627.

Reddy, B.S., L.A. Cohen, G.D. McCoy, P. Hill, J.H. Weisburger, and E.L. Wynder. 1980. Nutrition and its relationship to cancer. *Adv. Cancer Res.* **32:** 237.

Russell, W.L., P.R. Hunsicker, G.D. Raymen, M.H. Steele, K.F. Stelzner, and H.M. Thompson. 1982. Dose response for ethylnitrosurea-induced specific-locus mutagens in mouse spermatogonia. *Proc. Natl. Acad. Sci. U.S.A.* **73:** 3589.

Shimkin, M.B., J.H. Weisburger, E.K. Weisburger, N. Gubareff, and V. Suntzeff. 1966. Bioassay of 29 alkylating chemicals by the pulmonary-tumor response in strain A mice. *J. Natl. Cancer Inst.* **36:** 915.

Steinhoff, D., H. Weber, U. Mohr, and K. Boehme. 1983. Evaluation of amitrole (aminotriazole) for potential carcinogenicity in orally dosed rats, mice and golden hamsters. *Toxicol. Appl. Pharmacol.* **69:** 161.

Squire, R.A. 1981. Ranking animal carcinogens: A proposed regulatory approach. *Science* **214:** 877.

Surgeon General Report. 1982. The health consequences of smoking. In *Cancer,* chapt. 5, publ. no. DHHS (PHS) 82-50179. U.S. Government Printing Office, Washington, D.C.

Turnbull, B. and J.V. Rodricks. 1985. Assessment of possible carcinogenic risk to humans resulting from exposure to di(2-ethylhexyl)phthalate (DEHP). *J. Am. Coll. Toxicol.* **4:** 111.

Weisburger, E.K. 1982. N-2-Fluorenylacetamide and derivatives. In *Carcinogens in industry and the environment* (ed. J. Sontag), p. 583. Marcel Dekker, New York.

Weisburger, J.H. 1985. Definition of a carcinogen as a potential human carcinogenic risk. *Jpn. J. Cancer Res. (Gann)* **76:** 1244.

Weisburger, J.H. and G.M. Williams. 1987. Testing procedures to define carcinogens as human cancer risks. In *Human risk assessment: The role of animal selection and extrapolation* (ed. M.V. Roloff). Monsanto Company, St. Louis, Missouri. Raven Press, New York.

Williams, G.M. 1985. Genotoxic and epigenetic carcinogens. In *Safety evaluation and regulation of chemicals 2.* (ed. F. Homburger), p. 251. Karger, Basel.

————. 1986. Epigenetic effects of butylated hydroxyanisole. *Food Chem. Toxicol.* **24:** 1163.

Williams, G.M. and J.H. Weisburger. 1985. Carcinogenicity testing of drugs. *Prog. Drug Res.* **29:** 155.

————. 1987. Chemical carcinogens. In *Casarett and Doull's toxicology: The basic science of poisons,* 3rd edition (ed. J. Doull et al.), p. 99. Macmillan, New York.

Williams, G.M., B. Reiss, and J.H. Weisburger. 1985. A comparison of the animal and human carcinogenicity of environmental, occupational and therapeutic chemicals. *Adv. Mod. Environ. Toxicol.* **12:** 207.

Wynder, E.L. 1983. Tumor enhancers: Underestimated factors in the epidemiology of lifestyle-associated cancers. *Environ. Health Perspect.* **50:** 15.

Wynder, E.L., G.A. Leveille, J.H. Weisburger, and G.E. Livingston, eds. *Environmental aspects of cancer: The role of macro and micro components of foods.* Food and Nutrition Press, Westport, Connecticut.

COMMENTS

SWENBERG: You mentioned linear no-threshold models. Most of the agencies are not using those anymore. Rather, they utilize multistage models. Unfortunately, they then use the upper 95% confidence limit, which is again a linear term.

WILLIAMS: I don't know which agencies you are referring to. I can tell you that here, in New York State, the last time a carcinogen was banned it was on the basis of a linear no-threshold model.

SWENBERG: I don't think there is a scientific basis for that in a multistage process such as cancer.

WILLIAMS: I guess my point would be that there's not much basis for the use of either model.

SWENBERG: I think you're right.

PITOT: In your list of human carcinogens, you indicated that estrogens in liver are promoting agents, for which there is good evidence, both experimental and clinical. Asbestos also exhibits promoting activity, although it may be a cocarcinogen as well. The point is that you left out of that list two of the critical factors in human carcinogenesis: one is diet and the other is cigarette smoke. The effects of both of these are much more due to their promoting action than to their initiating activity.

WILLIAMS: I would be the last one to dispute the role of tobacco and diet in human cancer. You make a valid point. I think we all agree that promotion occurs in humans. What I was trying to say is that among the group of chemicals judged by the IARC to cause cancer in humans, there is not a synthetic chemical that acts as a promoting agent in animals to cause cancer.

PITOT: Except estrogen.

WILLIAMS: Again, I was talking about the human effect. Certainly, in animal models, enhancement of tumor development is produced by estrogen; whether that is related to the human carcinogenicity I think is unclear, but it may be. In the case of diethylstilbestrol, where it is vaginal adenocarcinomas, I don't think that has anything to do with promoting activity. Most likely, diethylstilbestrol exerts an effect on differentiation of the genital tract and probably a persistent effect on the endocrine system in the affected individuals.

PITOT: The epidemiology of hepatic lesions induced in the human by synthetic estrogen contraceptives is very similar to the action of these agents in rodent hepatocarcinogenesis. They are reversible, they produce lesions that are histologically identical, and their natural history is essentially the same as it is in the rat.

WILLIAMS: I am just not sure how clear that is. The problem is that the epidemiology really is so meager. Millions of women have used oral contraceptives, but the number of cases of liver adenomas is only in the hundreds at most. The circumstantial evidence is there, but, really, it's difficult to understand why there wouldn't be more cases if estrogens were really operating as a liver carcinogen in humans.

WEINSTEIN: You began by saying that there is no rational reason to do threshold and dose-response extrapolations between species for genotoxic agents.

WILLIAMS: For the DNA-reactive carcinogens, I do not see any way of estimating any safe level of exposure. Therefore, my approach would be either complete elimination or, if the chemical is an indispensable material in some way, reduction of exposure to the absolute minimum technologically possible. But I don't feel comfortable enough with the use of any mathematical model to say that a safe level of exposure to a DNA-reactive carcinogen can be calculated. On the other hand, I was also trying to say in my presentation that I think we might be able to do that for non-DNA-reactive carcinogens.

MAGEE: What is a DNA-reactive carcinogen?

WILLIAMS: It is a compound that reacts covalently with DNA, chemically forming adducts.

SWENBERG: I think we have to be very careful in making strong generalizations on even your DNA-reacting compounds, because the fact of the matter is, we really have very little data on low-dose effects. The number of chemicals for which we have molecular dosimetry data that cover more than two orders of magnitude can be counted on one hand. When we get into risk assessment, we are frequently talking four to six orders of magnitude below the lowest dose that produced tumors. The fact of the matter is that I don't know of any agent that has induced adducts at a level below 1 per 10^9 nucleotides that has been associated with a carcinogenic response. You said that you believe that there is no level of a genotoxic agent that is safe. We do not really have evidence to support or refute such a statement. Techniques are advancing that will allow us to measure adducts many more orders of magnitude lower than we have ever been able to before. This will permit the needed modeling to be done. I think that we should have a moratorium in the meantime, until we get some data to discuss.

CONCLUDING DISCUSSION

PITOT: In several earlier discussions at this conference, there was emphasis on the "reversibility" of the stage of tumor promotion. In the two systems that have been best studied in the rodent, epidermal and hepatic carcinogenesis, reversibility of lesions and altered function during the stage of tumor promotion has been clearly demonstrated. We have been confused in the past by always requiring that a promoting agent induce the malignant transformation. It is now clear from model systems of multistage hepatocarcinogenesis that lesions will appear during the stage of promotion, then disappear on removal of the promoting agent, and reappear on its reapplication. A similar effect has, I believe, been shown in the skin system. It therefore seems reasonable that multistage carcinogenesis must have at least three phases: initiation, promotion, and progression. Previously, we have tended to combine the latter two, but Dr. Weinstein has suggested, as did Dr. Slaga in his presentation at this conference, that some chemicals act primarily to bring cells into the stage of progression. Like initiation, progression appears to involve later genetic changes, which can be considered irreversible.

The reversibility of promotion, whether demonstrable as an altered rate phenomenon, such as in Dr. Boutwell's earlier experiments with skin, or in the reversibility of lesions occurring during this stage, indicates that chemicals acting during the stage of promotion may exhibit a different level of risk to the human population. Complete carcinogens cause cells to traverse all three stages of carcinogenesis, but some chemicals act primarily, if not exclusively, during the stage of promotion. Phenobarbital, despite its recently reported effects in some short-term, DNA-damaging tests, acts primarily, if not exclusively, during the promotion stage of hepatocarcinogenesis. The promoting action of TCDD and asbestos may appear to be irreversible, but these agents remain in the organism for extended periods, even a lifetime, indicating that their pharmacokinetic properties result in this appearance of irreversibility. Thus, the reversible aspects of the stage of tumor promotion should now become a factor in our consideration of the mechanisms of carcinogenesis and of the risk of agents acting primarily at this stage.

WEINSTEIN: I'm not sure that that provides any reassurance that these compounds are going to be safer because for every one of them that we are considering, there will be prolonged and repeated exposure, and many of them do accumulate in body fats. So, we hear of a mouse liver assay for halogenated organics as being discounted for the kinds of reasons you mentioned. These are the very compounds that do accumulate and remain there for long periods of time.

PITOT: But many promoting agents do not remain in the organism for prolonged periods (e.g., phenobarbital, saccharin, and CCl_4). With the reversibility of

Banbury Report 25: Nongenotoxic Mechanisms in Carcinogenesis
© Cold Spring Harbor Laboratory. 0-87969-225-1/87. $1.00 + .00

the promoting effects of these agents, it is certainly conceivable that a short exposure to such chemicals in industry with subsequent removal of the worker from exposure for a time, with reasonable precautions during exposure periods, may be applicable in certain instances.

WILLIAMS: I agree entirely with what Dr. Weinstein and Dr. Pitot have said about our knowledge of the causes of human cancer. Most of these probably relate to life-style factors, smoking and diet. However, I construe that as support for the position that I was making, namely, that synthetic chemicals that are not DNA-reactive have not been prominently involved in the causation of human cancer. We are continuously exposed to agents of this type (BHA, BHT, etc.). What I was trying to bring out was an explanation for why these have not caused cancer in humans and how we can use that knowledge to perhaps arrive at a way of assessing similar agents. The reason I agreed to talk on risk assessment is that I think that the two suggestions that have been made, Jim (Swenberg) said declare a moratorium and Dr. Weinstein said do more research, are truly impractical. Regulators have to decide almost every day on chemical substances of this type, and they cannot simply defer it until we "know more." What I was trying to get at is how we can best utilize the information that we have. My present conclusion is that current knowledge is telling us that agents pose different kinds of risks and that we can make judgments based on that.

WEINSTEIN: I disagree. As I told you, if I had to serve as a regulator this afternoon, I would not use your guidelines because I don't see any factual basis for them. I think humans are sensitive to "nongenotoxic agents." Your own Institute is committed to the principle, with breast cancer and colon cancer, where the major determinants are not genotoxic. There may be genotoxic agents there as well.

WILLIAMS: In those instances as with cigarette smoking, the people at risk are people who smoke two packs a day, not somebody who has a cigarette every other day. With dietary fat, it is the American population which consumes 40% of its calories as fat, not the Japanese population which consumes 15 or 20%. So, I think, even in the human situation we have evidence that these promoting effects have quite steep dose-response effects.

WEINSTEIN: Give me the evidence for the steep dose response.

WILLIAMS: Cigarette smoking. I just told you.

WEINSTEIN: It's linear with respect to the number of cigarettes smoked.

WILLIAMS: The slope is very steep.

WEINSTEIN: Do you have shallow slopes that are well established for a promoter?

WILLIAMS: I was showing the data that we have acquired on BHA over a dose range greater than two orders of magnitude. Those data show in the effective range a very steep slope and then no effect. Henry Pitot showed data for phenobarbital exactly like that earlier in the week.

WEINSTEIN: The benzo[a]pyrene dose-response curve is curvilinear.

SWENBERG: What happens if you take it four more orders of magnitude, which is what the risk assessment is based on?

WEINSTEIN: Lower? I don't know. Nor do you know on BHA.

SWENBERG: That's the way the risk assessments are going.

WEINSTEIN: Yes. Since there are no hard facts in that range, don't make assumptions.

SWENBERG: One way or the other.

WEINSTEIN: That's right, one way or the other. That's why if I were to buy your arguments, I would go to a NOEL (no-observed-effect level) approach for initiators also because I don't see the distinction. But if you do go to the NOEL approach, I would like to know how you arrive at the appropriate safety factor.

WILLIAMS: I am puzzled by your repeated assertion that you don't see the difference because, to me, there is a big difference between TPA and BHA. TPA has its own cellular receptors, and when it binds to them, it initiates a cascade of reactions that you are more familiar with than I am. But BHA does not have a receptor and it doesn't operate, so far as we know, through any process like that.

WEINSTEIN: Do you think bile acids are involved in colon cancer as promoters?

WILLIAMS: That's an old trick, trying to change the subject.

WEINSTEIN: No, it's right on the subject. The point is that there are agents that have receptors that will work in the range of 10^{-8} molar because receptors for these factors tend to have that affinity. For agents that don't, you will need a bigger dose, and they will work indirectly. But once they generate the signal, it can operate through the same mechanism. That's what I presume.

COHEN: But then, if you're exposed to a lower dose, is that relevant to any risk?

WEINSTEIN: The dose response will be different, but people are going to eat more BHA than they are going to eat TPA.

WILLIAMS: But not enough.

WEINSTEIN: How do you know?

WILLIAMS: To determine that, we should begin to try to do some kind of metabolic or biochemical epidemiology. That was part of the basis for my discussion of BHT, that we know in animal models that there are certain measurable effects that occur at high doses. We know that those are not occurring in humans at the lower dose. Now, where I would endorse very emphatically what you said is to go further with BHT and BHA and find out whether, at the doses that we are allowing to be used today, any of the biochemical alterations that occur at promoting and nonpromoting doses in the animal model are produced in humans. I have, in fact, proposed this to companies who are involved in manufacturing agents of this type. Unfortunately, there is a problem in conducting such studies. Many of the biochemical effects produced by promoters are also produced by other xenobiotics, such as ethanol. The companies are concerned that if they undertake a study on workers exposed to a promoter, some individual may have two shots of whiskey the night before, causing his parameters to go up. The subject would then show the alterations that were to be ascribed to the promoting activity of the chemical. This individual would look like he is at risk, and there would be a problem. What it is going to require, I guess, is almost putting people in a metabolic ward, to get them away from other extraneous influences, so that the effect of alteration of a single component in the environment can be studied.

WEINSTEIN: It's probably worth it. That's how we solve other human diseases. We don't just work on some animal model; we eventually go into the human and we dig deep and we find out what is going on there. Now, I'll give you a specific example on dose. TPA at 10^{-8} molar induces ornithine decarboxylase and the expression of a number of cellular genes. Maybe they're involved in the response. Let's assume they are. If you want to do the same thing with deoxycholic acid, which your group has implicated in colon cancer, you've got to go to 1 millimolar. But the colon sees 1 millimolar concentrations.

WILLIAMS: The thrust of what I was trying to say is that it's worthwhile doing the science. When you argue that there are no possible distinctions between different types of promoters, or whatever, I think that in fact discourages manufacturers from undertaking this kind of research.

REITZ: It seems to me one of the most fundamental differences between direct DNA-damaging agents and ones that produce either indirect DNA damage or effects that stimulate compensatory regeneration is in the very nature of genetic material. DNA is really a unique component of the cell, and if you pluck the nucleus out of the cell the cell cannot replace it. But, if you affect a ribosome, a protein molecule, or a small cofactor, the cell has a finite capacity to compensate for this type of alteration. So, at the cellular level, we could expect a fundamental difference in the implications of damaging genetic material versus indirect effects on nongenetic components. To me, that underlies the basis for a very real distinction between those types of actions.

BUTTERWORTH: Ray Tennant said that he thought that regulatory policy should be based on the best science available. Although the regulators do rely on the scientific community, they are sensitive to those that claim the greatest risk. This conservative position is understandable when dealing with public health issues. For the complicated area of chemical carcinogenesis the most conservative posture is that one employ the maximum tolerated dose (no matter how unrealistically high), followed by calculations of risk based on linear low-dose extrapolation models (no matter how many orders of magnitude values from the various models differ from one another). This stand has now become dogma. A response often heard is that this is only prudent and that no one is hurt by this position. Whenever dogma supersedes science, there are casualties. Let me point out a few.

First of all, the field of genetic toxicology is hurt. I have been in meetings where, in order to justify the use of linearized risk models, there is tremendous pressure to assign genotoxic activity to a known carcinogen. The genotoxicity data base will be searched for positive responses at the expense of a more objective view of all the data. A spurious positive result can be enough to get a plus in the summary table for genotoxicity. From there, it is easy for the popular literature to pigeonhole the chemical as just another genotoxic carcinogen. I fear that the quote that someone placed on the board is too true: "A nonmutagen is a substance which has been submitted to too few mutagenicity tests." The undue pressure on the field of genetic toxicology to prove that it can detect any carcinogen is creating a credibility crisis.

The second casualty is in the generation of new and valuable data. In fact, it does not matter how much effort is spent by industry in generating basic information on the mechanism of action of a particular chemical; it will have no effect on the outcome of regulatory policy. An individual at this conference told me of the great deal of time and money that was spent by his company on mechanistic studies for a chemical discussed at this meeting. When the research was presented to the regulators, it was simply ignored in the risk-assessment process. So, there is no incentive to do mechanistic work.

The third area where we are hurt is in the development of new and valuable products. I submit that, if a dose greater than 1000 mg/kg/day of an agent is employed in a long-term bioassay, the data are uninterpretable, particularly in extrapolating to potential low-dose effects in human beings. Dr. Weinstein asked Dr. Scribner if he knew what the meaning of induced hyperplasia was. I suggest that we don't know the meaning of the bioassay where doses in excess of 5% saccharin in the diet (3000 mg/kg/day) were required to produce tumors. My friends in the pharmaceutical industry tell me that it is a very bad situation to find that a promising new drug is nontoxic. Such massive doses are then required in order to reach the mandatory maximum tolerated dose that some adverse effect often appears in the animals in the course of the unrealistic study.

The fourth area that is compromised is in the development of better methods for safety evaluation. This conference illustrates how complex the area of nongenotoxic mechanisms in carcinogenesis can be. We learned that many chemicals may be acting through specific receptors. Species-specific effects are often dramatic for nongenotoxic carcinogens. I think that more effort should be placed in comparing receptors and responses in the rodent versus the human. Manufacturers are already switching to alternatives for di(2-ethylhexyl)phthalate for which there are no carcinogenicity data. Genotoxicity data will be of little value for this class of agents that are not DNA-reactive. Newer and better tests are required for nongenotoxic carcinogens. Induced hyperplasia is another endpoint that came up throughout this conference and deserves much more attention.

To a great extent, the Government controls which safety tests will be required, how they will be interpreted, and where money will be directed in developing new tests. If their posture is cool toward nongenotoxic mechanisms, then that area will not be fostered. In the end, it is good science that is hurt by letting dogma direct policy.

Author Index

Anderson, R.L., 277

Barrett, J.C., 311
Beer, D.G., 41
Berezesky, I.K., 69
Bhatt, T., 215
Boreiko, C.J., 287
Brand, K.G., 205
Bursch, W., 91
Butterworth, B.E., 119, 257

Cerutti, P.A., 325
Chenicek, K.J., 25
Cohen, S.M., 55
Cook, J.C., 247
Coombs, M., 215

de Camargo, J., 165
DiGiovanni, J., 25
Dold, K.M., 247
Doolittle, D.J., 355

Ellwein, L.B., 55

Farber, E., 179

Ghoshal, A., 179
Goldsworthy, T.L., 119

Goyer, M.M., 1
Greenlee, W.F., 247

Heck, H. d'A., 233
Hendrich, S., 41

Johansson, S.L., 55

Kruszewski, F.H., 25

Laconi, E., 85
Loury, D.J., 119

McCarthy, K.L., 355

Newberne, P.M., 165

O'Connell, J.F., 11
O'Neill, C., 215
Osborne, R., 247
Oshimura, M., 311

Parzefall, W., 91
Pitot, H.C., 41
Punyarit, P., 165

Rajalakshmi, S., 85
Rao, P.M., 85
Reitz, R.H., 107
Ricci, P.F., 1
Roe, F.J.C., 189
Ross, L., 247
Rotstein, J.B., 11
Rushmore, T., 179

Sarma, D.S.R., 85
Schulte-Hermann, R., 91
Scribner, H.E., 355
Short, B.G., 151
Sivak, A., 1
Slaga, T.J., 11
Suphakarn, V., 165
Swenberg, J.A., 151

Tanaka, N., 311
Tennant, R.W., 339
Trump, B.F., 69
Tsutsui, T., 311

Vasudevan, S., 85

Wachsmuth, E.D., 137
Williams, G.M., 367

Yamasaki, H., 297

Subject Index

A23187. *See* Calcium
Acetic acid, 22
Acetone, 16–17, 27, 31
Acetylaminofluorene (AAF), 177, 357–358
Actin, 71–72
Actinomycin D, 252
AD$_5$, as peroxidation block, 180–184
Adaptation, hepatocyte, 94–97
Adenosine triphosphatase (ATP), 42, 330
Adrenal gland
   and diet, 194–199
   spontaneous tumor incidence, 153
Aflatoxin B$_1$ (AFB$_1$), 170–173, 185
Age, and carcinogenesis, 151–157
Ah-receptor, 247–253
ALD, 138
Aldrin, 122–123, 166
Alkaline elution, 180, 182, 262, 328–329
Alkaline phosphatase, 357
Alkaline sucrose density gradient, 180
Alkalinization, 74, 76
Alkanes, 13
Allopurinol, 57
Ames assay, 1, 17, 36, 62, 260
Amiloride, 74
Amino acids, 55, 57
Aminopyrine, demethylation of, 93
3-Amino-1,2,4-triazole, 262
11-Aminoundecanoic acid, 342, 345
Amitrole, 312, 316–319
Aneuploidy, 4, 18, 264–265, 311, 313–316
Angiotensinogen, 92

Anthralin, 12–13, 26, 28–29, 32–33, 303–304, 325
Anthraquinone, 28
Anthrones, 25–35. *See also* Anthralin; Chrysarobin
Antibiotics, and cell proliferation, 140–141
Antioxidants, 14, 55, 57, 170, 180
Aplysiatoxins, 12–13, 25
Apoptosis, 72, 91–102. *See also* Cell death
Arachidonic acid hydroperoxides, 328–329
Aromatic amines, 55
Aromatic hydrocarbons. *See* Hydrocarbons
Arsenicals, 312
Asbestos, 211–212, 215, 227, 264, 311–316
Ascorbate, 58
Ascorbic acid, 58
Autooxidation, 28, 33–34
Autoradiography, of [^{3}H]thymidine, 57, 62, 87–88, 93, 108
   in cell culture, 222–226, 262–266, 362
   in kidney, 137–146
   in liver, 123–127, 166–168
5-Azacytidine, 42, 312

Benzene, 312, 318, 342, 344
Benzidine, 55
Benzo(a)pyrene, 120, 251
Benzo(e)pyrene, 13, 26, 317
Benzoyl peroxide, 11–18, 25, 30, 32–33, 304–305, 325, 327
Benzyl acetate, 342, 345
Bidens pilosa, and silica, 227

Bile acids, 304–305
Biphenyl, 55, 57
Bisphenol A, 342
Bladder. *See* Urinary bladder
Blebs. *See* Cell injury
BR-931, 261
Brain, spontaneous tumor incidence, 152
Bromocriptine, 197
7-Bromomethylbenz(a)anthracene, 13, 26
Butylated hydroxyanisole (BHA), 3–4, 36, 46, 55, 57, 170–173, 181, 303–304, 372, 383–384
Butylated hydroxytoluene (BHT), 39, 57, 121–122, 126, 181, 304, 372, 384
Butyl benzyl phthalate, 342, 345
N-Butyl-*N*-(4-hydroxybutyl) nitrosamine (BBN), 55–56
4-Butyl (nitrosamino)-1-butanol (NBBN), 277–278

Calcification
  and diet, pheochromocytoma, 197–199
  dystrophic, 70
  metastatic, 198
Calcium
  -free media, 71
  intra-, extracellular, 71
  ionophore A23187, 14, 17, 73
  ions, 55, 59, 69–77, 182–184, 329–331
    in calculi, 233, 239–241
  phosphate, 70
  salts, 56, 58–59
  urinary, 59, 277–278
Calmodulin, 72
Cancer hazard, 367–375
Cancer precursor cells, 206. *See also* Hepatocarcinogenesis
Caprolactam, 342
Carbon tetrachloride (CCl$_4$), 95, 120, 124–125, 181, 357, 381
Carcinogenesis. *See also* Tumors
  cell injury, 69–77
  and cytotoxicity, 107–115
  epidermal (skin), 44–47. *See also* Skin
    human keratinocytes, 247–253
  foreign body, "solid state," 205–212
  human, 367–375
    exposure control, 374, 375
    safety factor, 375
  liver. *See* Hepatocarcinogenesis
  mathematical model, 55, 60–61, 267. *See also* Cytotoxicity
  urinary bladder. *See* Urinary bladder
Carcinogens
  classification, 368
  complete, 44–46, 314, 381

dermal. *See* Skin
DNA-reactive, 367–375, 382. *See also* Genotoxic
  potency, 369
  threshold, 370
epigenetic, 367–375
genotoxic, 1–5, 18, 107, 151, 189, 325–331
hepatic. *See* Hepatocarcinogenesis
human, 367–375
incomplete, 44–46
nongenotoxic, 1–5, 91–94, 107, 119, 121, 126, 154, 156, 165–173, 185, 277, 311–319
nonmutagenic mechanisms, 318
pseudo-, pseudoanti-, 189–199
renal. *See* Nephrotoxicity
Carnitine acetyltransferase, 262
Carnitine palmitoyltransferase, 262
Catalase, 33, 262, 329
Cefsulodin, 141–142
Cell
  -cell communication, 17, 210, 289, 297–305
    dye-transfer method, 297–299
    electrical coupling, 297–299
    junctional, 297–305
    metabolic cooperation, 297–299
    recognition, 303
    selective, 302–305
  culture
    BALB/c-3T3 cells, 291–293, 298–305
    bronchial epithelial, 73
    C3H/10T1/2 cells, 287–293, 299, 328–329
    and DEHP, 260–262
    Ehrlich ascites tumor cells (EATC), 71–72
    in foreign body carcinogenesis, 207–209
    and human cells, 249–252
    mouse lymphoma (L5178Y), 341–342
    and silica, 222–223
    stimulus for cell division, 215
    Syrian hamster embryo, 301
  death (killing), 69–77, 172–173, 185. *See also* Apoptosis
  density, 288
  differentiation, 70, 211
    squamous, 74
    terminal, 70, 73–74
  division, 60–62, 70–73. *See also* Autoradiography; Cell proliferation; Cell replication; DNA
    compensatory, 107–115
  injury, 69–77
    acute, 69, 74, 185
    blebs, 71–73, 76
    and carcinogenesis, 74–76

chronic, 69
ion regulation/deregulation, 69–77
lethal, 70, 76
necrosis, 76, 137–146
neoplasia, 69
regeneration, 76, 139–141, 145
sublethal, 70, 76
intracellular buffering, 70
proliferation, 57, 70, 151–157
in kidney, 137–146
in liver, 87–89, 91–102, 180, 185
in urinary bladder, 60–63
proximal tubular, 71–72
transformation. See Transformation
turnover. See Autoradiography
Cephaloridine, 138–142
Chemical. See also Carcinogens
ingestants, inhalants, 212
noncarcinogenic, 340
nongenotoxic noncarcinogens, 342
Chloracne, 252–253
Chlorine, 69–70
Chlorobenzoic acid, 327
Chloroform, 107–110, 124, 125, 129, 166
Choline
-deficient diet, 87–88, 166, 170–172
-methionine diet, 179–185
Chromosome
aberrations, 207–208, 211, 313–316, 341
imbalance, 210
nondisjunction, 311
Chrysarobin, 25–34
mutagenicity, 36–37
toxicity, 32
Chrysophanic acid, 28–29. See also
1,8-Dihydroxy-9,10-anthraquinone
Cigarette smoke, 55. See also Tobacco
Cinnamyl anthranilate, 342, 344
Ciprofibrate, 269
Citrus oil, 13
Clastogenic, 340
action of peroxides, 326–331
agents, 44
Clofibrate, 45, 92, 262, 269
Cocarcinogenesis, 280–281, 314
Colcemid, 312
Communication, intracellular. See Cell-cell
communication
Croton oil, 13, 215–220
Cyclic AMP, 74, 247
Cycling, estrus and overfeeding, 196
Cyclohexamide, 252
Cyclophosphamide, 62
Cyproterone acetate, 92–96, 99
Cytochalasin, 71
Cytochrome P-450, 97

Cytoplasmic alkalinization, 74
Cytoskeleton, 69, 72, 76–77
Cytosol, 72
rat, hepatic, 29, 34
Cytostasis, 144
Cytotoxicity, 151–157
computer model, 107–115

Decanoylperoxide, 327
Deoxyribonuclease, 97
Deoxyribonucleic acid. See DNA
Dermis. See Epidermis
Desferrioxamine, 329
Dexamethasone, 250
Diacylglycerol (DAG), 12, 70, 74, 299
1,2-Dibromo-3-chloropropane, 2
Dichlorobenzene, 154
Dichlorodimethylpropynyl benzamide (DCB),
166
Dichlorodiphenyltrichloroethane (DDT), 92,
122–123, 303–304, 372
Dichloromethane, 2–3
Dieldrin, 122–123
Diene conjugates, 184
Diet
deficiency, 165–166. See also Choline
and fibers, unpolished seeds, 217–219
imbalance, 179
lipotrope deficiency, 185
overfeeding, 189–199
and hormones, 196
and neoplasia, 193–195
Diethylhexyladipate (DEHA), 262, 342, 345
Diethylhexylphthalate (DEHP), 2–3, 92, 122,
257–270, 342–344
Diethylnitrosamine (DEN, DENA), 41, 43–46,
86–88, 143–146, 263
Diethylstilbestrol (DES), 264–265, 311–319,
373
Differentiation. See Cell
Difluromethylornithine, 14
Diglycidylresorcinol ether, 2
15,16-Dihydro-11-methylcyclopenta[a]-
phenanthren-11-one, 217–221
1,8-Dihydroxy-9,10-anthraquinone, 28, 33–34.
See also Chrysophanic acid
1,8-Dihydroxy-3-methyl-9-anthrone. See
Chrysarobin
7,12-Dimethylbenzanthracene (DMBA),
15–16, 27, 32–33, 43, 45, 327
Dimethylhydrazine, 120
Dimethylnitrosamine (DMN), 150, 357–358
Dimethyl terephthalate (DMT), 233, 342,
345
Dinitrotoluene (DNT), 121
Dioxins, 2, 291. See also TCDD

DNA, 2, 73–74, 97, 107–115, 151
  adducts, 120
  alterations, 179–185
  breakage, 328–331
  and DEHP, 257–270
  methylation, 318
  replicative synthesis (RDS), 119–130
  in tumor promotion,
    liver, 44, 46, 85–87, 93–95, 99. *See also*
      Hepatocarcinogenesis
    skin, 11–13, 18, 37. *See also* Skin
    urinary bladder, 55–56, 61. *See also*
      Urinary bladder
  unscheduled synthesis (UDS), 340, 355–363
Dyes, 342, 345

Ehrlich ascites tumor cells (EATC), 71–72
Electrical coupling, in cell-cell
    communication, 297–298
Electron microscopy, 58
Electrophiles, 56
Enamide, acylated, 180
Endoplasmic reticulum (ER), 69, 77
Environmental Protection Agency (EPA),
    3–5
Enzyme, inducers and promoters, 165, 168
Enzyme-altered foci (EAF). *See*
    Hepatocarcinogenesis
Epidermal carcinogenesis. *See also* Skin
  human keratinocytes, 247–253
    glucocorticoids, 251–252
    growth factor (EFG) receptor, 248–249
Epinephrine, 74
Epithelium
  hamster tracheal, 74
  proximal tubular, 71, 73. *See also*
    Nephrotoxicity
  urinary bladder. *See* Urinary bladder
Epoxide hydratase, 97
Esophageal cancer, 15, 227
Estradiol esters, 92, 312–313
Estrus cycling, and overfeeding, 196
Ethidium bromide, 37
Ethinylestradiol, 122
L-Ethionine, 43, 312
Ethoxylated dodecyl alcohol, 342
Ethoxyquin, 57
Ethylene dibromide, 2
2-Ethylhexanol (2-EH), 258, 264
Ethylhydroxyethylnitrosamine (EHEN), 154,
    277–278
Ethylmorphine, demethylation of, 93
Ethylnitrosourea (ENU), 11, 15–18
4-Ethyl-sulfonylnaphthalene-1-sulfonamide,
    and urinary bladder calculi, 233
Euphorbia latices, 13

FANFT, 56, 60–61
Fibers, mineral, 311, 314, 316, 326. *See also*
    Asbestos; Silica
Fibroblasts, fibrosis, in foreign body
    carcinogenesis, 206, 208, 212
β-oxidation, 94
Filaggrin, 18
Fluorescent probes, 71, 74
1-Fluoro-2,4-dinitrobenzene, 13
Foci
  preneoplastic. *See* Hepatocarcinogenesis
  and transformation, 287–293
Food and Drug Administration (FDA), 3–5,
    347
Foreign body carcinogenesis, 205–212
  human, 211
  initiation, 207–208
  preneoplasia, 206–207
  promotion/progression, 208–209
  reaction, 206–208
Formaldehyde, 74, 151
Free radicals, 12, 14–16, 25, 34, 151,
    180–185
Furosemide, 59

Gap junctions, 297–305
Gasoline, unleaded, 125–126, 129,
    154–155
Gemfibrozil, 268
Gene regulation, 77
Genome errors, 211
Genotoxicity, 119–130. *See also* Carcinogen;
    Cell culture
  of DEHP, 257–270
  epigentic, 367–375
  genotoxic and epigenetic mechanisms,
    311–319, 340
  in regulatory decisions, 339–348
  in short-term in vitro and in vivo test
    systems, 340–341, 356–362
Gentamicin, 125, 140–142
Giant cells, kidney, 142
Glomerulonephritis, progressive (PGN),
    191–192
Glucocorticoids, 251–252
Glucose-6-phosphatase, 42, 97–98
Glucose-6-phosphate dehydrogenase, 28,
    97–98
Glucuronyl transferases, 97
γ-Glutamyl transferase (GGT), 18, 86–89,
    97–102, 357. *See also*
    Hepatocarcinogenesis
Glutathione (GSH), 170–173, 330
  conjugates, 98
  transferase, 97–98
Glycerol aldehyde phosphate (GAP), 98

Glycerol aldehyde phosphate (GAP)
dehydrogenase, 98
Glycogen, 144
phosphorylase, 98
synthetase, 98
Glycolysis, 71–72, 98
Glycosylation, 85–86
Growth factor, 327, 330
epidermal, 247–253

Hamamelis water (witch hazel), 342
HEMA, in cell culture, 222–223
Hepatocarcinogenesis, 41–47, 85–89,
143–144, 179, 185
cell proliferation, 87–89, 91–102, 179
cell replication, 119–130
and chloroform, 108
complete, 44–46
and diet, 170–172, 179–185
foci, preneoplastic, enzyme-altered, 41–47,
86–92, 95, 97, 99, 100, 120, 129,
257–258, 263–265
phenotypic remodeling, 97–102
reversibility, 41–47, 101–102
human, 91–92, 156, 165
hyperplasia, 88, 93, 102, 120–121,
126–130
incomplete, 44–46
initiation, 41–47, 86–89, 97, 180, 183
Kupffer cells, 360–361
liver growth, 91–102
mouse, 165–173
tumor inducers, 166
nodules, 86–89, 97, 124
progression, 42–47, 88
promotion, 41–47, 85–89, 91–92, 95–100,
129, 165–173
tumor incidence, 44–45, 152, 155–157,
167
tumor promoters, 87–89, 92
and UDS, 356–363
Hexachlorobenzene (HCB), 92
Hexachlorocyclohexane, as liver tumor
promoter, 87–88
Hexachlorohexane (HCH), 92, 96, 122, 125
Hormones, 91–94, 151, 319, 327, 330
and diet, 189–190, 196
Hydrocarbons
aromatic, 12, 25, 29, 217, 249
chlorinated, 154–155
Hydrocephalus, 190
Hydrogen
ions, 69–71, 74
peroxide, 12–14, 16–17, 327–328
Hydrolysis, phospholipase-mediated, 70
Hydroperoxides, 325–331

Hydroxyapatite, 72
Hydroxyperoxy-arachidonic acid (HPETE),
328–331
1-Hydroxysafrole, 43, 46
Hydroxyurea, 261
Hypercalcemia, 198
Hyperkeratinization, 248
Hyperplasia, 265–267, 355. See also Foreign
body; Hepatocarcinogenesis; Skin;
Urinary bladder
Hypocalcemia, 198
Hypolipidemic agents, 121, 206, 257–270
Hypoxanthine phosphoribosyl transferase,
316

Immunosurveillance, 206
Inflammation
and initiation, 210
and promotion, 325–326, 330
Initiation, 107, 288. See also Foreign body;
Hepatocarcinogenesis; Skin; Urinary
bladder
Inositoltriphosphate (InsP$_3$), 74, 77
Iodoacetic acid, 12, 72
Iodoform, 125
Ions, 55, 58–59
regulation/deregulation. See Cell injury
Isoleucine, 55, 57

Keratinocyte, 12–15, 32–33, 247–253
Keratoacanthomas, 18
Kidney, 71–72, 108. See also Nephrotoxicity
Kinase. See Protein kinase C; Pyruvate
kinase L

Labeling index. See Autoradiography
Lactinol, 198
Lactose, 198
Lauroyl peroxide, 12, 13
LDH, 138
Leucine, 55, 57
Leukemia, monocytic, 195
Lindane, 303–304
Lipid peroxidation. See Peroxidation
Liver carcinogenesis. See
Hepatocarcinogenesis
Lung tumors, 74, 107
and diet, 195
Lymphoreticular system, and diet, 195
Lyngbyatoxin, 13
Lysosomes, 138

Macrophages, 325
in foreign body carcinogenesis, 206, 208,
210
Magnesium, 199, 278

Mammary gland
  spontaneous tumor incidence, 152
  tumors and diet, 194–197
Mannitol, 198, 342
Mathematical model
  cytotoxicity, computer model, 107–115
  dose response of DNA-reactive carcinogens,
    370
  urinary bladder, 60
Maximum tolerated dose (MTD), 339
MDH, 138
Melamine, 342, 345
Membrane, 77, 85–86, 151. *See also* Plasma
    membrane
  enzymes of the brush border, 138
  homeostasis, 85
  in promotion, 210
  transport, 77
DL-Menthol, 342
Mercurials, 71
Mercuric chloride, 71–73, 149
Mesothelioma, 311, 314
Methionine. *See* Choline
Methylcholanthrene, 288–292, 302
Methylclofenapate, 262, 269
N-Methyl-*N*-nitro-*N* '-nitrosoguanidine
    (MNNG), 15, 17–18, 177, 252, 277,
    289–292, 331
N-Methyl-*N*-nitrosourea (MNU), 56
Mezerein, 17, 26, 28–29
Microanalysis, 70, 72
Microinjection, 291, 299
Microtubules, 72
Millipore filters, in foreign body
    carcinogenesis, 205, 209
Mitochondria, 69, 72
Mitosis. *See* Autoradiography; Cell division
Monoclonal origin, 207
Mono(ethylhexyl)phthalate (MEHP), 258–261,
    264
Monosaccharides, 198
Monosodium aspartate, 57
Mutagenicity, 1, 17, 36–37, 50–51, 55, 119,
    124–125, 312. *See also* Cell culture
  of DEHP, 258–262
  short-term tests, 313,341
Myocardial degeneration, and overfeeding,
    191
10-Myristoylanthralin, 29

Nafenopin, 87–88, 92, 96, 122
National Toxicology Program, 2, 125,
    153–156, 258–262, 339–342, 347–348
Neoantigens, in foreign body carcinogenesis,
    206
Neoplasia. *See* Tumors

Nephrotoxicity, 119–130, 314
  and α2μ-globulin, 154
  and cell turnover, 137–146
  and chlorinated hydrocarbons, 154–155
  giant cells, 142
  hyperplasia, 143
  nephrocalcinosis, 198–199
  and nitrilotriacetate, 277–281
  and overfeeding, 190–193
  spontaneous tumors, 152
Nicotinamide-adenine-dinucleotide (NAD), 330
Nitric acid, and silica fibers, 216
Nitrilotriacetate, 233, 277–281
Nitrilotriacetic acid, 3
P-Nitroanisole, 169
Nitrobenzoic acid, 327
N-[4-(5-nitro-2-furyl)-2-thiazoyl]formamide.
    See FANFT
4-Nitroquinoline-*N*-oxide, 15
Nitrosamines, 212, 227
N-Nitrosodiethylamine (DEN). *See*
    Diethylnitrosamine
N-Nitrosomorpholine (NNM), 99, 143
No-observed-effect-levels (NOELs), 370, 383
Nuclear magnetic resonance (NMR), 59
Nucleic acid synthesis, 85
Nucleotide
  biosynthesis, pyrimidine, 85, 89
  pools, 85–87, 89
  uridine, 85–86, 89

Oncogene, 76, 151, 155–157, 208, 302, 325
  proto-, 208
Oncoviruses, in foreign body carcinogenesis,
    206
Ornithine decarboxylase (ODC), 12, 13, 15,
    16, 26, 30–32, 34, 330
Orotic acid, as tumor promoter, 85–89
Overfeeding. *See* Diet
Oxidation, 262,
  β-oxidation, 13, 361
  prooxidation states and promotion, 326–328
4,4'-Oxydianiline, 2

Palmitoyl-CoA oxidase, 361
Palytoxin, 12, 13
Pancreas
  and diet, 194–195
  spontaneous tumor incidence, 152–153
Papilloma, 11–12, 14–16, 18, 25, 27, 30, 32,
    34, 47, 57, 60, 105
Parathyroid
  hyperplasia, 191, 198
  spontaneous tumor incidence, 153
PAS-haemalum, 139
PDBu, 28–29, 34

Pentachloroethane, 125, 129, 154–155
Perchloroethylene, 124–125, 129, 154–155
Pericytes, 207, 211
Peroxidase, 317
Peroxidation, lipid, 170–173, 179–183, 262
Peroxides, 325–331
Peroxisomal β-oxidation, 13, 361
Peroxisome proliferating compounds, 44, 46.
    See also Hypolipidemic agents
Peroxisome proliferation, 257
Pesticides, 165–168
pH, 55, 58–59, 71–72
Phalaris canariensis, and silica fibers,
    215–228
Phenobarbital (PB), 41–47, 57, 87–88,
    91–102, 121–122, 166–170, 303–304,
    381
    and unscheduled DNA synthesis, 357–358
Phenolic compounds, 13
Pheochromocytoma, and calcium absorption,
    197–199
Phorbol agents, esters, 12–13, 25–26, 29–35,
    63, 74, 76, 88, 249, 325
    in cell-cell communication, 298–300, 305
    in promotion, 327–330
    receptors, 25–27, 32, 34
Phosphate, and diet, 199
Phospholipids, 12, 70, 73
    diacylglycerol (DAG), 12, 70, 74
Phospholipidase, 73
    -mediated hydrolysis, 70
Phosphotidylinositol (PI), 70
    pathway, 73–74, 76
Physcion anthrone, 27–28
Pituitary, 194–197
Plasma membrane, 69–73, 329
Plastics, in foreign body carcinogenesis, 205
Platinum, *cis*-, 142–145
Pluripotentiality, in foreign body
    carcinogenesis, 206
Poly(ADP)ribosylation, 42, 330–331
Polyamine synthesis inhibitor, 14
Polyarteritis, and overfeeding, 191
Polybrominated biphenyls (PBB), 2, 92, 122,
    342–346
Polychlorinated biphenyls (PCB), 92
Polyhydroxymethyl methacrylate, in cell
    culture, 222–224
Polyols, 198
Polyvinyl chloride acetate (PVCA), 205
Potassium, 55, 71–72
    cyanide (KCN), 72
Progesterone, 92
Progression, 153. *See also* Foreign body;
    Hepatocarcinogenesis; Skin
Prolactin, -omas, 196–197

Promoters, tumor, 4, 69–77, 288–293,
    346–348, 372. *See also* Foreign body;
    Hepatocarcinogenesis; Skin; Urinary
    bladder
    antipromoters, 180
    genotoxic oxidant, 325–331
Promotion, 4, 69–77, 288–293, 346–348, 381.
    See also Foreign body;
    Hepatocarcinogenesis; Skin; Urinary
    bladder
    antipromoters, 180
    in cell-cell communication, 297–305
    genotoxic oxidant, 325–331
    and phorbol esters, 330
    short-term screen test, 303
Prostaglandin, 328
    synthesis inhibitors, 14
Protease inhibitors, 14
Protein kinase C (PKC), 12, 16, 25, 74,
    76–77, 299, 327
Pyruvate kinase L, 97–98

Redox cycles, 33
Regulatory policy, 339, 343, 381–386
Renal toxicity. *See* Nephrotoxicity
Replicative DNA synthesis (RDS). *See* DNA
Reproductive performance, 196
Reserpine, 342, 344–348
Respiration, 71–72
Ribonuclease, 92
Risk, 1–3, 5, 17, 91, 157, 239–240, 355–356,
    374–375

Saccharin, 2–4, 58–59, 233, 381, 386. *See
    also* Sodium saccharin
Salmonella, assay, 37, 50, 119, 124–125, 235,
    341–342
Sarcoma
    in foreign body carcinogenesis, 206, 211
    in skin, 217
Schistosomiasis, 211–212
Serine dehydrogenase (SDH), 98
Serum alanine transaminase, 121
Serum glutamic pyruvic transaminase (SGPT),
    167–169, 357
Signal transduction, 77
Silica fibers, biogenic, 215–228
    size, 220–221, 227
Sister chromatid exchange (SCE), 260,
    340–342
Skin
    carcinogenesis, multistage, 11–19, 25–35,
    55–56
    hyperplasia, 11–17, 32, 34
    initiation, 11–12, 14–18, 217
    progression, 11, 14–19

Skin (continued)
  promotion, 11–18, 25–35
    genotoxic effects, 18, 29–30
    inhibitors, 14
    mechanisms, 14, 25–35
    and peroxides, 327
    promoters, 11–18, 25–35, 218
    responses, 12–18, 25–35
    and silica fibers, 215–228
    spontaneous tumor incidence, 152
    toxicity, 32
Sodium
  arsenate, 318
  arsenite, 318
  ascorbate, 55–59
  bicarbonate, 57, 59
  bisulfite, 312
  citrate, 57
  cyclamate, 56
  erythorbate, 57
  (2-ethylhexyl) alcohol sulfate, 342, 345
  hippurate, 59
  ions, 55, 69–71, 77
  lauryl sulfate, 13
  o-phenylphenate, 55, 57
  orthophenylphenol (SOPP), 107–108, 110
  -proton carrier, 74, 76–77
  -proton exchange, 74, 76
  saccharin, 55–63
  salts, 55–59
Sorbitol, 198
S-phase. See Autoradiography; DNA;
    Genotoxicity
Spontaneous tumors. See Tumors
Stem cells, in foreign body carcinogenesis,
    207
Steroids, 87–88, 91
  anti-inflammatory, 14
  contraceptive, 91
  sex, 123
Superoxide, 325–331
  dismutase, 33
Syrian hamster embryo assay, 301

Tannic acid, 124
Teleocidins, 12–13, 25, 28–29
Terephthalic acid, 233–241
2,3,7,8-Tetrachlorodibenzo-p-dioxin (TCDD),
    2–4, 29, 34, 43–44, 46, 92, 122,
    247–253, 263, 290–293, 317, 342–346,
    381
Tetrachloroethylene. See Perchloroethylene
12-O-Tetradecanoylphorbol-13-acetate (TPA),
    12, 14–17, 25–34, 74, 289–292,
    298–301, 304, 317, 325, 328, 383–384

Theiler's Original mouse strain, 216–221
Thiobarbituric acid (TBA), 171–173
Thorotrast, 91
Thymidine. See Autoradiography
Thyroid, 317, 319
  and diet, 194
  spontaneous tumor incidence, 153
  -stimulating hormone (TSH), 155
Titanium dioxide, 342
Tobacco, 13, 325, 372, 382
Tolerance induction, to nephrotoxins, 139,
    145
Transformation, 60, 257, 287–293, 311–319.
    See also Cell culture
  and cell-cell communication, 299–305
  frequency, 288
  SHE assay, 312, 313
Transforming growth factor-β (TGF-β),
    73–74, 327
Transplantation, 41, 69, 209
  antigens, 206
Trichloroethylene (TCE), 123–125, 129,
    154–155, 357–358
Triglyceride, 183
1,2,3-Trihydroxyanthraquinone, 37
Trimethylpentane (TMP), 122, 125–128
Tris (2-ethylhexyl) phosphate, 342, 345
Trolox-C, 181
Tryptophan, 57
Tubulin, 71
Tumor
  promoters. See Promoters
  spontaneous, 151–153, 347

Unleaded gasoline. See Gasoline
Uracil, 55, 57
Urethane, 15
Uridine diphosphate glucose, 98
Uridine diphosphate glucuronic acid, 98
Urinary bladder,
  calculi, 55, 57, 233–241
  carcinogenesis, 55–63, 233–241
  cell
    cycle, 60–62
    proliferation, 57, 60–63, 233
  human, 55
  hyperplasia, 57, 60–62
  initiation, 55–56, 60–62
  mathematical model, 60
  and nitrilotriacetate, 277–281
  promotion, 55–58, 62, 280–281
  and sodium orthophenylphenol (SOPP),
    107–108, 110
  transformation, 60–61
  ulceration, 62–63

urine, 55, 58–60, 62
   calcium, 59, 277–279
   growth factors, 60, 63
   zinc, 277–279
   urothelium, 56, 62
Urine. *See* Urinary bladder
Uterine tumors, 197

Vascularization, in foreign body
   carcinogenesis, 208
Vinblastine, 71
Vincristine sulfate, 312

Vitamin D deficiency, 198
Vitamin E, 39

Wy-14, 643, 43, 46, 122, 261, 269

Xanthine oxidase, 37, 328, 330
X-ray, 212
   microanalysis, 71–72
Xylitol, 198

Zinc, in renal toxicity, 277–279

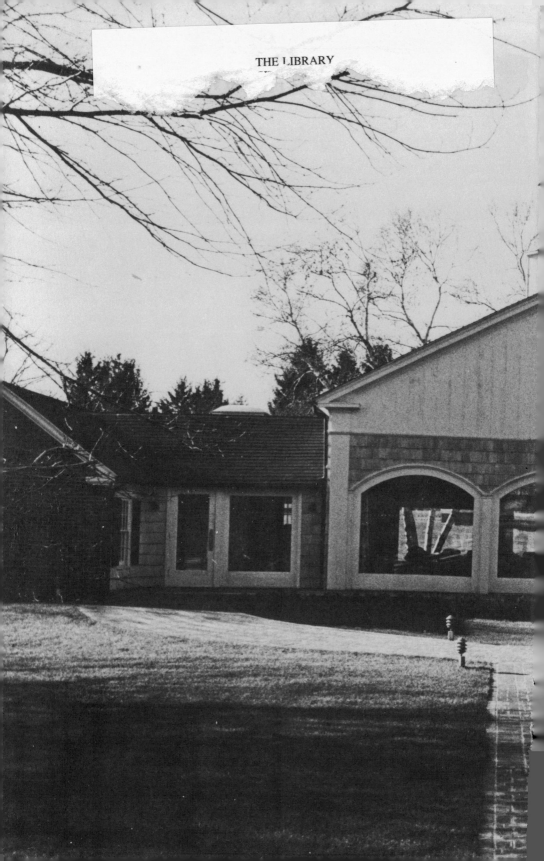